ALLE · ZEIT · WACH · 1842

G.F. Placidi L. Dell'Osso G. Nisticò
and H.S. Akiskal (Eds.)

Recurrent Mood Disorders

New Perspectives in Therapy

With a Foreword by Sir J. Eccles

Springer-Verlag
Berlin Heidelberg New York
London Paris Tokyo
Hong Kong Barcelona
Budapest

Prof. GIAN FRANCO PLACIDI

Prof. LILIANA DELL'OSSO

Clinica Psichiatrica
Università di Pisa
Via Roma, 67
I-56100 Pisa, Italy

Prof. GIUSEPPE NISTICÒ

Chair of Pharmacology
Department of Biology
University of Rome "Tor Vergata"
Via della Ricerca Scientifica
I-00133 Rome, Italy

Prof. HAGOP S. AKISKAL

Department of Psychiatry,
University of California at San Diego
La Jolla, CA 92093-0603, USA

With 82 Figures and 95 Tables

ISBN-13: 978-3-642-76648-0 e-ISBN-13: 978-3-642-76646-6
DOI: 10.1007/978-3-642-76646-6

Library of Congress Cataloging-in-Publication Data. Recurrent mood disorders : new perspectives in therapy/G.F. Placidi ... [et al.] (eds). p. cm. Includes bibliographical references and index. ISBN-13: 978-3-642-76648-0 1. Affective disorders—congresses. I. Placidi, G.F. (Gian F.) [DNLM: 1. Affective Disorders—therapy. 2. Affective Disorders, Psychotropic Drugs—therapeutic use. WM 207 R311 1993] RC537.R427 1993 616.85'27-dc20 DNLM/DLC for Library of Congress 92-48355

Softcover reprint of the hardcover 1st edition 1993

Typesetting: Macmillan India Ltd., Bangalore-25

21/3130/SPS-543210 — Printed on acid-free paper

Foreword

The Human Person

At the present time there is much publication on human consciousness. It is mostly devoted to "what is" questions, rather loosely discussed, and it is not very fruitful. I prefer to start with "how" questions. For example, how does the whole range of mental events come to be expressed in actions? And how does the whole range of neural events lead to mental experiences, as in perceptions and memories? These "how" questions are basic to the dualist concepts of the mind–brain problem.

I maintain that two propositions are central to any attempt at understanding ourselves and our relationship to the world, including other selves: first the certainty that one exists as a unique self-conscious being, and second the certainty that the material world exists, including one's body and brain.

Problems relating to the experienced uniqueness of each self are neglected in contemporary philosophy. Presumably this neglect arises from the pervasive materialism that is blind to the fundamental problems arising in spiritual experience. It will be my task to concentrate on the most extraordinary event in the world of our experience, namely the coming to be of each of us as a unique self-conscious being. It is a miracle forever beyond science.

SIR JOHN ECCLES

Sir John Eccles graced our symposium as Honorary President and delivered the opening address, from which these remarks are derived (Eds).

Preface

Current evidence indicates that over two-thirds of mood disorders pursue a recurrent or chronic course. Yet much of the progress recorded in the field of mood disorders and their treatment has been in research into the acute phase of the illness. Hence there is a need for a volume that specifically addresses the special clinical problems encountered in the recurrent forms of these disorders.

This book derives from the proceedings of an international symposium held in Monte Carlo on March 23–25, 1990. We thank the authors for updating their contributions since that time.

The various chapters embrace a wide range of topics, including etiology, course, and long-term treatment, integrative reviews, results of recent investigations, and clinical reports. In this respect, the contributions reflect current concepts, research, and clinical practice. We have endeavored to build a bridge between neurobiology and psychology and have covered both the psychotherapeutic and the psychopharmacologic aspects of mood disorders. Since the focus is on recurrent disorders, generous space has been allocated to prophylaxis and long-term treatment, especially new approaches.

Pisa, Italy	G.F.P.
Pisa, Italy	L.D.
Rome, Italy	G.N.
San Diego, USA	H.S.A.

May 1993

Contents

List of Contributors

Aguglia, E., Istituto di Clinica Psichiatrica, Università degli Studi di Trieste, via s. Cilino, 16, I-34126 Trieste, Italy

Akiskal, H.S., Department of Psychiatry, University of California at San Diego, La Jolla, CA 92093-0603, USA

Allegranti, I., Istituto di Clinica Psichiatrica, Università degli Studi di Trieste, via s. Cilino, 16, I-34126 Trieste, Italy

Altamura, A.C., Dipartimento di Clinica Psichiatrica, Università degli Studi di Milano, I-20122 Milano, Italy

Amado-Boccara, I., Service Hospitalo-Universitaire de Santé mentale et de thérapeutique, N.E. 75007 0294, Hôpital Public Agréé S.S. No. 1032, 1 Rue Cabanis, F-75674 Paris Cedex 14, France

Angst, J., Research Department, Psychiatric University Hospital, P.O. Box 68, CH-8029 Zürich, Switzerland

Bartalena, L., Istituto di Endocrinologia, Università degli Studi di Pisa, viale del Tirreno, 64, I-56100 Tirrenia (Pisa), Italy

Battini, S., Instituto di Clinica Medica II, Università degli Studi di Pisa, via Roma, 67, I-56100 Pisa, Italy.

Bertoli, M., Clinica Medica, Università di Pisa, via Roma, 67, I-56100 Pisa, Italy

Bianchi, M.L., Istituto di Psichiatria, Università degli Studi di Milano, Ospedale San Paolo, I-20135 Milano, Italy

Bionda, A., Instituto di Clinica Medica II, Università degli Studi di Pisa, via Roma, 67, I-56100 Pisa, Italy

Bogetto, F., Istituto di Clinica Psichiatrica II, Università degli Studi di Torino, via Cherasco, 15, I-10100 Torino, Italy

Bonelli, G., Istituto di Clinica delle Malattie Nervose e Mentali, Università degli Studi di Siena, piazza Duomo, 1, I-53100 Siena, Italy

Buffa, G., Ospedale Fatebenefratelli, viale Montenero, 15, I-20135 Milano, Italy

Cappa, C., Istituto di Clinica Psichiatrica II, Università degli Studi di Torino, via Cherasco, 15, I-10100 Torino, Italy

Carlson, G.A., Department of Psychiatry, South Campus-Putnam Hall, S.U.N.Y. at Stony Brook, Stony Brook, NY 11794-8790, USA

Casacchia, M., Clinica Psichiatrica, Università degli Studi L'Aquila, I-00198 Roma, Italy

Cassano, G.B., Istituto di Clinica Psichiatrica, Università degli Studi di Pisa, via Roma, 67, I-56100 Pisa, Italy
Castrogiovanni, P., Istituto di Clinica Psichiatrica, Università degli Studi di Pisa, via Roma, 67, I-56100 Pisa, Italy
Cataldo, S. de., Clinica Psichiatrica, Università degli Studi L'Aquila, I-00198 Roma, Italy
Cogrossi, S., Ospedale San Raffaele, Dipartimento di Scienze Neuropsichiche, via Prinetti 29, I-20127 Milano, Italy
Conte, G., Istituto di Psichiatria, Università degli Studi di Milano, Ospedale San Paolo, I-20135 Milano, Italy
Conti, G., Istituto di Clinica Psichiatrica, Università degli Studi di Trieste, via S. Cilino, 16, I-34126 Trieste, Italy
Corsini, G.U., Istituto di Farmacologia, Università di Pisa, via Roma, 55, I-56100 Pisa, Italy
Dalmotto, M., Istituto di Clinica Psichiatrica II, Università degli Studi di Torino, via Cherasco, 15, I-10100 Torino, Italy
Dal Pino B. Instituto di Clinica Medica II, Università degli Studi di Pisa, via Roma, 67, I-56100 Pisa, Italy
Dell'Osso, L., Istituto di Clinica Psichiatrica, Università degli Studi di Pisa, via Roma, 67, I-56100 Pisa, Italy
Deltito, J.A., Anxiety and Depression Clinic, Cornell University Medical College, New York Hospital (Westchester Division), 21 Bloomingdale Road, White Plains, New York, NY 10605, USA
De Maio, D., Ospedale Fatebenefratelli, viale Montenero, 15, I-20135 Milano, Italy
De Vanna, M., Istituto di Clinica Psichiatrica, Università degli Studi di Trieste, via S. Cilino, 16, I-34126 Trieste, Italy
Di Figlia, C., New York State Psychiatric Institute, 722 West 168th Street, New York, NY 10032, USA
Di Muro, A., Istituto di Clinica Psichiatrica, Università degli Studi di Pisa, via Roma, 67, I-56100 Pisa, Italy
Dorigo, D., Ospedale Fatebenefratelli, viale Montenero, 15, I-20135 Milano, Italy
Dunner, D.L., University of Washington School of Medicine and Harborview Medical Center, Seattle, WA, USA
Fieve, R.R., New York State Psychiatric Institute, 722 West 168th Street, New York, NY 10032, USA
Frank, E., Department of Psychiatry, University of Pittsburgh School of Medicine, Western Psychiatric Institute and Clinic, 3811 O'Hara Street, Pittsburgh, PA 15213, USA
Freer, P., Istituto di Clinica Psichiatrica, Università degli Studi di Pisa, via Roma, 67, I-56100 Pisa, Italy
Gasperini, M., Ospedale San Raffaele, Dipartimento di Scienze Neuropsichiche, via Prinetti 29 I-20127 Milano, Italy
Geisler, A., Department of Pharmacology, University of Copenhagen, Juliane Maries Vej 20, DK-2100 Copenhagen, Denmark

Gianetti, S., Dipartimento di Clinica Psichiatrica, Università degli Studi di Milano, via F. Sforza, 35, I-20122 Milano, Italy
Hamer, T., Department of Psychiatry, University of Pittsburgh School of Medicine, Western Psychiatric Institute and Clinic, 3811 O'Hara Street, Pittsburgh, PA 15213, USA
Hirschfeld, R.M.A., Mood, Anxiety, and Personality Disorders, Research Branch, Division of Clinical Research, National Institute of Mental Health, Perklawn Building, Room 10c-24, 5600 Fishers Lane, Rockville, MD 20857, USA
Invernizzi, G., Dipartimento di Clinica Psichiatrica, Università degli Studi di Milano, via F. Sforza, 35, I-20122 Milano, Italy
Johnson, F.N., Department of Psychology, University of Lancaster, Bailrigg, Lancaster LA1 4YF, UK
Kupfer, D.J., Department of Psychiatry, University of Pittsburgh School of Medicine, Western Psychiatric Institute and Clinic, 3811 O'Hara Street, Pittsburgh, PA 15213, USA
Laviani, M., Ospedale Fatebenefratelli, viale Montenero, 15, I-20135 Milano, Italy
Loo, H.Y., Service Hospitalo-Universitaire de Santé mentale et de thérapeutique, N.E. 75007 0294, Hôpital Public Agréé S.S. No. 1032, 1 Rue Cabanis, F-75674 Paris Cedex 14, France
Lucca, A., Dipartimento di Scienze Neuropsichiche, Ospedale San Raffaele, via Prinetti, 29, I-20127 Milano, Italy
Lucini, V., Dipartimento di Scienze Neuropsichiche, Ospedale San Raffaele, via Prinetti 29, I-20127 Milano, Italy
Luly, P., Dipartimento di Biologia, Università degli Studi di Roma "Tor Vergata", I-00173 Roma, Italy
Magnani, N., Istituto di Clinica delle Malattie Nervose e Mentali, Università degli Studi di Siena, piazza Duomo, 1, I-53100 Siena, Italy
Maj, M., Istituto di Psichiatria, Università degli Studi di Napoli, largo Madonna delle Grazie, I-80138, Napoli, Italy
Mancuso, M., Istituto di Clinica delle Malattie Nervose e Mentali, Università degli Studi di Siena, piazza Duomo, 1, I-53100 Siena, Italy
Maremmani, I., Istituto di Clinica Psichiatrica, Università degli Studi di Pisa, via Roma, 67, I-56100 Pisa, Italy
Martini, G., Istituto di Clinica Psichiatrica II, Università degli Studi di Bologna, via S. Luca, 9/2, I-40135 Bologna
Mauri, M.D., Dipartimento di Clinica Psichiatrica, Università degli Studi di Milano, via F. Sforza, 35, I-20122 Milano, Italy
Meltzer, H.L., New York Psychiatric Institute, 722 West 168th Street, New York, NY 10032, USA
Mendelewicz, J., University Clinic of Brussels, Department of Psychiatry, Erasme Hospital, Free University of Brussels, Route de Lennik 808, B-1070 Brussels, Belgium
Meschi, M., Istituto di Clinica Psichiatrica, Università degli Studi di Pisa, via Roma, 67, I-56100 Pisa, Italy

Mørk, A., Department of Pharmacology, University of Copenhagen, Juliane Maries Vej 20, DK-2100 Copenhagen, Denmark
Nardini, M., Istituto di Clinica delle Malattie Nervose e Mentali, Università degli Studi di Siena, piazza Duomo, 1, I-53100 Siena, Italy
Nassi, R., Istituto di Clinica Psichiatrica, Università degli Studi di Pisa, via Roma, 67, I-56100 Pisa, Italy
Nisticò, G., Istituto di Farmacologia Clinica e Patologia Toracica, Università degli Studi di Reggio Calabria, Policlinico Mater Domini, via Campanella, I-88100 Catanzaro, Italy
Pacini, L., Dipartimento di Biologia, Università degli Studi di Roma "Tor Vergata", I-00173 Roma, Italy
Pasquini, C., Clinica Medica, Università di Pisa, via Roma, 67, I-56100 Pisa, Italy
Pellegrini, L., Istituto di Clinica Psichiatrica, Università degli Studi di Pisa, via Roma, 67, I-56100 Pisa, Italy
Peselow, E.D., New York University School of Medicine, New York, NY, USA
Petrini, M., Istituto di Farmacologia, Università di Pisa, via Roma, 55, I-56100 Pisa, Italy
Placidi, G.F., Istituto di Clinica Psichiatrica, Università degli Studi di Pisa, via Roma, 67, I-56100 Pisa, Italy
Platman, S.R., Psychiatry and Behavioral Medicine, Homewood Hospital Center, 3915 Nth. Charles St, Baltimore, MD 21218, USA
Rapisarda, V., Clinica Psichiatrica, Università degli Studi di Catania, viale A. Doria, 6, I-95100 Catania, Italy
Ravizza, L., Istituto di Clinica Psichiatrica II, Università degli Studi di Torino, via Cherasco, 15, I-10100 Torino, Italy
Sacchetti, E., Istituto di Psichiatria, Università degli Studi di Milano, Ospedale San Paolo, I-20135 Milano, Italy
Scherillo, P., Ospedale S. Raffaele, Dipartimento di Scienze Neuropsichiche, via Prinetti 29, I-20127 Milano, Italy
Schou, M., The Psychiatric Hospital, 2 Skovagervej, DK-8240 Risskov, Denmark
Smeraldi, E., Dipartimento di Scienze Neuropsichiche, Ospedale San Raffaele, via Prinetti, 29, I-20127 Milano, Italy
Sorge, G.A., Clinica Psichiatrica, Università degli Studi di Catania, viale A. Doria, 6, I-95100 Catania, Italy
Spagnolini, M., Istituto di Clinica Psichiatrica II, Università degli Studi di Torino, via Cherasco, 15, I-10100 Torino, Italy
Spinedi, A., Dipartimento di Biologia, Università degli Studi di Roma "Tor Vergata", I-00173 Roma, Italy
Stefanelli, A., Clinica Medica, Università di Pisa, via Roma, 67, I-56100 Pisa, Italy
Stratta, P., Clinica Psichiatrica, Università degli Studi L'Aquila, I-00198 Roma, Italy

Taddei, M., Clinica Medica, Università di Pisa, via Roma, 67, I-56100 Pisa, Italy
Torta, R., Istituto di Clinica Psichiatrica II, Università degli Studi di Torino, via Cherasco, 15, I-10100 Torino, Italy
Tuoni, M., Istituto di Clinica Medica, Università di Pisa, via Roma, 67, I-56100 Pisa, Italy
Vaglini, F., Istituto di Farmacologia, Università di Pisa, via Roma, 55, I-56100 Pisa, Italy
Virzi, A., Clinica Psichiatrica, Università degli Studi di Catania, viale A. Doria, 6, I-95100 Catania, Italy
Volterra, V., Istituto di Clinica Psichiatrica II, Università degli Studi di Bologna, via S. Luca, 9/2, I-40135 Bologna, Italy
Weller, E.B., The Ohio State University, 473 W. 12th Avenue, Columbus, Ohio 43210, USA
Weller, R.A., The Ohio State University, 473 W. 12th Avenue, Columbus, Ohio 43210, USA
Zanardi, R., Ospedale San Raffaele, Dipartimento di Scienze Neuropsichiche, via Prinetti 29, I-20127 Milano, Italy

Etiologic Aspects

Toward a Psychobiology of Affective Recurrences: Interaction of Biological and Psychological Factors

H.S. Akiskal

Introduction

As Memphis is the home of the blues, where I have conducted much of my research on mood disorders, I would like to begin with the following Memphis Slim (1968) song because it provides a very important insight into the nature of mood states:

My mama had them
Her mama had them
Now I've got them too

I've got something
Something you just don't learn in school
You'll never find them in no books
You just got to inherit the blues.

When I'm sad and lonely
Even when I am happy too
All of a sudden
I find myself singing the blues
That's why I know I was born with them.

Slim, who died recently in Paris where he had lived for over 20 years, was one of the most famous blues musicians of all times. He tells us that the blues have a three-generation family history; he also notes that more women have it. He then boldly states that the environment has relatively little to do with the blues that hit a person on a recurrent basis, that they are not learned, and that they supervene even when everything is going well. All of these observations lead him to conclude that one is born with the blues – that the blues are inherited. Of course Slim is talking metaphorically, not just about the blues as a clinical entity but about the blues as a frame of mind, a form of music, and blues as talent. All the same, these insights in a song composed in the 1960s are remarkable, because in those days American psychiatry – with few exceptions (e.g., Winokur et al. 1969) – ignored familial-heredity factors in mood disorders.

Today, of course, we know that family history for mood disorders and being a female are two of the main risk factors for mood disorders (Weissman and Klerman 1977; Boyd and Weissman 1981; Gershon et al. 1982). Precise quantification of these two risk factors has come after several million dollars of

Table 1. Major risk factors for clinical depression (Summarized from Akiskal 1988)

Familial affective loading
Young female
Aversive life circumstances
Addictive disorders
Somatic disease and its treatment

rigorous research in the United States and elsewhere (Table 1). In the process, we have learned about other risk factors. Our understanding of pathogenetic mechanisms, whereby these risk factors operate to produce the final common pathway of depression (Akiskal and McKinney 1973) is limited. In particular, we are uncertain whether these risk factors operate independently from one another. This chapter discusses several lines of research that may shed some light on this question and proposes hypotheses on how selected risk factors might interact in giving rise to recurrence in mood disorders. In doing so, I will focus on primary depressive illness and refer largely to those research papers that specifically illustrate these issues. This chapter is updated from previous attempts at integration (e.g., Akiskal 1986, 1988, 1990); a more exhaustive review of the literature can be found in other published work (Whybrow et al. 1984).

Depression as a Psychobiologic Final Common Pathway

My interest in an interactional model of mood disorders developed during my training at the Wisconsin Primate Laboratory in Madison (Akiskal and McKinney 1973). The experimental paradigm being investigated in this laboratory was the response of infant monkeys to separation from their peers (McKinney and Bunney 1969). The "protest" stage – characterized by behavioral agitation ostensibly in search for the lost object – was universal. However, no more than one of three animals progressed to the stage of behavioral "despair", characterized by profound psychomotor inhibition. The investigations of Rene Spitz (1942) and John Bowlby (1961) on human infants provided comparable – somewhat lower – rates. It is customary to invoke psychosocial explanations to account for the occurrence of these phenomena, yet it would appear that – at least in monkeys – the predisposition to the "depressive" stage is limited to certain genetic strains. Similar considerations also appear relevant to Seligman's (1975) "learned helplessness" model. Although it is generally believed that the absence of instrumental responses to escape aversive contingencies in dogs and rats is based on past instances when such effort had proven useless, current data seem to indicate that the propensity to such "learning" can be considerably enhanced by selective breeding of animal strains that exhibit such inclinations (Henn and McKinney 1987).

The experimental and clinical data reviewed thus far favor the conclusion that aversive environmental contingencies – whether based on past history or

Table 2. Clinical evidence for midbrain derangement in primary depressive illness (Updated from Akiskal and McKinney 1973)

Seasonality	Anhedonia
Cyclicity	Decreased libido
Diurnal variation	Appetite disturbances
Early AM awakening	Autonomic disturbances
Hypersomnia	

current contingencies – are most potent in inducing depressive-like behaviors in those who are genetically vulnerable to such behaviors. This and related considerations have led us to the formulation of a multifactorial model of mood disorders in which familial-hereditary factors play an important role in the pathogenetic chain, which culminates in the final common pathway of limbic-diencephalic dysfunction clinically manifest as depressive illness (Akiskal and McKinney 1973). Familial, of course, is not synonymous with genetic. Evidence strongly in favor of genetic contributions has come from several strategies. Thus, the largest adoption study conducted to date (Wender et al. 1986) supports the view that heredity plays a dominant role across a broad range of clinical severity. Similar conclusions were reached using twin data (Kendler et al. 1992). However, it is in the most recurrent forms of mood disorders that we find the largest difference in monozygotic-dizygotic concordance (Bertelsen et al. 1977), as well as the highest familial loading for mood and related disorders (Gershon et al. 1982; Bland et al. 1986; Musetti et al. 1989).

It is beyond the scope of this chapter to discuss in detail evidence for limbic-diencephalic disturbances in depression. Suffice it to mention that over the 15 years since our postulation of such disturbances (Akiskal and McKinney 1973), sleep neurophysiological (Reynolds et al. 1987) and neuroendocrine (Nemeroff and Loosen 1987) abnormalities that support them have accumulated in the scientific literature. Although the specificity of these disturbances to clinical depression leaves much to be desired, cumulatively, they give credence to the notion that midbrain homeostatic mechanisms are disrupted in this illness. I wish to point out that I do not regard these laboratory perturbations as the underlying biologic causes of depressive illness, but merely as the biologic counterpart of the symptomatology that we observe in the clinic (Table 2).

It is entirely possible that the specificity of putative biologic markers for depressive illness is limited to specific subtypes – as, for instance, Carroll (1985) would argue. In addressing this heterogeneity of mood disorders, I will attempt to clarify how selected putative clinical and biologic risk factors interact in giving rise to the various recurrent patterns of mood disorders.

Precipitating Factors

A popular view of depression is that it arises understandably from aversive life circumstances, especially losses. Although the majority of individuals exposed to such circumstances do not sink into morbid despair, those predisposed to mood disorders may do so at such times. The lifetime risk for clinically significant depression is estimated somewhere between 5% and 10% (Regier et al. 1988) and, as expected, the proportion of those exposed to "exit" type life events decompensating into clinical depression does not exceed these figures (Clayton 1979; Lloyd 1980b). Furthermore, history of previous depressive episodes has been found to be a stronger predictor of depression than the characteristics of the stressors and their social context (Warheit 1979). Indeed, the likelihood that bereavement would produce clinical depression with melancholic clinical and biologic (e.g., neuroendocrine) features is significantly increased in those with past episodes of depression (Roy et al. 1988). Other factors that could hypothetically mediate the depressant effect of losses include concurrent (nonloss) life events, inadequate social support, deficient social skills, and personality.

Biologic stressors, too, appear insufficient alone to produce clinical depression. For instance, in reserpine-induced depressions (Goodwin and Bunney 1971), two-thirds of cases represent "pseudodepressions" secondary to the sedative side effects of the drug, which reverse as medication is discontinued; melancholia persisting autonomously despite withdrawal of the offending chemical occurs in the remaining third and is largely limited to those with past personal history of or predisposition for depression.

Thus, neither psychosocial events nor biologic events appear to be sufficient causes for the occurrence of clinical depressions; the likelihood of exerting a depressant influence depends on predisposing factors. What about the precipitation of hypomania or mania? The relevance of life events – especially losses – in manic episodes is suggested by Ambelas' work (1987). Obviously, such losses can easily result from premorbid cyclothymic or hyperthymic dysregulation in mood (Akiskal et al. 1977). The best known precipitants of hypomania – and to a lesser extent, mania – are drugs and physiological procedures that increase the CNS level of catecholamines. These include the tricyclic antidepressants, the monoamine oxidase inhibitors, ephedrine, L-dopa, cocaine, amphetamine-like drugs, REM deprivation, and total sleep deprivation (Akiskal 1983; Wehr et al. 1987). These factors, which often represent medically or self-administered treatments – and, in the case of REM deprivation, possibly a manifestation of the cyclothymic's decreased need for sleep – are more consistent in producing a switch from depression to hypomania than from euthymia to hypomania. Thus, the pharmacological switch appears largely limited to individuals with a bipolar diathesis – best measured as a function of personal or family history of mania (Sultzer and Cummings 1989). The same applies generally to postpartum affective episodes, whether manic, mixed, or retarded depressive. Another class of precipitating circumstances that has received attention is seasonality, which again appears largely relevant to bipolar II disorder or depressions with bipolar diathesis (Akiskal and Mallya 1987; White et al. 1990).

The evidence reviewed thus far suggests that environmental circumstances may determine the precipitation of initial episodes and the timing of subsequent recurrences. These and related considerations also indicate that "endogenous" depressive (or melancholic) episodes often arise from what initially appear to be more "reactive" or precipitated illnesses (Kraepelin 1921; Akiskal et al. 1978).

Developmental Antecedents

In a reformulation of classic psychoanalytic tenets borrowed from Bowlby (1961), Brown and Harris (1978) have hypothesized that these environmental circumstances – especially losses – could act as potent agents in initiating affective episodes in women who lack social support in raising young children and who have lost their mothers in childhood. In other words, they have attempted to argue that what individually appear to be nonspecific factors could, when considered jointly, impart some specificity to the pathogenetic role of selected psychosocial variables in depression. However, cumulative retrospective evidence has been generally inconclusive regarding the specificity of childhood loss to adult mood disorders (Lloyd 1980a). Even if present, the specificity of such loss for clinical depression appears rather dubious. Thus, Bowlby in his subsequent reformulation (1977) on the consequences of early loss subsumes a large spectrum of adult personality disturbances with mood instability and acting-out behavior.

While failing to specifically relate adult depression to childhood loss, the available research evidence does suggest several interesting links in line with Bowlby's revised formulation. For instance, we now know from the work of Perris (1966) that unipolar depressives who experienced developmental object loss have an illness onset 10 years earlier than those depressives without such loss. Moreover, other research (Levi et al. 1966) suggests that suicide attempts are more common in depressed subjects who have sustained early separations. Finally, work conducted at the University of Tennessee (Akiskal et al. 1978) has shown that early losses are associated with the adult occurrence of "unstable" characterological attributes (such as immaturity, hostile dependency, manipulativeness, impulsiveness, and low threshold for alcohol and drug abuse), rather than overt mood disorders. These findings illustrate how breaks in early object relations can be relevant to certain clinical aspects of depression. While not causing depressive illness, developmental loss might modify the clinical expression of the adult disorder. The characterological propensity toward hostile dependency may prepare a fertile soil of interpersonal friction that facilitates a depressive onset earlier than that determined by innate genetic factors; such friction may, in effect, create the life events that trigger the depression.

Another possible mechanism whereby early losses can influence the occurrence of adult depression is the creation of conditions favorable to the development of character traits associated with what Seligman (1975) refers to as "learned helplessness" or the self-denigrating depressive mental schemata described by Beck (1967). It is reasonable to assume that situations wherein the individual has failed to master a series of tasks can lead to subsequent helplessness when that individual is faced with similar situations. This viewpoint is concordant with research at the Wisconsin Primate Laboratory (Harlow 1974) that demonstrated that coping skills are developed in the context of the contact comfort provided by caring and loving parental objects; conversely, the loss of such contact comfort often precludes the development of environmental exploration and of coping skills in general. Thus, early separations from parent(s), without adequate substitute(s), may prevent the emergence of a sense of mastery of the environment. Such children may become insecure adults who feel unable to face the challenge of new situations. The mere presence of parents, however, is obviously insufficient protection against the trait of helplessness; developing a sense of mastery would require suitable role models and the opportunity to cope with a series of life events of increasing complexity. Such formulations, while plausible, need to be verified by prospective studies in clinical populations.

Arguing against the proposed relationship between childhood loss and depression is the fact that history of such loss is not present in two-thirds of adult depressives (Lloyd 1980a). Furthermore, childhood parental deprivation does not appear to exert specific formative influence on depressive illness. It is nevertheless likely that, given specific genetic predisposition to mood disorder, the experience of being raised in an unstable early home might contribute to the development of unstable personality disturbances. University of Tennessee work (Akiskal et al. 1978, 1985) suggests that these embrace a spectrum of characterological disturbances, including what North American psychiatrists refer to as "borderline" features. Thus, having affectively ill parents represents a double jeopardy, i.e., the possibility of inheriting the biologic predisposition to affective dysregulation and developmental disruption arising from having an affectively ill parent.

Research conducted at the Karolinska Institute in Sweden (Asberg et al. 1987) further suggests that affectively labile individuals, who often have low cerebrospinal fluid (CSF) indices of serotonin function, are more likely to die from violent suicides; this eventuality is not necessarily linked with a clinically diagnosable mood disorder. Actually, such serotonergic deficits have been hypothesized by van Praag et al. (1987) as being generic to a large class of psychopathological entities – including bulimia, alcoholism, suicide, and violence against others – and clinically mediated by high impulsivity. Low central serotonergic function, though probably not specific to mood disorder, appears relevant to both men and women and in the presence of mood disorder might, hypothetically, color the affective clinical picture with characterological instability.

Pathoplastic Effect of Gender

Now, women are more likely to receive unstable characterological labels such as "borderline". They also seem more prone to depressive recurrences. It is customary to invoke psychosocial variables to account for this increased vulnerability; yet biologic factors appear at least equally relevant. Premenstrual emotional changes might represent one hormonally mediated factor that has a bearing on such vulnerability. Although this factor does not appear specific to mood disorder (Dalton 1984), it could color, accentuate, or determine the recurrence of affective experiences in those women suffering from such disorders (Parry 1989). Other biologic factors relevant to the vulnerability of women to depression include marginal hypothyroid indices – especially relevant to rapid cycling (Cowdry et al. 1983) – and an elevated level of the enzyme monoamine oxidase (Robinson et al. 1971). Being controlled by the X chromosome (Kochersperger et al. 1986), this enzyme might account in part for the anxious-depressive clinical picture, the "atypical" (hypersomnic-lethargic-bulimic) depressive coloring, and the relative selectivity of monoamine oxidase inhibitors observed in women (Davidson and Pelton 1986). It is also of interest that recent collaborative research (Perugi et al. 1990) between the University of Pisa and the University of Tennessee has shown that women are more likely to exhibit dysthymic or depressive temperaments and men hyperthymic temperaments. This, in part, could explain why more women have recurrent depressions, whereas the sex ratio in classic bipolar illness is about even.

Hypothesized Mediating Role of Temperament

It is, of course, still largely a mystery why in the same affective pedigree we observe patients with the gamut of affective and related disorders, i.e., predominantly manic forms of bipolar illness (bipolar I) and purely depressive forms (unipolar I), bridged by "soft" phenotypes with recurrent depressions and hypomania rather than mania (bipolar II or unipolar II), as well as the lesser or "subaffective" phenotypes of cyclothymic, hyperthymic, and depressive temperaments. As discussed elsewhere (Akiskal 1983), in some instances temperaments precede the overt expression of frank affective episodes. Other evidence (Akiskal 1986, 1988) suggests the hypothesis that the genetic potential to develop affective episodes might be transmitted as "subclinical" temperamental dysregulation in the form of cyclothymia, hyperthymia, or dysthymia. These temperamental propensities might interact with other risk factors – some independent, but more often resulting from their social or physiological repercussions – to bring about major affective breakdowns (Fig. 1). Whereas depression that arises in the absence of such propensities begins later in life, depressive conditions arising from temperamental substrates typically begin much earlier in life and tend to pursue a more recurrent course (Musetti et al. 1989). A tendency towards early relapse and/or chronicity has also been reported in "double depressives", i.e., those with major depressive episodes coexisting with dysthymic traits (Keller et al. 1983).

Factors relevant to the expression of the different bipolar forms are beyond the scope of this chapter. Suffice it to mention that high rates of recurrence – as represented by rapid-cycling forms – is favored when bipolar disorder coexists with thyroid abnormalities (Extein and Gold 1986; Cowdry et al. 1983) and there has been prolonged exposure to tricyclic antidepressants (Kukopoulos et al. 1980; Wehr and Goodwin 1987); repeated object loss which commonly occurs in bipolars with cyclothymic temperament (Akiskal et al. 1977) could, likewise,

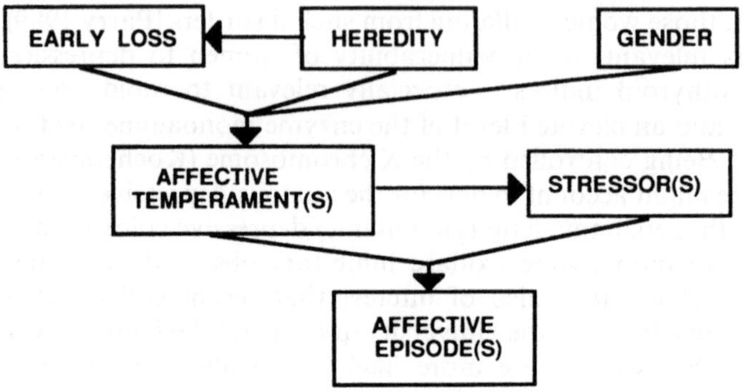

Fig. 1. A proposed pathogenic chain in recurrent mood disorders based on Akiskal (1986)

"kindle" the brain (Post 1992). It is finally tempting to return where I began: given talent, artistic expression, and eminence could represent one of the "social phenotypes" of the soft or subbipolar spectrum (Akiskal and Akiskal 1988).

Acknowledgment. Parts of this chapter previously appeared in Akiskal HS (1989) New insights into the nature and heterogeneity of mood disorders (J Clin Psychiatry 50 [suppl 5]: 6–12) and are reproduced here by permission of Physicians Postgraduate Press, Memphis.

References

Akiskal HS (1983) The bipolar spectrum: new concepts in classification and diagnosis. In: Grinspoon L (ed) Psychiatry update: the American psychiatric association annual review. American Psychiatric Press, Washington DC, pp 271–292

Akiskal HS (1986) A developmental perspective on recurrent mood disorders: a review of studies in man. Psychopharmacol Bull 22: 579–586

Akiskal HS (1988) Personality as a mediating variable in the pathogenesis of mood disorders: implications for theory, research and prevention. In: Helgason T, Daly RD (eds) Depressive illness: prediction of course and outcome. Springer, Berlin Heidelberg New York, pp 131–146

Akiskal HS (1990) An integrative perspective on recurrent mood disorders. In: Becker J and Kleinman A (eds) Psychosocial Aspects of Depression. Lawrence Erlbaum Associates, Inc, Hillsdale, pp 215–235

Akiskal HS, Akiskal K (1988) Re-assessing the prevalence of bipolar disorders: clinical significance and artistic creativity. Psychiatr Psychobiol 3: 29s–36s

Akiskal HS, Mallya G (1987) Criteria for the "soft" bipolar spectrum: treatment implications. Psychopharmacol Bull 23: 68–73

Akiskal HS, McKinney WT Jr (1973) Depressive disorders: toward a unified hypothesis. Science 182: 20–29

Akiskal HS, Djenderedjian AM, Rosenthal RH et al (1977) Cyclothymic disorder: validating criteria for inclusion in the bipolar affective group. Am J Psychiatry 134: 1227–1233

Akiskal HS, Bitar AH, Puzantian VT et al (1978) The nosological status of neurotic depression: a prospective three- to four-year examination in light of the primary-secondary and unipolar-bipolar dichotomies. Arch Gen Psychiatry 35: 756–766

Akiskal HS, Chen SE, Davis GC et al (1985) Borderline: an adjective in search of a noun. J Clin Psychiatry 46: 41–48

Ambelas A (1987) Life events and mania. A special relationship? Br J Psychiatry 150: 235–240

Asberg M, Schalling D, Traskman-Bendz L et al (1987) Psychobiology of suicide, impulsivity, and relapsed phenomena. In: Meltzer HY (ed) Psychopharmacology – the third generation of progress. Raven, New York, pp 655–668

Beck AT (1967) Depression – causes and treatment. University of Pennsylvania Press, Philadelphia

Bertelsen A, Harvald B, Hauge M (1977) A Danish twin study of manic-depressive disorders. Br J Psychiatry 130: 330–351

Bland RC, Newman SC, Orn H (1986) Recurrent and nonrecurrent depression. A family study. Arch Gen Psychiatry 43: 1085–1089

Bowlby J (1961) Childhood mourning and its implications for child psychiatry. Am J Psychiatry 118: 481–498

Bowlby J (1977) The making and breaking of affectional bonds: 1. Aetiology and psychopathology in the light of attachment theory. Br J Psychiatry 130: 201–210

Boyd JH, Weissman MM (1981) Epidemiology of affective disorders: A re-examination and future directions. Arch Gen Psychiatry 38: 1039–1046

Brown GS, Harris T (1978) Social origins of depression. Tavistock, London

Carroll BJ (1985) Dexamethasone suppression test: a review of contemporary confusion. J Clin Psychiatry 46(2, 2): 13–24

Clayton PJ (1979) The sequelae and nonsequelae of conjugal bereavement. Am J Psychiatry 136: 1530–1534

Cowdry RW, Wehr TA, Zis AP, Goodwin FK (1983) Thyroid abnormalities associated with rapid-cycling bipolar illness. Arch Gen Psychiatry 40: 414–420

Dalton K (1984) The premenstrual syndrome and progesterone therapy. Year Book, Chicago

Davidson JRT, Pelton S (1986) Forms of atypical depression and their response to antidepressant drugs. Psychiatry Res 17: 87–95

Extein I, Gold MS (1986) Psychiatric applications of thyroid tests. J Clin Psychiatry 47 [Suppl 1]: 13–16

Gershon ES, Hamovit J, Guroff JJ et al (1982) A family study of schizoaffective, bipolar I, bipolar II, unipolar and normal control probands. Arch Gen Psychiatry 39: 1157–1167

Goodwin F, Bunney WE Jr (1971) Depressions following reserpine: a re-evaluation. Semin Psychiatry 3: 19–53

Harlow HF (1974) Learning to love. Aronson, New York

Henn FA, McKinney WT Jr (1987) Animal models in psychiatry. In: Meltzer HY (ed) Psychopharmacology – the third generation of progress. Raven, New York, pp 687–695

Keller MB, Lavori PW, Endicott J et al (1983) Double depression: two-year follow-up. Am J Psychiatry (1983) 140: 689–694

Kendler KS, Neale MC, Kessler RC et al. (1992) A population-based twin study of major depression in women. Arch Gen Psychiatry 49: 257–266

Kochersperger LM, Parker EL, Siciliano M et al (1986) Assignment of genes for human monoamine oxidases A and B to the X-chromosome. J Neurosci Res 16: 601–616

Kraepelin E (1921) Manic-depressive insanity and paranoia. (Translated by Barclay RM, Robertson GM.) Livingstone, Edinburgh

Kukopoulos A, Reginaldi D, Laddomada P et al (1980) Course of the manic-depressive cycle and changes caused by treatments. Pharmacopsychiatria 13: 156–167

Levi LD, Fales CH, Stein M et al (1966) Separation and attempted suicide. Arch Gen Psychiatry 15: 158–164

Lloyd C (1980a) Life events and depressive disorder reviewed: I. Events as predisposing factors. Arch Gen Psychiatry 37: 529–535

Lloyd C (1980b) Life events and depressive disorder reviewed: II. Events as precipitating factors. Arch Gen Psychiatry 37: 541–548

McKinney WT Jr, Bunney WE Jr (1969) Animal model of depression. Arch Gen Psychiatry 21: 240–248

Musetti L, Perugi G, Soriana A et al (1989) Depression before and after age 65. A re-examination. Br J Psychiatry 155: 330–336

Nemeroff CB, Lossen PT (eds) (1987) Handbook of clinical psychoneuroendocrinology. Guilford, New York

Parry BL (1989) Reproductive factors affecting the course of affective illness in women. Psychiatr Clin North Am 12: 207–220

Perris C (1966) A study of bipolar (manic-depressive) and unipolar recurrent depressive psychoses. II. Childhood environment and precipitating factors. Acta Psychiatr Scand 194 [Suppl]: 45–57

Perugi G, Musetti L, Simonini E et al (1990) Gender mediated clinical features of depressive illness: The importance of temperamental differences. Br J Psychiatry 157: 835–841

Post RM (1992) Transduction of psychosocial stress into the neurobiology of recurrent affective disorder. Am J Psychiatry 149: 999–1010

Regier DA, Boyd JH, Burke JD et al (1988) One-month prevalence of mental disorders in the United States. Based on five epidemiological catchment area sites. Arch Gen Psychiatry 45: 977–986

Reynolds CF, Gillin JC, Kupfer DJ (1987) Sleep and affective disorders. In: Meltzer HY (ed) Psychopharmacology – The third generation of progress. Raven, New York, pp 647–654

Robinson DS, Davis JM, Nies A et al (1971) Relation of sex and aging to monoamine oxidase activity of human brain, plasma and platelets. Arch Gen Psychiatry 24: 536–539

Roy A, Gallucci W, Avgerinos P et al (1988) The CRH stimulation test in bereaved subjects with and without accompanying depression. Psychiatr Res 25: 145–156

Seligman MD (1975) Helplessness: on depression, development and death. Freeman, San Francisco

Slim M (1968) Born with the blues. Shreveport, Jewel Records, 5004

Spitz R (1942) Anaclitic depression: an inquiry into the genesis of psychiatric conditions in early childhood. Psychoanal Study Child 2: 313–342

Sultzer DL, Cummings JL (1989) Drug-induced mania – causative agents, clinical characteristics and management. A retrospective analysis of the literature. Med Toxicol Adverse Drug Exp 4: 127–143

van Praag HM, Kahn RS, Asnis GM et al (1987) Denosologization of biological psychiatry or the specificity of 5-HT disturbances in psychiatric disorders. J Affective Disord 13: 1–8

Warheit GJ (1979) Life events, coping, stress, and depressive symptomatology. Am J Psychiatry 136: 502–507

Wehr TA, Goodwin FK (1987) Can antidepressants cause mania and worsen the course of affective illness? Am J psychiatr 144: 1403–1411

Wehr TA, Sack DA, Rosenthal NE (1987) Sleep reduction as a final common pathway in the genesis of mania. Am J Psychiatry 144: 201–204

Weissman MM, Klerman GL (1977) Sex differences and the epidemiology of depression. Arch Gen. Psychiatry 34: 98–111

Wender PH, Kety SS, Rosenthal D et al (1986) Psychiatric disorders in the biological and adoptive families of adopted individuals with affective disorders. Arch Gen Psychiatry 43: 923–929

White DM, Lewy AJ, Sack RL et al (1990) Is winter depression a bipolar disorder? Compr Psychiatry 31: 196–204

Whybrow PC, Akiskal HS, McKinney WT Jr (1984) Mood disorders: toward a new psychobiology. Plenum, New York

Winokur G, Clayton P, Reigh T (1969) Manic-depressive illness. Mosby, St Louis

New Genetic Findings in Recurrent Mood Disorders

J. Mendlewicz

Affective disorders, and in particular, manic depression, have been the subject of many classic genetic studies. Table 1 summarizes concordance rates for manic depression in twin studies of manic-depressive probands (Mendlewicz 1988). Table 1 concordance rates are consistently higher in monozygotic (MZ) than dizygotic pairs, but they do not reach the 100% value in MZ pairs, indicating that nongenetic (environmental) factors may also be operating in this illness and interacting with the genetic predisposition. Such interactions between nature and nurture can be best examined through the use of more sophisticated strategies such as the adoption method and the new linkage analyses. The adoption method has been applied to manic depression with conclusive results demonstrating the necessary presence of important genetic factors in the etiology of the illness (Table 2; Mendlewicz and Rainer 1977). More recent linkage studies with classic genetic markers such as color blindness and G6PD deficiency have provided consistent evidence of the presence of a major single gene located on the distal end of the long arm of the X chromosome in bipolar manic depression (Mendlewicz 1986, 1988) despite the fact that this type of inheritance has not been observed in all families studied (Mendlewicz 1988). In addition, using the DNA recombinant method in molecular genetic studies of manic depression, a close linkage has recently been demonstrated between manic depression and factor IX (hemophilia B) on the distal end of the long arm of chromosome X in a new set of pedigrees (Mendlewicz et al. 1987), as illustrated in Fig. 1. Conversely, the localization of a gene situated on the distal

Table 1. Concordance rates for manic-depressive illness in twins

Study	Concordance rate (%)	
	Monozygotic	Dizygotic
Rosanoff et al. (1934)	69.6	16.4
Kallmann (1954)	92.6	23.6
Da Fonseca (1959)	71.4	38.5
Harvald and Hauge (1965)	50.0	2.6
Kringlèn (1967)	33.3	0.0
Bertelsen (1977)	58.0	17.0
Torgersen (1986)	75.0	17.0

From Mendlewicz (1988)

Table 2. Diagnosis of parents for normal adoptees and nonadoptees.

	Normal adoptees ($n = 24$)						Poliomyelitis ($n = 20$)		
	Adoptive parents			Biologic parents			Biologic parents		
	Male	Female	Total	Male	Female	Total	Male	Female	Total
Bipolar	0	0	0	0	0	0	0	0	0
Unipolar	1	2	3	1	0	1	3	1	4
Schizoaffective	0	0	0	0	0	0	0	0	0
Cyclothymic	1	0	1	0	0	0	0	0	0
Affective spectrum	2	2	4	1	0	1	3	1	4
Percentage	10	10	10	5	0	2	15	5	10
Schizophrenic	0	1	1	0	0	0	0	0	0
Alcoholism	0	0	0	1	2	3	1	0	1
Sociopathy	0	0	0	2	1	3	0	0	0
Other	0	0	0	0	1	1	0	0	0
All psychopathology	2	3	5	4	4	8	4	1	5
Percentage	9	14	11	18	18	18	20	5	12

From Mendlewicz and Rainer (1977)

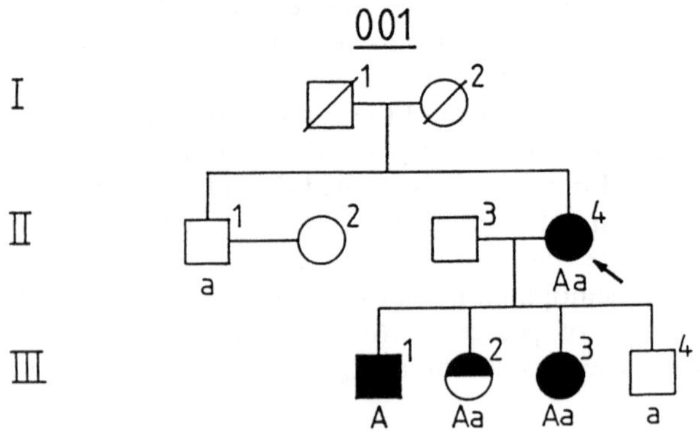

Fig. 1. Pedigrees indicating linkage between manic depression and factor IX, from Mendlewicz et al. 1987

part of the short arm of chromosome 11 has also been reported in one family originating from the old Amish community (Egeland et al. 1987), but this chromosomal linkage has not yet been confirmed in other pedigrees (Detera-Waldeigh et al. 1987; Hodgkinson et al. 1987; Michael et al. 1988), using the same chromosomal probes in informative families selected in different geographical areas. Furthermore, a recent reevaluation of the linkage relationship between chromosome 11p loci and the gene of bipolar affective disorder in the old order Amish provided supplementary data on the original core pedigree and on a new extension of the Amish family (Kelsoe et al. 1989). The newly extended family showed lod scores to be considerably weakened, indicating that a single locus linked to INS and HRAS1 was unlikely to be the sole causal factor for affective disorder. Furthermore, genetic probes on the long arm of the X chromosome have suggested the presence of a major locus for manic depression between ST 14 and factor IX genes (Mendlewicz 1989). Thus, these new chromosomal linkage findings reveal the existence of several distinct genetic forms of bipolar illness, with at least two potential different chromosomal locations, one on the tip of the long arm of the X chromosome and the other (if confirmed by other groups) on the short arm of chromosome 11, as illustrated in Figs. 2 and 3. Other pedigrees of bipolars have been reported not to show linkage with the above genetic markers (Mendlewicz 1988). These results provide strong support for the hypothesis of molecular heterogeneity in the genetic etiology of bipolar manic-depressive illness. The application of molecular genetics such as the use of various RFLP and polymerase chain reaction (PCR) for gene amplification will provide new powerful tools for data banking of genetic material. The data originating from the behavioral studies in inbred strains of rats could also provide through chromosomal segregation studies relevant important information on specific candidate genes and chromosomal markers of neurobiologic interest such as the gene for tyrosine hydroxylase (TH)

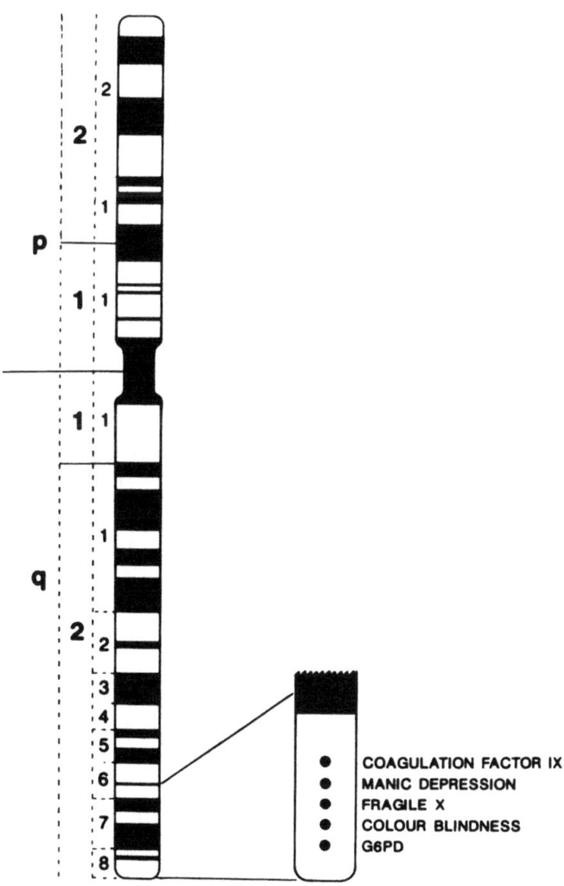

Fig. 2. Chromosome X

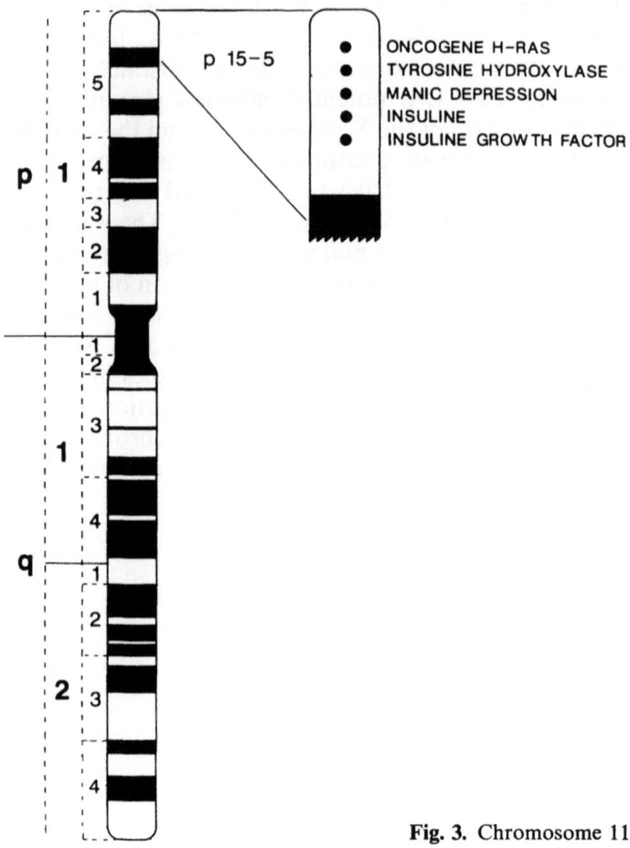

Fig. 3. Chromosome 11

in the 11q region of chromosome 11 (Grima et al. 1985) and the 3 GABA receptor gene in the Xq 28 region of chromosome X (Schofield et al. 1987), two potential candidate genes in manic-depressive illness to be explored in man. Chromosomal rearrangement studies are also to be studied in psychiatric disorders, because these observations could help targeting new chromosomal probes in specific chromosomal regions of interest as exemplified by the single reports of sex chromosome anomalies in some bipolar patients (Caroff 1978; Pascalis et al. 1985) and by recent observations of a translocation between chromosome 11 (long arm) and chromosome 9 in a family with affective illness (Potkin et al. 1989). The discovery of linkage in mental disorders, apart from clarifying the mode of genetic transmission and allowing for studying the interaction between genes and other factors in complex behaviors, will also ultimately lead to the isolation, sequencing, and cloning of the mutant genes and thus help provide some rationale for etiologic and preventive therapeutic approaches.

References

Caroff SN (1978) Klinefelter's syndrome and bipolar affective illness: a case report. Am J Psychiatry 135: 748–749

Detera-Waldeigh SD, Berretini WH, Goldin LR, Boorman D, Anderson SB, Gershon ES (1987) Close linkage of C-Harvey-ras-1 and the insulin gene to affective disorder is ruled out in three North American pedigrees. Nature 325: 806–808

Egeland JA, Gerhard DS, Pauls DL, Sussex JS, Kidd KK, Allen CR, Hostetter AM, Housman DE (1987) Bipolar affective disorders linked to DNA markers on chromosome 11. Nature 325: 783–787

Grima B, Lamoureux A, Blanot F, Faucon Biguet N, Mallet J (1985) Complete coding sequence of rat tyrosine hydroxylase mRNA. Proc Natl Acad Sci USA 82: 617–621

Hodgkinson S, Sherrington R, Gurling H, Marchbanks R, Reeders S, Mallet J, McInnes M, Petursson H, Brynjolfson J (1987) Molecular genetic evidence of heterogeneity in manic-depression. Nature 325: 805–806

Kelsoe JR, Gings EI, Egeland JA, Gerhard DS, Goldstien AM, Bale SJ, Pauls DL, Long RT, Kidd KK, Conte G, Housman DE, Paul SM (1989) Re-evaluation of the linkage relationship between chromosome 11p loci and the gene for bipolar affective disorder in the old order Amish. Nature 342: 238–243

Mendlewicz J (1986) X-linked transmission of affective illness: current status and new evidence. Shagass C, Josiassen R, Bridger W, Weiss K, Stoff D, Simpson G (eds) Biological psychiatry, vol 7. Elsevier, Amsterdam, pp 46–48

Mendlewicz J (1988) Population and family studies in depression and mania. Br Psychiatry 153 [Suppl 3]: 16–25

Mendlewicz J (1989) Molecular genetics studies in affective disorders. Plenary session: progress in biological research of mood and anxiety disorders. VIIIth World Congress of Psychiatry, 12–19 Oct 1989, Athens, Greece (plenary lecture)

Mendlewicz J, Rainer JD (1977) Adoption study supporting genetic transmission in manic-depressive illness. Nature 268: 327–329

Mendlewicz J, Simon P, Charon F, Brocas H, Legros S, Vassart G (1987) A polymorphic DNA marker on X chromosome and manic-depression. Lancet 1230–1232

Michael G, McKeon P, Humphries P (1988) Linkage analysis of manic depression in an Irish family using H-ras-1 and INS DNA markers. J Med Genet 25: 634–637

Pascalis G, Teyssier JR, Carre-Pigeon F (1985) Présence d'un xq-fra chez un maniaque: situation du géne de la P.M.D. sur le bras long. Ann Med Psychol (Paris) 146(6): 594–595.15. S G

Potkin, Bunney WE, Wasmuth J, Smith M, Deantonio M (1989) Translocation of chromosome 9 and 11 in a family with manic-depressive illness. Biological aspects of non-psychotic disorders. (WFSBP) Regional congress. 2–7 April 1989 (Jerusalem, Israel)

Schofield PR, Darlison MG, Fujita N, Burt DR, Stefpenson FA, Rodriguez H, Rhee LM, Ramachandran J, Reale V, Glencorse TA, Seeburg PH, Barnard EA (1987) Sequence and functional expression of the $Gaba^A$ receptor shows a ligand-gated receptor super-family. Nature 328 (6127): 221–227

Recent Findings on Thyroid Function in Depression

G.F. Placidi, L. Bartalena, M. Meschi, L. Pellegrini, and L. Dell'Osso

Historical Overview

It has been generally agreed that mood disturbances are quite common in patients with thyroid dysfunctions. Depressive symptoms are very frequent in hypothyroid patients although manic episodes may be occasionally observed. On the other hand, it has been reported that depressive patients may show some clinical symptoms of hypothyroidism (Gold et al. 1981; McGaffe et al. 1981); treatment with thyroid hormones may have beneficial effects on these patients.

Depression shares many symptoms with hypothyroidism (Table 1). Animal studies have demonstrated that tricyclic antidepressants (TCA) may be less

Table 1. Symptoms of depression and hypothyroidism (modified from Nemeroff, 1989)

Symptoms	Depression	Hypothyroidism
Depressed mood	+	+
Loss of interest or pleasure	+	+
Weight gain	+	+
Appetite decrease	+	+
Sleep increase	+	+
Constipation	+	+
Decreased libido	+	+
Anergia, fatigue	+	+
Decreased concentration	+	+
Suicidal ideation	+	+
Delusions	+	+
Weight loss	+	−
Appetite increase	+	−
Sleep increase	+	−
Goiter	−	+
Cold intolerance	−	+
Brittle hair	−	+
Loss of eyebrow hair	−	+
Thickened, dry skin	−	+
Bradycardia	−	+
Cardiac failure	−	+
Delayed reflexes	−	+

effective in the presence of hypothyroidism (Avni et al. 1967) and that the administration of small amounts of triiodothyronine (T3) or thyrotropin-releasing hormone (TRH) to depressives enhance the effectiveness of TCA.

The above data, together with the observation of increased baseline thyrotropin (TSH) levels and/or enhanced TSH response to TRH in some depressed patients (Gold et al. 1981; Wilson and Jefferson 1985), led to the hypothesis that depressives might be subclinical primary hypothyroids.

The evaluation of the hypothalamus-pituitary-thyroid (HPT) axis in depressives, however, has provided controversial results which do not easily fit with this hypothesis. Normal serum total thyroxine (TT4), free T4 (FT4) and free T3 (FT3) values have been reported by Takahashi et al. (1974), Kierkegaard et al. (1978), Linnoila et al. (1982) and Undén et al. (1986) in bipolar and unipolar, neurotic and reactive depression, whereas increased thyroid hormone concentrations were found by Dewhurst et al. (1969), Whybrow et al. (1972), Hatotani et al. (1977), Loosen and Prange (1980), Kirkegaard and Faber (1981) and Maes et al. (1989).

However, most authors observed a decrease in serum total T3 (TT3) and FT3 values (Kirkegaard et al. 1975; Nordgreen and Sheele 1976; Linnoila et al. 1979; Kjellman et al. 1983; Loosen et al. 1983b; Joffe et al. 1985; Orsulak et al. 1985; Rubin et al. 1987), with a concomitant increase in serum reverse T3 (rT3) concentration (Linnoila et al. 1979; Kirkegaard and Faber 1981; Linnoila et al. 1982, 1983; Kjellman et al. 1983; Undén et al. 1986). Different methodological approaches in the selection of patients and in psychotropic treatment may explain such controversial findings.

Conflicting results for serum TSH changes in depressed patients have also been reported. Normal (Dewhurst et al. 1969; Loosen et al. 1977; Kirkegaard et al. 1978; Loosen and Prange 1980; Linkowski et al. 1981; Orsulak et al. 1985; Marchesi et al. 1988), decreased (Weeke and Weeke 1978; Goldstein et al. 1980; Targum et al. 1982; Kjellman et al. 1983; Undén et al. 1986; Rubin et al. 1987; Roy et al. 1988; Maes et al. 1989), and increased baseline levels in the morning (Tollefson et al. 1985), particularly in rapid cycling bipolar patients (O'Shanick and Ellinwood 1982; Cowdry et al. 1983) have been reported.

When only relatively insensitive TSH radioimmunoassays were available, the evaluation of TSH secretion necessarily had to rely on the results of the stimulation test with TRH.

So far more than 60 studies on about 2000 patients have documented a diminished or blunted TSH response to TRH in 25%–30% of depressed patients. In about half of the patients the blunted response may also persist after recovery from depression; so it remains unclear if this abnormality is state- or trait dependent. Alternatively, it is possible that the normalization of the neuroendocrine regulatory mechanisms may be particularly slow in some patients.

As for the possibility of differentiating subtypes of depression by TRH test, controversial results have been reported. Some authors have considered the TSH response to TRH a useful tool to discriminate between unipolar and bipolar depressives, since most unipolar depressives (77%) and few bipolar depressives (17%) show a blunted TSH response (Kirstein et al. 1982). Other authors, however, failed to find any difference between unipolar and bipolar depressives (Loosen and Prange 1982).

The impairment of TSH secretion in depressives has been related to a desensitization of the thyrotroph due to down-regulation of the TRH receptors following excessive TRH stimulation (Kjellman et al. 1984). In fact chronic low-dose TRH administration causes a reduction in the nocturnal serum TSH surge (Spencer et al. 1980) and TRH levels in the cerebrospinal fluid of depressed patients are high (Kirkegaard et al. 1979; Banki et al. 1988). However, no correlation has been reported between cerebrospinal fluid TRH concentration and the TSH response to TRH (Kirkegaard et al. 1979; Banki et al. 1988). Furthermore, the normal TSH response to TRH elicited in two thirds of the patients suggests a mechanism operating at suprapituitary level.

On the contrary, the absence of the nocturnal TSH surge in central hypothyroidism in man (Caron et al. 1986) or after hypothalamic lesion in animals (Fukuda and Greer 1975), and the observation that the administration of TRH to animals produces behavioral effects similar to those determined by TCA drugs (Ogawa et al. 1984) suggest that hypothalamic TRH secretion may be reduced in major depression. In this case the blunted TSH response to exogenous TRH administration found in one third of the patients remains to be explained.

Other hormones and/or neurotransmitters have been involved in the changes of TSH secretion in depression.

Cortisol is known to reduce TSH secretion (Bartalena et al. 1990; Re et al. 1976; Duick and Wahner 1979; Brabant et al. 1987); alterations in cortisol secretion have been found in about 50% of depressives (Stokes and Sikes 1988), though their relation to the changes in TSH secretion is controversial (Agren and Wide 1982; Targum et al. 1982; Roy et al. 1988).

Dopamine also plays an inhibitory role in the basal TSH secretion and after TRH (Sowers et al. 1982). The role of this neuromediator is otherwise uncertain, as are the suggestions of some authors of increased noradrenergic or decreased serotoninergic activities (Roy et al. 1988; Maas et al. 1987). The role of somatostatin and melatonin, both having an inhibitory action on TSH secretion, still await adequate confirmation.

Unresolved Issues

There are several theoretical and methodological problems concerning the clinical application of the TRH test:

1. A blunted TSH response is not specific to depression; it has been found in alcoholism, in borderline and panic disorders, in mania, anorexia nervosa, dysthymic disorder, and schizophrenia (Loosen et al. 1983a; Calloway et al. 1984; Prange et al. 1987).
2. The test-retest reproducibility of TSH blunting is not documented.

3. Not much is known about the persistence of TSH blunting in the same patient evaluated prospectively and/or during a recurrent depression.
4. Very few studies have evaluated the correlation between TSH blunting and the length and severity of illness, prior antidepressant drug treatment, or subtypes of depression.
5. It is hard to explain why a blunted TSH response to TRH is present in only 30% of depressed patients and little is known about the underlying mechanisms and the role of other neurotransmitters.
6. The TRH test represents a pharmacological stimulus which may not strictly reflect changes occurring in the physiological TSH secretion. Indeed TSH secretion shows circadian variations, with the highest serum concentrations in the late evening or early morning (Patel et al. 1972; Vanhaelst et al. 1972; Azukizawa et al. 1976; Weeke and Laurberg 1976; Brabant et al. 1986; Caron et al. 1986; Evans et al. 1986; Greenspan et al. 1986; Bartalena et al. 1987).

Personal Contribution

The nocturnal serum TSH surge is abolished in hyperthyroids and in patients under chronic thyroxine treatment, whereas it is maintained in patients with mild primary hypothyroidism. The lack of nocturnal serum TSH surge in patients with structural alterations of the hypothalamus and pituitary is often correlated with central hypothyroidism, despite normal serum levels of morning TSH. Recently, it has been reported that the nocturnal serum TSH surge is also not present in patients who have undergone major surgery; this is as a consequence of the surgery-associated stress, with increased serum cortisol concentrations. It would therefore appear that the evaluation of the nocturnal serum TSH surge may provide relevant information concerning the pituitary–thyroid axis.

Only very few studies have evaluated the nocturnal serum TSH surge in depressives, employing relatively insensitive TSH radioimmunoassays (Weeke and Weeke 1978; Goldstein et al. 1980; Kjellman et al. 1984; Rubin et al. 1987; Sack et al. 1988; Souêtre et al. 1989).

In order to evaluate the HPT function in depression, a clinical study was carried out in which the nocturnal serum TSH surge was measured by means of an ultrasensitive immunoradiometric assay in 15 depressed females, untreated for at least 2 months, and 15 healthy females with no present or past history of psychiatric or thyroid disorders (Bartalena et al. 1990). A significant decrease in both TT3 and FT3 and T4 levels was observed in depressives, whose serum rT3 concentration was significantly increased. FT4 values were subnormal in two patients and low–normal in five. Positive thyroglobulin and/or thyroid peroxidase autoantibody tests were found in two depressives and in two controls.

Serum cortisol levels both in the morning and, in particular, at night were significantly increased in depressives; five patients (33%) had supranormal values at night. Mean morning TSH values did not differ in the two groups

(1.3 ± 0.2 mU/L in depressives and 1.4 ± 0.1 mU/L in controls, ±standard error of mean), whereas mean night values were significantly reduced in depressives (1.5 ± 0.3 mU/L vs 3.1 ± 0.3 mU/L, $p < 0.0005$). At variance with the control group, morning and night TSH values did not differ in depressives. The nocturnal serum TSH surge was abolished in 14 out of 15 depressed patients. The mean peak TSH value after TRH administration in depressives was significantly lower than in controls (7.8 ± 1.6 mU/L vs 11.4 ± 1.0 mU/L, $p < 0.05$, Fig. 1).

Of six patients with subnormal (<0.4 mU/L) morning TSH values, the nocturnal TSH surge was abolished in all six and TSH response to TRH was blunted in five out of six (Fig. 2). Conversely, the TRH test provided normal results in all the nine patients with normal morning TSH concentration,

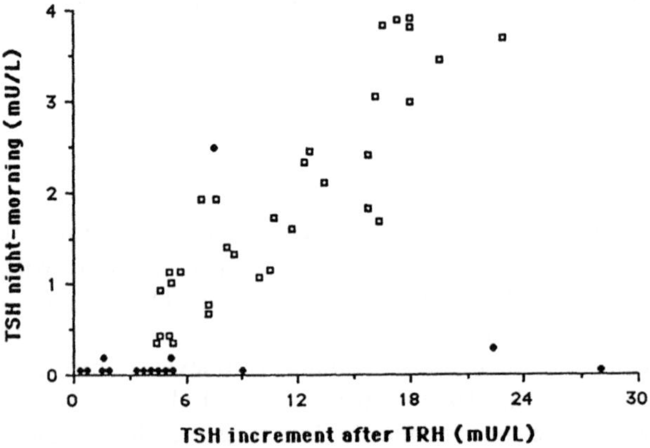

Fig. 1. Relationship of TSH response to TRH with the nocturnal TSH peak. □, Controls; ◆, depressed

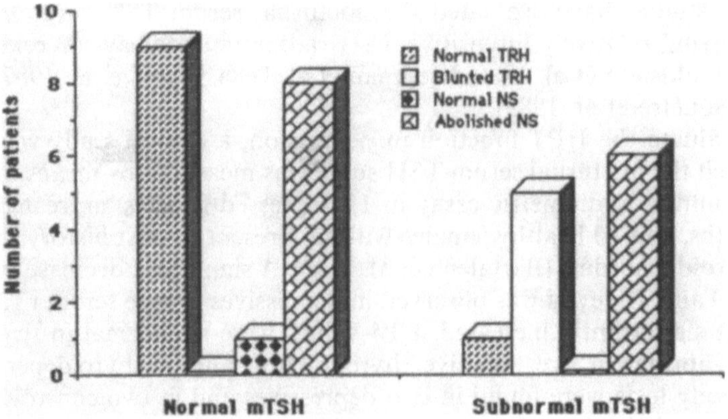

Fig. 2. Mean serum TSH concentrations at night and in the morning and mean TSH (MTSH) peak value after TRH administration

although the nocturnal TSH surge was maintained in only one of them. The baseline TSH values in the morning were reduced marginally in only 40% of the patients, who, with one exception, also showed blunted TSH responses to TRH.

Thus, on the basis of these parameters (morning measurement and TSH response to TRH), TSH secretion would have been considered to be normal in more than 60% of patients. However, all these patients showed, with one exception, a lack of the nocturnal serum TSH surge. This phenomenon has been described by few authors, although the use of conventional and relatively insensitive radioimmunoassays, instead of the ultrasensitive immunoradiometric assays employed in the present study, might have prevented the detection of small changes in serum TSH levels. Furthermore, our report emphasizes the dissociation between the response to TRH and the nocturnal surge of the hormone, in that the supraphysiological stimulation determined by 200 μg TRH could still elicit a TSH response, even in patients in whom the physiological nocturnal TSH surge had already been abolished.

No correlation could be found between the TSH values at night or after TRH stimulation and the total or the single Hamilton Rating Scale for Depression (HRSD) item score, and no differences were detected among bipolar and unipolar depressives.

Concluding Remarks

We found an inverse relationship between night cortisol and TSH levels suggesting that cortisol may be at least in part responsible for this phenomenon.

The observation in our series that baseline prolactin (PRL) levels were not reduced and the PRL response to TRH was even enhanced, tends to indicate that an excessive dopaminergic activity is unlikely to play a major role in the pathogenesis of the observed changes in TSH secretion.

The observation of a significant reduction in serum sex hormone-binding globulin and ferritin concentrations in the depressed patients (four patients of this series having subnormal serum levels of the former protein) suggests the occurrence of a certain degree of hypothyroidism at the tissue levels.

The most significant finding of this study, in agreement with Rubin's recent results at UCLA, is that the assessment of the nocturnal serum TSH surge is essential to unveil the profound derangement of TSH secretion that occurs in major depression.

The evaluation of the nocturnal serum TSH peak, abolished in the large majority of depressives, appears to be a more sensitive and physiological tool than the TRH test to study the abnormalities of the HPT axis. The TRH test is abnormal in only 25% of the depressives and represents a pharmacological stimulus still eliciting a normal response in depressed patients with abolished nocturnal peak.

The finding that low–normal or reduced serum thyroid hormone levels are associated with inappropriately normal morning TSH values and the abolition of the nocturnal TSH surge suggests that some degree of central hypothyroidism occured in several depressed patients.

As regards the clinical significance, although these findings appear quite promising, further studies involving a larger number of patients are needed to evaluate (1) the specificity or not of TSH derangement in depression and (2) the persistence of this abnormality in the same patients evaluated prospectively and/or during recurrent depressive episodes.

References

Ågren H, Wide L (1982) Pattern of depressions reflected in pituitary-thyroid and pituitary-adrenal endocrine changes. Psychoneuroendocrinology 7: 309–327

Avni J, Edelstein EL, Khazan N, Sulman FG (1967) Comparative study of imipramine, amitriptiline and their desmethyl analogues in hypothyroid rats. Psychopharmacologia 10: 426–430

Azukizawa M, Pekary AE, Hershman JM, Parker DC (1976) Plasma thyrotropin, thyroxine and triiodothyronine relationships in man. J Clin Endocrinol Metab 43: 533–542

Banki CM, Bissette G, Arato M, Nemeroff CB (1988) Elevation of immunoreactive CSF TRH in depressed patients. Am J Psychiatry 142: 1526–1531

Bartalena L, Martino E, Falcone M, Buratti L, Grasso L, Mammoli C, Pacchiarotti A, Aghini-Lombardi F, Balzano S, Pinchera A (1987) Evaluation of the nocturnal serum thyrotropin (TSH) surge, as assessed by TSH ultrasensitive assay, in patients receiving long term L-tyroxine suppression therapy and in patients with various thyroid disorders. J Clin Endocrinol Metab 65: 1265–1271

Bartalena L, Martino E, Placidi GF, Falcone M, Pellegrini L, Dell'Osso L, Pacchiarotti A, Pinchera A (1990) Nocturnal serum thyrotropin (TSH) surge and the TSH response to TSH-releasing hormone: dissociated behavior in untreated depressives. J Clin Endocrinol Metab 71: 650–655

Brabant C, Ranft U, Ocran K, Hesch RD, Von Zur Muhlen A (1986) Thyrotropin – an episodically secreted hormone. Acta Endocrinol (Copenh) 112: 315–322

Brabant G, Brabant A, Ranft U et al. (1987) Circadian and pulsatile thyrotropin secretion in euthyroid man under the influence of thyroid hormone and glucocorticoid administration. J Clin Endocrinol Metab 65: 83–88

Calloway SP, Dolan RJ, Fonagy P, Desouza VF, Wakeling A (1984) Endocrine changes and clinical prophiles in depression: II. The thyrotropin-releasing hormone test. Psychol Med 14: 759

Caron PJ, Nieman LK, Rose SR, Nisula BC (1986) Deficient nocturnal surge of thyrotropin in central hypothyroidism. J Clin Endocrinol Metab 62: 960–964

Cowdry RW, Wehr TA, Zis AP, Goodwin FK (1983) Thyroid abnormalities associated with rapid cycling bipolar illness. Arch Gen Psychiatry 40: 414

Dewhurst KE, El Kabir DJ, Harris GW, Mandelbrote BM (1969) Observations on the blood concentrations of thyrotrophic hormone (TSH) in schizophrenia and the affective states. Br J Psychiatry 115: 1003–1007

Duick DS, Wahner HW (1979) Thyroid axis in patients with Cushing's syndrome. Arch Intern Med 139: 767–772

Evans PJ, Weeke J, Jones MK, Woodhead JS, Scanlon MF (1986) The circadian variation of thyrotropin in patients with primary thyroidal disease. Clin Endocrinol (Oxf) 24: 343–348

Fukuda H, Greer MA (1975) The effect of basal hypothalamic deafferentation on the nyctohemeral rhythm of plasma TSH. Endoccrinology 97: 749–752

Gold PW, Goodwin FK, Wehr T, Rebar R (1977) Pituitary thyrotropin response to thyrotropin-releasing hormone in affective illness: relationship to spinal fluid amine metabolites. Am J Psychiatry 134: 1028–1031

Gold MS, Pottash ALC, Extein I (1981) Hypothyroidism and depression: evidence from complete thyroid function evaluation. JAMA 245: 1919–1922

Goldstein J, Van Cauter E, Linkowski P, Vanhaelst L, Mendlewicz J (1980) Thyrotropin nyctohemeral pattern in primary depression: differences between unipolar and bipolar women. Life Sci 27: 1695–1703
Greenspan SL, Klibanski A, Schoenfels D, Ridgway EC (1986) Pulsatile scretion of thyrotropin in man. J Clin Endocrinol Metab 63: 661–668
Hatotani N, Nomura J, Yamaguchi T, Kitayama J (1977) Clinical and experimental studies of the pathogenesis of depression. Psychoneuroendocrinology 2: 115–130
Joffe RT, Blank DW, Post RM, Uhde TW (1985) Decreased triiodothyronines in depression: a preliminary report. Biol Psychiatry 20: 922–925
Kirkegaard C, Faber J (1981) Altered serum levels of thyroxine, triiodothyronines and diiodothyronines in endogenous depression. Acta Endocrinol (Copenh) 96: 199–209
Kirkegaard C, Norlem N, Lauridsen UB (1975) Protirelin stimulation test and thyroid function during treatment of depression. Arch Gen Psychiatry 32: 1115–1118
Kirkegaard C, Bjørum N, Cohn D, Lauridsen UB (1978) Thyrotropin-releasing hormone (TRH) stimulation test in manic-depressive illness. Arch Gen Psychiatry 35: 1017–1021
Kirkegaard C, Faber J, Hummer L, Rogowski P (1979) Increased levels of TRH in cerebrospinal fluid from patients with endogenous depression. Psychoneuroendocrinology 4: 227–235
Kjellman BF, Ljunggren JG, Beck-Friis J, Wetterberg L (1983) Reverse T3 levels in affective disorders. Psychiatry Res 10: 1–9
Kjellman BF, Beck-Friis J, Ljunggren JG, Wetterberg L (1984) Twenty-four-hour serum levels of TSH in affective disorders. Acta Psychiatr Scand 69: 491–502
Kristen L, Gold MS, Extein I, Martin D, Pottash ALC (1982) Clinical correlates of the TRH infusion test in primary depression. J Clin Psychiatry 43: 191–194
Linkowski P, Brauman H, Mendlewicz J (1980) Prolactin secretion in women with unipolar and bipolar depression. Psychiatry Res 3: 265–271
Linkowski P, Brauman H, Mendlewicz J (1981) Thyrotropin response to thyrotropin-releasing hormone in unipolar and bipolar affective illness. J Affective Disord 3: 9–16
Linnoila M, Lamberg BA, Rosberg G, Karonen SL, Welin MG (1979) Thyroid hormones and TSH, prolactin and LH response to repeated TRH and LRH injections in depressed patients. Acta Psychiatr Scand 59: 536–544
Linnoila M, Lamberg BA, Potter WZ, Gold PW, Goodwin FK (1982) High reverse T3 levels in manic and unipolar depressed women. Psychiatry Res 6: 271–276
Linnoila M, Cowdry R, Lamberg BA, Makinen T, Rubinow D (1983) CSF triiodothyronine (rT3) levels in patients with affective disorders. Biol Psychiatry 18: 1489–1492
Loosen PT, Prange AJ (1980) Thyrotropin-releasing hormone (TRH): a useful tool for psychoneuroendocrine investigation. Psychoneuroendocrinology 5: 63–80
Loosen PT, Prange AJ (1982) The serum TRH response to TRH in psychiatric patients: a review. Am J Psychiatry 139: 405–415
Loosen PT, Prange AJ, Wilson IC, Lara PP, Pettus C (1977) Thyroid-stimulating hormone response after thyrotropin-releasing hormone in depressed, schizophrenic and normal women. Psychoneuroendocrinology 2: 479–486
Loosen PT, Wilson IC, Dew BW (1983a) Thyrotropin-releasing hormone (TRH) in abstinent alcoholic men. Am J Psychiatry 140: 1145–1149
Loosen PT, Kistler K, Prange A (1983b) Use of TSH response to TRH as an independent variable. Am J Psychiatry 140: 700–703
Maas JM, Koslow SH, Davis J, Martin K, Frazer A, Bowden CL, Berman N, Gibbons R, Stokes P, Landis H (1987) Catecholamine metabolism and disposition in healthy and depressed subjects. Arch Gen Psychiatry 44: 337–344
Maes M, Vandewoude M, Maes L, Schotte C, Cosyns P (1989) A revised interpretation of the TRH results in female depressed patients: I: TSH responses. Effects of severity of illness, thyroid hormones, monoamines, age, sex hormonal, corticosteroid and nutritional state. J Affective Disord 16: 203–213
Marchesi C, Chiodera P, De Risio C, Dasso' L, Govi AM, De Ferri A, Piagneri B, Minelli R, Bianconi L, Gnudi A, Coiro V (1988) Dopaminergic control of TSH secretion in endogenous depression. Psychiatry Res 25: 277–282
McGaffe J, Barnes MA, Lippmann S (1981) Psychiatric manifestations of hyperthyroidism. Am Fam Physican 23: 129–133

Nordgreen L, Von Scheele C (1976) Myxedema madness without myxedema. Acta Med Scand 199: 233–236
Ogawa J, Mizuno S, More A, Nukina I, Ota Z, Yamamoto M (1984) Potential antidepressive effects of thyrotropin-releasing hormone (TRH) and its analogues. Peptides 5: 743
Orsulak PJ, Crowley G, Schlesser MA, Giles D, Fairchild C, Rush AJ (1985) Free triiodothyronine (T3) and thyroxine (T4) in a group of unipolar depressed patients and normal subjects. Biol Psychiatry 29: 1047–1054
O'Shanick GJ, Ellinwood EH (1982) Persistent elevation of thyroid-stimulating hormone in women with bipolar affective disorder. Am J Psychiatry 139: 513
Patel YC, Alford FP, Burger HC (1972) The 24-hour plasma thyrotropin profile. Clin Sci 43: 71–77
Prange AJ, Garbutt JC, Loosen P (1987) The hypothalamic–pituitary–thyroid axis in affective disorders. In: Meltzer HY (ed) Psychopharmacology: the third generation of progress. Raven, New York, pp 629–636
Re RN, Kourides IA, Ridgway EC, Weintraub BD, Maloof F (1976) The effect of glucocorticoid administration on human pituitary secretion of thyrotropin and prolactin. J Clin Endocrinol Metab 43: 338–346
Roy A, Karoum F, Linnoila M, Pickar D (1988) Thyrotropin-releasing hormone test in unipolar depressed patients and controls: relationship to clinical and biologic variables. Acta Psychiatr Scand 77: 151–159
Rubin RT, Poland RE, Lesser IM, Martin DJ (1987) Neuroendocrine aspects of primary endogenous depression: IV. Pituitary–thyroid axis activity in patients and matched control subjects. Psychoneuroendocrinology 12: 333–347
Sack DA, James SP, Rosenthal NE, Wehr TA (1988) Deficient nocturnal surge of TSH secretion during sleep and sleep deprivation in rapid cycling bipolar illness. Psychiatry Res 23: 179–191
Souetre E, Salvati E, Belugou JL et al. (1989) Circadian rhythms in depression and recovery: evidence for blunted amplitude as the main chronobiological abnormality. Psychiatry Res 28: 263–278
Sowers JR, Catania RA, Hershman JM (1982) Evidence for dopaminergic control of circadian variations in thyrotropin secretion. J Clin Endocrinol Metab 54: 673–675
Spencer CA, Greenstadt MA, Wheeler WS, Kletzkiy OA, Nicoloff JT (1980) The influence of long-term low-dose thyrotropin-releasing hormone infusions on serum thyrotropin and prolactin concentration in man. J Clin Endocrinol Metab 51: 771–775
Stokes PE, Sikes CR (1988) The hypothalamic–pituitary–adrenocortical axis in major depression. Endocrinol Metab Clin North Am 17: 1–18
Takahashi S, Kondo H, Yoshimura M, Ochi Y (1974) Thyrotropin responses to TRH in depressive illness: relation to clinical subtypes and prolonged duration of depressive episodes. Folia Psychiatr Neurol Jpn 28: 355–365
Targum SD, Sullivan AC, Byrnes SM (1982) Neuroendocrine interrelationships in major depressive disorders. Am J Psychiatry 139: 282–286
Tollefson G, Valentine R, Hoffmann N, Garvey MJ, Tuason VB (1985) Thyroxine binding and TSH in recurrent depressive episodes. J Clin Psychiatry 46: 267–272
Unden F, Ljunggren JG, Kjellman BF, Beck-Friis J, Wetterberg L (1986) Twenty-four-hour serum levels of T4 and T3 in relation to decreased TSH serum levels and decreased TSH response to TRH in affective disorders. Acta Psychiatr Scand 73: 358–365
Vanhaelst L, Van Cauter E, Degaute JP, Goldstein J (1972) Circadian variations in serum thyrotropin levels in man. J Clin Endocrinol Metab 35: 479–484
Weeke A, Weeke J (1978) Disturbed circadian variation of serum thyrotropin in patient with endogenous depression. Acta Psychiatr Scand 57: 281–289
Weeke J, Laurberg P (1976) Diurnal TSH variations in hypothyroidism. J Clin Endocrinol Metab 43: 32–37
Whybrow PC, Coppen A, Prange AJ, Noguera R, Bailey JE (1972) Thyroid function and the response to liothyronine in depression. Arch Gen Psychiatry 26: 242–245
Wilson WH, Jefferson JW (1985) Thyroid disease behavior and psychopharmacology. Psychosomatics 26: 481–492

Cognitive Aspects of Depression: An Experimental Study

I. Amado-Boccara and H. Loo

Introduction

Depression can alter mental and cognitive functions, but it is often difficult to define in a clinical presentation if the problems it faces concern only concentration or if there are also memory and learning defects. Moreover, it is difficult to establish a link between cognitive impairment and specific depressive symptoms. What are the implications of mood, anxiety, or psychomotor retardation? This experimental work intends to analyze cognitive problems in depression and to establish a link between cognitive problems and major symptoms of depression.

Several cognitive defects have already been shown in the literature. Depressed people have difficulty in performing tasks requiring effortful processing (for tasks requiring sustained attention, e.g., recall of unrelated items). With easier tasks (such as recall of categorized words), depressed people perform as well as controls (Weingartner and Silbermann 1982; Roy-Byrne and Weingartner 1986). There are also some defects in short-term memory (Sternberg and Jarvik 1976), but other authors with the same kind of tasks concluded that depressed people have problems transferring information from short- to long-term storage (Henry et al. 1973). With an abstract reasoning task, difficulty was demonstrated in focused thinking, with perseveration (Silbermann et al. 1983). All the studies insist on the difficulties of attention and concentration.

However, the literature shows no evidence of depression impacting on automatic memory (Roy-Byrne and Weingartner 1986) and knowledge memory (Wolkowitz and Weingartner 1988).

Some research has analyzed cognitive tasks related to specific symptoms in the depressive pathological condition. Psychomotor retardation provokes difficulties in memory, attention, and concentration (Wildlocher 1983), and in an experimental study, prolongation of the speech pause time in a standardized talk was described (Ghozlan and Wildlocher 1987). Anxiety seems to provoke a defect in concentration and lower performances in intellectual tasks (Watts and Sharrock 1985). Mood can also alter the context in which information is encoded or retrieved (Fogarty and Hemsley 1983; Breslow et al. 1981). Most of the cognitive problems are correlated with the severity of depression (Silbermann et al. 1983).

Presentation of the Study

The study includes inpatients who have a major depressive disorder (in the DSM-III-R) with a score higher than 25 in the Montgomery and Asberg scale. The sample consisted of seven 30- to 60-year-old inpatients. We excluded severe depressive pathological conditions with mutism or acute anxiety, atypical depression or psychosis, organic brain disease, recent or chronic use of alcohol, and electroconvulsive therapy during the last 6 months. The control sample was matched in terms of sex, level of education, and age with the depressive patients sample.

Depressive symptoms were evaluated by many scales for diagnosis and severity of depression: Montgomery and Asberg, and Hamilton depression scales; psychomotor retardation was assessed by *l'échelle de ralentissement dépressif de Wildlocher* (scale of psychomotor retardation); anxiety was evaluated by the Hamilton anxiety scale and the hospital anxiety depression of Zygmond and Snaith. The patients had been drug-free for 8 days (only 50 mg oxazepam was authorized). Clinical and psychometric evaluation was carried out at the beginning of the hospitalization. The battery of tasks was divided into two parts, and the patients were tested in the morning on 2 consecutive days. The presentation of the task battery was divided into two main parts. The first one dealt with attention and alertness. It contained the letter cancellation test (J. Poitrenaud), which consists of rows of letters randomly interspersed with a designated target letter. The patient must cross out all the target letters. The performance is the time for completion. It tests concentration and visuomotor tracking and includes a rapidity factor. The trail-making test is a visuomotor tracking test in which a patient must draw lines to connect consecutively numbered circles (for part A of the test) and then the same amount of numbered and lettered circles (for part B). The score is the time to connect the circle. The mental control test and digit span are extracted from the Wechsler Memory Scale (1945). The first one explores concentration and mental tracking. It consists of reverse counting and doing simple mental counting operations as fast as possible. The digit span tests how many bits of information a person can repeat in order and reverse. It also explores immediate memory. The Stroop control test measures the ease with which a patient can shift his perceptual set to conform to changing demands. With card A, the patient must read color names; with card B, the patient must design the color which is printed; with card C, each color name is printed in a different color than its name. The score for each card is the time for reading the color as fast as possible. This test is also a stress test because it supposes an interference of two sensorial perceptions and an inhibition of the semantic one giving the preference to the visual one (for card C). The second part of the tasks deals with memory and learning. It contains the logical memory test and the paired associate learning test (Wechsler Memory Scale). The first one explores the comprehension and repetition of two short texts read by the observer. The second one consists of a repetition of one word from a pair of items. This pair of words can be easy to retain (with categorized words) or difficult (with unrelated items). This part contains also the working memory test

(Signoret): this notion established by Baddeley (1986) can link memory and concentration. Working memory is an active memory which contains three dynamic operations. One immediate or auditive memory; in this section the information encoded can be transformed in a more easy one to be retained. The last operation is a transfer of this information from short-term memory to long-term memory to be stored. This concept implies the existence of a control unit to supervise and distribute attention for the manipulation and the choice of information which must be stored. The working memory test consists of three words read by the subjects and recalled after having done reverse counting during a variable time.

The selective learning and recall test (Signoret from Buschke and Fuld 1974) is a recall of ten-word list with six successive trials, the observer giving only the items forgotten from the second to the sixth trial. There are two scores: one for the total number of items repeated and one for items learned (repeated in two successive trials).

Results of the Experiment

The first result concerns attention tasks for depressed people and controls (Table 1). For the statistical analysis a nonparametric Mann-Whitney test was used. A significant difference was found for the trail-making test form B, the cancellation test, and the Stroop color test card B. Concerning memory and learning, no task demonstrated significant differences between the two populations.

Analysis of the Correlations. For statistical correlation a unilateral Spearman test was used.

Table 1. Results of attention tasks for depressed people and controls ($n = 7$)

Tasks	Mean value	Standard deviation
Trail-making test		
Part B		
C	70.18	22.13
D	93.57*	25.07
Cancellation		
C	65.81	7.02
D	55.14*	13.05
Stroop test		
Card B		
C	98.27	3.28
D	90.71*	11.6

Nonparametric Mann-Whitney test
* Significant difference between depressed (D) and controls (C) ($P < 0.05$)

Table 2. Correlations between different tasks

	Trail-making		Cancellation	Stroop		Mental control	Digit span	Logical memory	Associate learning	Visual reproduction	Selective Learning	
	PA	PB		CB	CC						Total score	Learning score
Trail-making PA	● ○	●	●									
PB		● ○	● ●	●	●	●		●		●		●
Cancellation			● ○		●	●		●		●		
Stroop CB				● ○	●	●		●	●	●		●
CC					● ○	●		● ●		●		○
Mental control						● ○	○ ○	● ●		● ●		
Digit span							● ○		○			
Logical memory								● ○	●	● ●		●
Associate learning									● ○		○	○ ○
Visual reproduction										● ○		
Selective learning												
Total score											● ○	
Learning score												● ○

○, positive correlation of depressed people; ●, positive correlation of control
$P < 0.05$ ● or ○; $P < 0.01$ ●● or ○○; $P < 0.001$ ●●● or ○○○
(Unilateral Spearman test)

Correlations Between Different Tasks (Table 2). For controls, concentration tasks were all correlated with one another, memory tasks were positively correlated with concentration tasks, and the cancellation test was positively correlated with attention and simple memory tests.

Correlations Established for the Working Memory Task (Table 3). The performances of this task were evaluated by measuring a score of interference errors (when people confuse two words) and errors of omission. These errors were found at different assessment times (3–18 s). So it appears that for depressed people all types of errors at different delay times are correlated with one another.

Correlations Between Different Kinds of Errors and Other Tasks (Table 4). For controls, errors of omission were positively correlated with attention and rapidity tasks. For depressed people, interference errors were negatively correlated with memory performances (precisely for logical memory and visual reproduction tasks).

Correlations Between Cognitive Tasks and Clinical Evaluations (Table 5). The selective learning test was positively correlated with the severity of depression. The Stroop color test was correlated with the two anxiety scales. For psychomotor retardation, most of the memory tasks were negatively correlated with the severity of retardation.

Table 3. Correlations between different errors for the working memory test

	Errors of omission	Interference errors	Sum of errors at 3 s	Sum of errors at 6 s	Sum of errors at 9 s	Sum of errors at 18 s
Errors of omission	● ○	◆ ○				
Interference errors		● ○				
Sum of errors at 3 s			● ○	●		○
Sum of errors at 6 s				● ○		○
Sum of errors at 9 s					● ○	○
Sum of errors at 18 s						● ○

○, positive correlation of depressed people; ●, positive correlation of control; ◆, negative correlation of control
$P < 0.05$ (Unilateral Spearman test)

Table 4. Correlations between omission and interference errors of working memory and other tasks

	Trail-making		Stroop		Cancellation	Mental control	Digit span	Logical memory	Associate learning	Selective learning
	PA	PB	CB	CC						
Sum of omission errors (at 3, 6, 9, 18 s)	◆ ⊖	◆	●		● ●					
Sum of interference errors (at 3, 6, 9, 18 s)		● ●			◆	◆		◆ ⊖		◆

⊖ negative correlation of depressed people
● positive correlation of control
◆ negative correlation of control
$P < 0.05$ ● ⊖ ◆ $P < 0.01$ ●● (Unilateral Spearman test)

Table 5. Correlation between clinical rating scales and tasks for depressed people

	MADRS	Hamilton depress.	Hamilton anxiety	Anxiety items from Zygmond and Snaith	*Ralentissement* Wildlocher
Trail-making PA					
PB					
Stroop CB					
CC			○	○	
Mental control					
Digit span					⊖
Logical memory					⊖
Associate learning					⊖
Visual reproduction					
Working memory, sum of interference errors					⊖
Selective learning	⊖				⊖

○, positive correlation for depressed people; ⊖, negative correlation for depressed people
$P < 0.05$
(Unilateral Spearman test)

Discussion

This study in seven patients investigated cognitive impairments found in depressed people and correlations established between all the tasks used and the depressive symptoms. The significant differences found for three concentration tasks mean that depressed patients seem to have trouble with some complex concentration tasks and with rapidity performance measured by the cancellation task only.

However, for very simple attention tasks (such as the trail-making test form A) or tasks which also have a memory factor with a more sophisticated mental treatment (such as the digit span or mental control test), depressed people perform like controls.

For the correlations between different tasks, the fact that for depressed people correlations between the concentration tasks were not established with homogeneity and the fact that memory tasks were not correlated with attention tasks indicate that mental treatment mechanisms do not seem to be homogeneous for depressed people. The second point is that they cannot be helped to resolve memory tests by their concentration abilities.

In the controls, attention tasks were positively correlated with the cancellation test. Therefore, they performed them with a rapidity component. The same phenomenon occurred with simple memory tests such as logical memory and visual reproduction, but this could not be found for depressed people.

Without this rapidity component, they cannot be helped by automatic processing to resolve some average complexity tasks as controls do.

Concerning correlations established for the working memory task, the existence of positive correlations at different assessment times for depressed people seems to reflect a difficulty to answer, whatever the delay is.

Regarding correlations between different kinds of errors and other tasks, the positive correlation between concentration tasks and errors of omission found for controls could reflect a distraction process. In contrast, the existence of a negative correlation for depressed patients between interference errors and memory performances would mean that there is perhaps a sort of mental conflict concerning the confrontation of different information before choosing the right solution. With regard to correlations between cognitive tasks and clinical evaluations, it seems that only the selective learning test, which is a difficult task, is positively correlated with the severity of depression. Thus, in this study we found no influence of the mood state on the cognitive test we used. However, for anxiety, as we expected, the Stroop test was correlated with the two anxiety scales. For psychomotor retardation, this symptom seems to have a great impact on complex tasks because all the correlations were only established for memory tasks. We did not find correlations between concentration tasks and psychomotor retardation.

Conclusion

The most important fact is that depressed people do not exhibit poor performance. Their cognitive problems are moderate, but they do have difficulty in achieving some tasks which depend on automatic processing for control. To resolve these tests, they must use more elaborated mental information processing than controls. Concerning the working memory test, we may think that for depressed people a mental conflict could exist when information is confronted to give the correct answer. This could perhaps be linked with mood brooding which requires retaining repetitive themes and is a major symptom of psychomotor retardation. The aim of this experimental study was to present some guidelines dealing with cognitive impairments in pathological depression. These preliminary results have to be confirmed by further studies. However, we can already say that we have some information about the qualitative aspect of cognitive defects in depression. Moreover, this study contributes to our knowledge of the link between clinical symptoms of depression and cognitive performance.

References

American Psychiatric Association (1987) Diagnosis and statistical manual of mental disorders, 3rd edn, revised. American Psychiatric Association, Washington DC
Baddeley A (1987) Working memory. Oxford Science Publications, Oxford
Breslow R et al. (1981) Contribution of the depressive perspective of memory function in depression. Am J Psychiatry 138(2): 227–230
Buschke H, Fuld P (1974) Evaluating storage, retention and retrieval in disordered memory and learning. Neurology 124: 1019–1025
Clement F (1966) Analyse de l'échelle de mémoire de Wechsler: facteurs qui influent sur ses résultats. Rev Psychol Appl 16(4): 197–244
Dyer F (1973) The stroop phenomenon and its use in the study of perceptual cognitive and response process. Mem Cognit 1(2): 106–120
Fogarty S, Hemsley D (1983) Depression and the accessibility of memories: a longitudinal study. Br J Psychiatry 142: 232–237
Ghozlan A, Widlocher D (1987) Epreuves cognitives et ralentissement psychomoteur dépressif. J Psychol Biol Ther 25: 14
Henry G et al. (1973) Influence of affective states and psycho-active drugs on verbal learning and memory. Am J Psychiatry 130: 966–971
Roy-Byrne P, Weingartner H (1986) Effortful and automatic cognitive processes in depression. Arch Gen Psychiatry 43: 265–267
Silbermann E et al. (1983) Thinking disorders in depression. Logic and strategy in an abstract reasoning task. Arch Gen Psychiatry 40: 775–780
Silbermann E et al. (1983) Processing of emotional properties of stimuli by depressed and normal subjects. J Nerv Ment Dis 171: 11–14
Sternberg D, Jarvik ME (1976) Memory functions in depression; improvement with antidepressant medication. Arch Gen Psychiatry 33: 219–224
Watts F, Sharrok R (1985) Description and measurement of concentration problems in depressed patients. Psychobiol Med 15: 317–326
Wechsler D (1945) A standardized memory scale for clinical use. (Traduction Centre de Psychologie Appliquée 1969, Paris.) J Psychol 19: 87–95
Weingartner H, Silbermann EK (1982) Models of cognitive impairment: cognitive changes in depression. Psychopharmacol Bull 18(2): 28–43
Widlocher D (1983) Le ralentissement dépressif. PUF, Paris (Coll Nodules)
Wolkowitz OM, Weingartner H (1988) Defining cognitive changes in depression and anxiety: a psychobiologic analysis. Psychiatr Psychobiol 3(3B): 131–138

Variability of Cognitive Patterns in Subjects with Mood Disorder

P. Scherillo, M. Gasperini, V. Lucini, and E. Smeraldi

Introduction

Cognitive patterns and their relationship with mood disorders have attracted much interest in psychiatric clinical research, beginning with Beck's etiopathogenetic hypothesis (Beck 1967). Some cognitive distortions in the view of oneself, the world and the future have been supported as being related to cognitive-personological patterns of subjects with mood disorders and as factors indicating vulnerability to depression (Blackburn et al. 1986; Hollon et al. 1986; Olinger et al. 1987). In addition, cognitive depressive patterns seem to affect specific courses of the illness (Eaves and Rush 1984) as well as the outcome of treatment (Simons et al. 1986; La Rue and Spar 1986; Pilkonis and Frank 1988).

Since the etiopathogenetic link between personality disorders and traits with mood disorders has not yet been solved, the mutual relationship between cognitive and personality traits seems to be a crucial point to take into account, even because particular cognitive-personality structures could be considered as subclinical manifestations of susceptibility to mood disorders (Pfhol et al. 1984; Koenigsberg et al. 1985; Gasperini and Provenza 1987; Coryell and Zimmerman 1989).

In a previous study (Gasperini et al. 1989) cognitive distortions measured by the Self-Control Schedule (SCS) (Rosenbaum 1980) and the Automatic Thoughts Questionnaire (ATQ) (Hollon and Kendall 1980), were found to be differently associated with Axis I and Axis II disorders in a group of subjects with mood disorders than in a control group. In fact, the cognitive pattern as measured by the ATQ appeared not to be related to Axis I or Axis II diagnoses: the mean total scores of ATQ were the same for the group of medical controls and the major recurrent depressives and bipolar patients, and did not depend on the presence of a personality disorder. On the other hand, the cognitive pattern as measured by the three subscales of the SCS appeared to be conditioned by Axis I diagnosis, since major recurrent depressives and bipolar patients always have worse SCS mean total scores than control subjects.

One of the aims of the present study was to analyze the possible influences of the absence/presence of any Axis II disorders in modifying the cognitive patterns, even related to early–late age of onset and different durations of the course of the illness.

Materials and Methods

Our sample included 68 subjects, all referred to our outpatient clinic for mood disorders (32 female and 36 male subjects). Of the patients 40 met the criteria for "major depression, recurrent" and 28 for "bipolar disorder" according to DSM III-R (American Psychiatric Association 1987). The mean current age (±standard deviation, SD) was 47.18 ± 12.8 years for major depression subjects and 49.96 ± 14.7 years for bipolar subjects. The mean age of onset was 37.4 ± 10.8 and 30.5 ± 11.3 years for the two polarity subjects.

Of the patients, 40 were on long-term treatment (of at least 24 months) with lithium salts (45% among major depressive subjects and 79% among the bipolar ones). All subjects were in normothymic phase as evaluated by clinical judgment with score levels less than 21 using the Hamilton Rating Scale for Depression (Hamilton 1960). They were assessed for their cognitive patterns by the use of the ATQ and SCS. The mean ATQ score was 63.22 ± 28.5 and the mean SCS score was 88.01 ± 24.0 and did agree with the results of previous studies (Dobson and Shaw 1986; Gasperini et al. 1989).

In addition, all subjects were assessed for Axis II diagnoses, according to DSM III-R criteria using the structured interview for personality disorders (SIDP) (Stangl et al. 1985) by senior psychiatrists whose interrater agreement of 0.80 had been previously tested. The Axis II was evaluated according to the absence/presence of specific personality disorders (PD) and to the classification of clusters.

We carried out some statistical analyses using the reg-linear model (Morabito and Marubini 1976) in which the ATQ and SCS mean scores were considered as dependent variables tested against other clinical features of interest. They were the sex, polarity, current age and onset and duration of the illness, as well as the total number of depressive/manic phases during the course of the illness. We included, as independent variables, whether or not the subjects were on lithium prophylaxis and the absence/presence of PD and clusters.

Results

The distributions of ATQ and SCS mean scores of our subjects according to the variables of interest are listed in Table 1.

Table 2 shows the results of the logistic analysis taking into account ATQ mean scores as dependent variable. The variable polarity and sex of probands did not result in significant differences in the distribution of ATQ mean scores. In other words, the total mean scores on ATQ did not differ in major depressed subjects when compared to bipolar subjects: they were 65.13 + 27.0 and 60.5 + 30.0, respectively. Similarly, female and male subjects did not show different ATQ scores (58.7 vs 65.1).

Table 1. Mean (+SD) ATQ and SCS scores in the sample according to the variables of interest

			Major recurrent depression (*n* = 40)		Bipolar disorder (*n* = 28)	
			Male	Female	Male	Female
Lithium treatment	PD present	ATQ	85.7 + 26.9	99.3 + 27.09	66.7 + 42.6	57.0 + 11.7
		SCS	124.0 + 26.9	97.0 + 12.2	84.8 + 11.7	85.0 + 17.1
		Onset	41.7 + 11.2	28.7 + 10.6	32.5 + 15.4	29.3 + 12.3
		Duration	8.3 + 7.0	3.3 + 2.08	11.0 + 9.3	8.7 + 11.6
		Episodes TOT	3.7 + 3.05	2.7 + 1.5	4.5 + 2.3	4.8 + 3.8
	PD absent	ATQ	62.7 + 24.7	34.6 + 0.5	55.1 + 23.8	64.0 + 32.0
		SCS	81.7 + 28.3	72.3 + 37.3	91.7 + 25.9	133.0 + 45.0
		Onset	39.2 + 11.5	29.0 + 9.0	32.6 + 10.6	29.0 + 8.2
		Duration	8.6 + 5.2	6.7 + 1.2	14.9 + 10.5	5.0 + 2.7
		Episodes TOT	4.0 + 1.12	3.7 + 1.5	3.8 + 1.4	2.0 + 0.7
No lithium treatment	PD present	ATQ	67.4 + 32.9	58.5 + 25.9	71.0 + 42.9	41.0 + 20.0
		SCS	91.0 + 6.1	86.0 + 30.1	91.4 + 25.7	75.0 + 15.2
		Onset	32.8 + 5.5	39.0 + 14.0	25.0 + 10.7	28.0 + 10.0
		Duration	12.0 + 7.5	7.5 + 11.1	21.6 + 12.7	0 + 0
		Episodes TOT	4.0 + 2.6	1.3 + 0.5	6.6 + 3.4	1.0 + 0.4
	PD absent	ATQ	67.3 + 22.5	51.3 + 16.4	–	–
		SCS	76.3 + 16.4	91.7 + 16.1	–	–
		Onset	36.7 + 10.4	48.5 + 9.7	–	–
		Duration	13.1 + 10.9	11.5 + 7.9	–	–
		Episodes TOT	4.8 + 4.8	1.3 + 0.5	–	–

Table 2. Logistic analysis: statistical significance of variables on ATQ mean scores

Variables	*t*	*p*
Sex	1.80	n.s.
Age at onset	4.44	0.0003
Duration of illness	1.74	n.s.
Polarity	−0.70	n.s.
Number of depressive/ manic episodes	−0.01	n.s.
Lithium prophylaxis (no/yes)	2.12	0.001
Personality disorder (absent/present)	3.34	0.0001

The variable age of onset was statistically significant ($t = 4.40$, $p = 0.005$) in modifying the mean ATQ scores. Early onset subjects, independently of their sex or polarity, showed cognitive patterns worse than late onset subjects.

On the other hand, the age of probands did not significantly condition the variability of ATQ. Neither the duration of illness nor the number of depressive and manic episodes seemed to condition different cognitivity patterns.

The presence of any PD was statistically significant in increasing the scores of ATQ. The worst ATQ cognitive patterns were significantly conditioned by the comorbidity of Axis I and II disorders.

In addition, some differences were shown in cognitive patterns among the subjects according to whether or not they were undergoing lithium treatment and whether or not they exhibited PD. In fact, even if the subjects on lithium treatment showed a lesser degree of cognitive distortions than subjects without lithium, the presence of any PD played a systematic effect in worsening their scores on ATQ (see Table 1: 55.75 vs 73.93).

Table 3 shows the results of the logistic analysis carried out on SCS measures as dependent variable. Polarity and sex did not significantly affect the differences in SCS distributions. Major depressed and bipolar subjects did not show significant differences in their SCS distributions (86.7 vs 89.5). Similarly no difference was shown according to sex (male: 87.6, female: 88.4).

The presence of any PD played a significant effect in conditioning worse cognitive SCS patterns ($t = 3.36$, $p = 0.001$). An opposite trend compared to ATQ was shown by SCS scores with respect to the age of onset: the worst behavioral cognitive patterns were shown by the late onset subjects.

The duration of illness conditioned a significant variability in SCS distribution: the longer the duration of illness the higher the SCS scores.

The cluster subclassification was not statistically significant in modifying the ATQ and SCS scores even for our example. Nevertheless, the specific cluster subjects showed some differences in their cognitive scores. In fact, cluster C subjects had the worst patterns both on ATQ and SCS (see Table 1). Specifically, cluster C was represented by compulsive and dependent PD which accounted for 42% and 35%. Cluster C showed higher scores both on ATQ and SCS than clusters B and A (ATQ: 73.5 vs 68.8 and 57.5; SCS: 103.0 vs 87.9 and 84.5).

Table 3. Logistic analysis: statistical significance of variables on SCS mean scores

Variables	*t*	*p*
Sex	0.90	n.s.
Age at onset	8.92	0.0000001
Duration of illness	3.32	0.005
Polarity	0.20	n.s.
Number of depressive/ manic episodes	−0.35	n.s.
Lithium prophylaxis (no/yes)	2.93	0.005
Personality disorder (absent/present)	3.36	0.001

Comments

The results of the present study support the interest on personality disorders in dealing with cognitivity patterns. The presence of specific personalities, such as compulsive and dependent seemed to be strongly associated with worse cognitive patterns both on ATQ and SCS scales. One important distinction in ATQ and SCS was provided by the results relating to age of onset and duration of illness.

In fact, the worst ATQ scores seemed to be clustered among early–late subjects and were not conditioned by long duration or several episodes of illness. This might be explained by the fact that a distorted cognitive pattern is present just at the onset of mood disorders and therefore representing a possible factor related strictly to mood tendency.

On the other hand, the SCS which represents a measure of behavioral cognitive manifestations was affected by the duration of illness and seemed to be worse in the late onset group. One possible explanation might be that as the SCS is a behavioral measure it has to be conditioned by the age and ability of subjects to adapt to consequences of long duration.

The results of this study are preliminary because of the small size of the sample and because we considered mean scores of ATQ and SCS independently of their possible subdimensions (Gasperini et al. 1989). Future research will be addressed to looking for relationships between specific cognitive dimensions and personality traits.

References

American Psychiatric Association (1987) Diagnostic and statistical manual of mental disorders, 3rd edn revised. American Psychiatric Association Washington

Beck AT (1967) Depression: clinical, experimental and therapeutic aspects. Harper and Row, New York

Blackburn IM et al. (1986) Cognitive style in depression. Br J Clin Psychol 25: 241–252

Coryell WH, Zimmerman BA (1989) Personality disorder in the families of depressed, schizophrenic, and never-ill probands. Arch. Gen. Psychiatry 146: 496–502.

Dobson KS, Shaw BI (1986) Cognitive assessment with major depressive disorders. Cognitive Ther Res 10: 13–29

Eaves G, Rush AJ (1984) Cognitive patterns in symptomatic and remitted major depression. J Abnorm Psychol 93: 31–40

Gasperini M, Provenza M (1987) The relationship between affective illness and personality disorders. Preliminary reports. In: Racagni G, Smeraldi E (eds) Anxious depression: assessment and treatment. Raven, New York

Gasperini M et al. (1989) Cognitive processes and personality disorders in affective patients. J Pers Disord 31: 63–71

Hamilton M (1960) A rating scale for depression. J. Neurol. Neurosurg. Psychiatry 23: 56–61

Hollon SD, Kendall PC (1980) Cognitive self-statements in depression: development of an automatic thoughts questionnaire. Cognitive Ther Res 4: 383–396

Hollon SD et al. (1986) Specificity of depressotypic cognitions in clinical depression. J Abnorm Psychol 95: 52–59

Koenigsberg HW et al. (1985) The relationship between syndrome and personality disorder in DSM-III: experience with 2462 patients. Am J Psychiatry 142: 207–212
La Rue A, Spar J (1986) Cognitive impairment in late-life depression: clinical correlates and treatment implications. J Affective Disord 11: 179–184
Morabito A, Marubini E (1976) A computer program suitable for fitting linear models when the dependent variable is dichotomous, polichotomous or censored survival and non-linear models when the dependent variable is quantitative. Comput Programs Biomed 5: 283–295
Olinger LJ et al. (1987) Nonassertiveness and vulnerability to depression: a cognitive perspective. Can J Behav Sci 19: 40–49
Pfhol B, Stangl D and Zimmerman M (1984) The implications of DSM-III personality disorders. J Affective Disorders 7: 309–318
Pilkonis PA, Frank E (1988) Personality pathology in recurrent depression: nature, prevalence, and relationship to treatment response. Am J Psychiatry 145: 435–441
Rosenbaum M (1980) A schedule for assessing self-control behaviors: preliminary findings. Behav Ther 11: 109–121
Simons AD et al. (1986) Cognitive therapy and pharmacotherapy for depression. Arch of Gen Psychiatry 43: 43–48
Stangl D et al. (1985) The structured interview for the DSM-III personality disorders (SIDP). Arch Gen Psychiatry 42: 591–596

Personality and Depression

R.M.A. Hirschfeld

Introduction

Clinical observers and theorists have written extensively on the relationship between personality and depression. Psychoanalytic theorists have described the depression-prone personality as one characterized by high dependency on others for support and approval, low frustration tolerance, and labile self-esteem (Chodoff 1972). Social learning theorists have emphasized constricted social skills and behaviors (Lewinsohn 1974), and other behavioral psychologists have focused on deficits in learning mastery (Seligman 1974). Cognitive theorists have described a pessimistic, negative perception of self and the world (Beck 1972).

In the last two decades, a great deal of empirical research has been done to elucidate the nature of the relationship between personality and depression. This research has followed substantial progress in our ability to measure reliably and validly aspects of personality and of specific diagnostic entities.

This paper will present three general models of the relationship between personality and depression, will review recent findings relevant to our elucidation of this relationship, and will identify unresolved questions to be addressed in the future. This presentation will focus on data derived from the author's investigation of personality and depression, as part of the NIMH Collaborative Program on the Psychobiology of Depression–Clinical Studies (Katz et al. 1979) (the "Psychobiology Collaborative Study") over a period of 15 years. In addition, data from a variety of other studies will be included.

Models

There are three basic ways in which personality and depression may relate, including (1) certain personality features may predispose to depressive episodes ("predisposition" hypothesis), (2) personality features may change as the result of depression, especially after a protracted or severe episode (the "complication" hypothesis), or (3) personality and depression may be interrelated, genetically or familially (the "spectrum" hypothesis).

Methodological Issues – State/Trait Phenomenon

Clinicians see patients when they are ill because that is when patients seek medical help. Researchers conduct investigations on patients when they are ill. This can influence many important assessments. For example, we have learned that sleep architectural measurements, neuroendocrinologic status, and a host of other biologic measures differ considerably if assessed during a period of psychiatric depressive illness in comparison with when the patient is free of illness. We have learned that we must be cautious about making claims of trait assessment when in fact we are measuring changeable state variables.

Is this true of personality measures of patients? We tested this in our study of nearly 1000 inpatients and outpatients who had been admitted with the least moderate to severe depression or mania to one of five major university centers in the United States. We administered a battery of 17 scales from self-report inventories of normal personality features. The battery assessed general personality measures (such as general activity levels and sociability), personality traits associated theoretically with depression (interpersonal dependency), and personality traits which had been empirically demonstrated to be related to depression (neuroticism and extraversion).

The 17 personality scales were divided into four clusters including one for emotional strength, one for interpersonal dependency, one for introversion, and a miscellaneous group. The personality battery was administered at intake and 1 year later.

When we examined the traits in patients who had remained ill throughout the 12-month period, there were no significant changes in their personality traits over this period of time. However, when we looked at the scale scores of patients who had *recovered fully* during this period, we found a striking change in all personality attributes, all in the direction toward normality upon recovery, and most at statistically significant levels (Hirschfeld et al. 1983).

This phenomena of a change from rather abnormal levels of personality traits to more normal ones upon recovery from depression has been replicated in a number of studies (Coppen and Metcalfe 1965; Ingraham 1966; Kerr et al. 1970; Bianchi and Ferguson 1977; Liebowitz et al. 1979; Frank et al. 1987; Reich et al. 1987).

These findings have convinced us that assessments of personality made during a depressive episode are likely to be significantly adversely influenced by the clinical state of depression. It also raised some concerns about clinical theory based upon observations of patients during depressive episodes. After all, the clinician views the patient's personality through the eyes and thoughts of the patient during a depressive episode, which contains extremely distorted self-perceptions.

More recently, self-report measures of personality have been shown to be influenced by anxiety also (Mavissakalian and Hamann 1988; Reich et al. 1987) and depression (Joffe and Regan 1988). In addition, the presence of depression has been shown to affect clinical assessments of personality *disorders*.

Post Recovery Assessment of Personality

To remove the effects of the clinical state of depression on assessment of personality, we restricted analyses to measures obtained at the 1-year follow-up evaluation on patients *fully recovered* from their depressive episodes.

The most marked differences in personality between controls (never ill relatives of psychiatric patients) and both unipolar and bipolar I patients for both sexes occurred in the emotional strength cluster. Patients who had recovered from either unipolar or bipolar depression were characterized by less emotional strength, more moodiness, and less ability to cope with stress. (Hirschfeld et al. 1983, 1986; Benjaminsen 1981).

In the interpersonal dependency cluster, the bipolar and unipolar women showed significantly higher levels of interpersonal dependency than did the controls. This was also true of both the bipolar and the unipolar men, but the differences were somewhat more modest.

In the extraversion/introversion cluster, there were several unexpected and interesting findings. Among the women, both bipolar and unipolar recovered women were significantly less extroverted and more introverted than were controls. Among the men, only the unipolar men were significantly introverted. However, the bipolar recovered men evidenced only normal levels of extroversion, and not increased levels. Thus, the notion of extroverted, perhaps "hypomanic" personality was not found in our sample.

Among the miscellaneous scales, all recovered patient groups in general were characterised by less energy and activity than were the control groups.

A recent study in Canada (Joffe and Regan 1988) using a self-report inventory for personality *disorders* (as contrasted with normal personality traits) similarly found a significant reduction in 6 of 11 DSM-III-R personality disorders including schizoid, avoidant, dependent, passive-aggressive, schizotypal, and borderline. Interestingly, there was an increase in the personality disorders scores upon recovery for histrionic, narcissistic, antisocial, and compulsive. In 6 of 11 DSM-III-R personality disorders, they found a significant reduction in the frequency of 6 of 11 personality disorders upon remission, including schizoid, avoidant, dependent, passive-aggressive, schizotypal, and borderline personality disorder.

In a recent study of patients with recurrent unipolar depression, Frank, Kupfer, and their colleagues (1987) replicated the findings from the Psychobiology Collaborative Study. Their control group included normals recruited from the community. In addition, these investigators found that personality scores assessed in the postrecovery period differed between groups divided on rapidity of response to tricyclic antidepressant medication (imipramine 150–300 mg/day) and psychotherapy (interpersonal psychotherapy). "Normal responders" who showed a clear-cut remission of symptoms within 8 weeks and who remained well for a subsequent 8 weeks were compared with "slow responders" who achieved remission after 8 but before 16 weeks. The normal responders had significantly higher levels of emotional strength and stability and were less interpersonally dependent. The two groups did not differ on extorversion scores.

Other studies, in general, have supported these findings. However, none of these studies is able to address the question of whether the personality features and differences found among these patients reflect true premorbid qualities of these patients. It may well be that these personality assessments are reflective of complications of depressive illness in these patients. Unfortunately, all of these studies are clinical and therefore began with patients in episodes. The only way to address this question is to perform assessments prior to the onset of a first episode of depression.

Preonset Assessment of Personality

Truly premorbid assessments require identification of a significantly large pool of high-risk subjects early enough in life so that they can be assessed prior to their first episode of depression and requires follow-up, usually for several years. For these methodological reasons, few investigators have done this.

In the Psychobiology Collaborative Study, nearly 500 relatives of patients with mood disorders were identified who had no history of mental disorder and who took the personality battery. During the subsequent 6-year follow-up, 29 people suffered their first episode of major depression (Hirschfeld et al. 1989). When these 29 first-onset relatives were compared with 370 relatives who continued to remain without mental illness, few differences emerged. With the exception of modestly lower emotional strength in the first-onset group. Interestingly though, the levels of the first-onset relatives were much more emotionally strong than were patients who recovered from either unipolar or bipolar depression.

When the sample was divided on the basis of age, differences emerged. Among the younger subjects (aged 17–30 years of age), none of the personality variables significantly discriminated between the first-onset and the never-ill group. However, among older subjects (aged 31–41 years of age), decreased emotional strength and increased interpersonal dependency were associated with the first onset of depression. These findings suggest that personality risk factors for depression may be different among different age cohorts. In general, the younger adults, both those who became ill and those who remained well, showed somewhat less emotional strength and more interpersonal dependency. Among the older group only the first-onset group showed decreased emotional strength.

Another study which included premorbid assessments was completed by Angst and Clayton (1986). In this study, increased aggressiveness and automatic lability were found among the subjects who went on to unipolar depression.

The difference in personality predictors among different age group cohorts is consistent with the temporal effects for depression that have been demonstrated in the Psychobiology Collaborative Study and by other investigators. It may be that there is an interaction between birth cohorts and personality factors such that personality factors are more predictive of onset in persons born just before and during World War II. In contrast, personality traits may not be risk factors for those born after World War II. The lack of influence of personality factors in the younger segment of our sample may be due to the more powerful and overriding influence of other risk factors, such as family loading for major affective disorder. Onset in adolescents and the early 20s may involve risk factors other than personality factors. However, as subjects mature into their 30s and 40s, personality features may become more important.

Interaction of Personality and Depression – Personality Disorders

This review and our experience in the Psychobiology Collaborative Study has revealed that personality factors may be involved in the predisposition to depression, but that the differences between those who go on to get depression and those who do not are modest. In addition, with the exception of the Frank and Kupfer findings of discrimination between normal and slow reaction response time to treatment, personality factors have, in general, not been helpful in predicting course. Perhaps a more fruitful area for investigation may be in the interaction between personality disorders and depression. Personality disorders are defined in the DSM-III-R as maladaptive and inflexible personality traits (i.e., enduring patterns of perceiving, relating to, and thinking about the environment and oneself) which are exhibited in a wide range of important social and personal contexts. Depression when it becomes chronic meets this description.

Depressive Personality Disorder

Depressive personality disorder may be conceptualized as being consistent with any of the three models: predisposition, complication, or spectrum. The distinction between predisposition and spectrum may sometimes be difficult to make definitively because depressive personality disorder may meet both models at the same time. Certainly depressive personality disorder may also result from incomplete resolution of a depressive episode.

Akiskal et al. 1980 have written articulately on the subject of depressive personality. In his scheme for chronic depression, two types are of particular interest: subaffective dysthymia and character spectrum disorder. Both of these may include characteristics described by Kurt Schneider, including gloomy, humorless; given to a tendency to dysphoria, introversion, and lethargy; given to worry, brooding, or pessimistic; preoccupied with inadequacy, failure, and negative events; self-critical, self-reproachful, and guilt-prone; skeptical, over-critical, or complaining.

At this time, the task force on the DSM-IV, which is in the process of revising the revision to DSM-III-R, is considering the introduction of depressive personality disorder into the nomenclature. The core clinical concept expressed in this depressive personality disorder is negative, highly critical evaluations of oneself and others in all aspects of life. Thus, it would be highly cognitive conceptually, although its expression would obviously have many behavioral and mood aspects.

A particularly problematic issue is the relationship of depressive personality disorder to dysthymia. Currently, dysthymia is considered to be a somewhat attenuated, more chronic version of major depression, and its defining criteria include primarily vegetative and to a lesser extent cognitive symptoms. They differ substantially from the modified Schneiderian criteria proposed by Akiskal that I mentioned that were described earlier. If dysthymia were redefined in as more temperamental rather than symptomatic fashion, depressive personality disorder and dysthymia might overlap considerably.

Perhaps they are, in fact, the same disorder and can be considered from several different vantages. From the point of mood disorders, it may be genetically, or at least familially related, and it may respond to the same treatments, both pharmacological and psychotherapeutic, that major depression does. From the personality disorder point of view, it is characterized by pervasive and maladaptive behaviors beginning in early adulthood and sustained through much of life. One particularly creative solution might be to consider this interaction between personality and depression as both a mood disorder and a personality disorder. This option is being considered.

Personality Disorders and Depression – Other Spectrum Models

Several spectrum models relevant to personality disorders and mood disorders have been proposed. The classic spectrum model is Kraepelin's, in which all forms of affective disorders have a subclinical temperamental basis. Only those people with more severe forms of the illness go beyond temperamental expression and become manifestly psychopathological.

George Winokur has proposed another model, described as "depressive spectrum disease." Depressive spectrum disease is based on the use of familial patterns to define subtypes of depressive disorders. Depressive spectrum disease is defined by the presence of alcoholism and/or antisocial personality in first-degree relatives of unipolar depressives; these disorders are believed to form a spectrum with depression. "Pure spectrum disease" in contrast, is defined by the absence of alcoholism and antisocial personality in relatives. A more restrictive definition of pure depressive disease requires the presence of a history of depression in the relatives. Patients with depression and no family history are classified as sporadic or nonfamilial depression.

The Akiskal spectrum proposal has been to divide patients with chronic depression into those with more personality disorder, alcoholism, sociopathy, and somatization from those more related to primary affective disorder. This model was described earlier.

Personality Disorder and Depression – Clinical Studies

In general, studies which use structured clinical interviews, both for personality disorders and for major depression, have found that in samples of depression rates of personality disorders range from 36% to 81% with most 50% (Pfohl et al. 1984; Reich and Troughton 1988; Shea et al. 1987; Zimmerman et al. 1988; Alnaes and Torgersen 1988a, b; Mavissakalian and Hamann 1988). The most common comorbid personality disorders are avoidant, dependent, compulsive, histrionic, and borderline. In general, patients with comorbid personality disorders when compared with patients with major depression alone have an earlier age of onset of depression, suffer from a more severe depression, report more marital disruption, have more episodes of depression, report more episodes of substance abuse, and make more suicide attempts (Charney et al. 1981; Friedman et al. 1983; Hope et al. 1983; Pfohl et al. 1984, 1987; Zimmerman et al. 1986; Docherty et al. 1987; Frank et al. 1987; McGlaushin 1987; Shea et al. 1987; Black et al. 1988).

Patients with comorbid personality disorders and depression, in general, have a worse outcome than depressed patients without comorbid personality. In general, the comorbid patients have more symptomatology, more rehospitalizations, worse social and occupational functioning, a poorer clinical course, and respond more poorly to treatment (Pfohl et al. 1984; McGlashin 1987; Black et al. 1988; Shea et al. 1990). Overall, these studies indicate that a cooccurrence of personality disorders and depression defines a more pernicious disease.

In general, patients with coexistent depression and major depression and personality disorders have a younger age of onset of depression, have worse marital relationships, respond more poorly to treatment, and have more familial alcoholism and sociopathy (Pfohl et al. 1984; Black et al. 1988; Alnaes and Torgersen 1988a, b; Reich and Troughton 1988).

This strongly suggests that the more important interaction is between personality disorders and depression than personality traits and depression, and that this is a more fruitful avenue for study and for clinical intervention.

Summary

The last decade has revealed a great deal to us about the conundrum of personality and depression. Most important is the profound influence of the clinical state of depression on the assessment of personality disorders. This simple observation has great implications in terms of theory and clinical practice. We simply cannot accept as accurate and valid measures self-perceptions of individuals while they are depressed. We must assess them either after they have recovered or optimally prior to their first onset of depression.

Following complete recovery from depression, both unipolar and bipolar patients are characterized in general by decreased emotional strength, modestly increased interpersonal dependency, and to some extent by introversion (unipolars only).

In the few studies that have been able to assess people prior to their first onset of depression, personality differences are much more modest (at least in relatives) and include modestly decreased emotional strength, and aggressiveness and autonormic lability in middle-aged adults and interpersonal dependency. We found no personality predictors for young adults. The interaction of personality disorder and depression appears to be a much more interesting and meaningful relationship than personality traits and depression.

We already have learned that this interaction has significant effects on prior clinical history, treatment response, and long-term course of the disorder. Our research efforts in the future must concentrate on this area.

References

Abramson LY, Seligman ME, Teasdale JD (1978) Learned helplessness in humans: critique and reformulation. J Abnorm Psychol 87: 49–74

Akiskal HS, Rosenthal TL, Haykal RF, Lemmi H, Rosenthal RH, Scott-Strauss A (1980) Characterological depressions. Clinical and sleep EEG findings separating "subaffective dysthymias" from "character spectrum disorders." Arch Gen Psychiatry 37: 777–783

Alnaes R, Torgersen S (1988a) DSM-III symptom disorder (Axis I) and personality disorders (Axis II) in an outpatient population. Acta Psychiatr Scand 78: 348–355

Alnaes R, Torgersen S (1988b) The relationship between DSM-III symptom disorders (Axis I) and personality disorders (Axis II) in an outpatient population. Acta Psychiatr Scand 78: 485–492

Angst J, Clayton P (1986) Premorbid personality of depressive, bipolar, and schizophrenic patients with special reference to suicidal issues. Compr Psychiatry 17: 511–532

Beck AT (1972) Depression: causes and treatment. University of Pennsylvania Press, Philadelphia

Benjaminsen S (1981) Primary non-endogenous depression and features attributed to reactive depression. J Affective Disord 3: 245–259

Bianchi GN, Fergusson DM (1977) The effect of mental state on EPI scores. Br J Psychiatry 131: 306–309

Black DW, Bell S, Hulbert J, Nasrallah A (1988) The importance of axis II in patients with major depression: a controlled study. J Affective Disord 14: 115–122

Charney DS, Nelson JC, Quinlan DM (1981) Personality traits and disorder in depression. Am J Psychiatry 138: 1601–1604

Chodoff P (1972) The depressive personality. Arch Gen Psychiatry 27: 666–667

Coppen A, Metcalf M (1965) Effect of a depressive illness on MPI scores. Br J Psychiatry 111: 236–239

Frank E, Kupfer DJ, Jacob M, Jarrett D (1987) Personality features in response to acute treatment and recurrent depression. J Pers Disord 1: 14–26

Friedman RC, Aronoff MS, Clarkin JF, Corn R, Hurt SW (1983) History of suicidal behavior in depressed borderline inpatients. Am J Psychiatry 140: 1023–1026

Hirschfeld RMA, Klerman GL, Clayton PJ, Keller MB, McDonald-Scott P, Larkin BH (1983a) Assessing personality: the effects of depressive state on trait measurements. Am J Psychiatry 140: 695–699

Hirschfeld RMA, Klerman GL, Clayton PJ, Keller MB (1983b) Personality and depression: empirical findings. Arch Gen Psychiatry 40: 993–998

Hirschfeld RMA, Klerman GL, Keller MB, Andreasen NC, Clayton PJ (1986) Personality of recovered patients with bipolar affective disorder. J Affective Disord 11: 81–89

Hirschfeld RMA, Klerman GL, Lavori P, Keller MB, Griffith P, Coryell W (1989) Premorbid personality assessments of first onset of major depression. Arch Gen Psychiatry 86: 345–350

Ingham JG (1966) Changes in MPI scores in neurotic patients: a three year follow-up. Br J Psychiatry 112: 931–939

Joffe RT, Regan JJ (1988) Personality and depression. J Psychiatr Res 22: 279–286

Katz MM, Secunda SK, Hirschfeld RMA, Koslow SH (1979) NIMH clinical research branch collaborative program on the psychobiology of depression. Arch Gen Psychiatry 36: 765–771

Kerr TA, Schapira K, Roth M (1970) The relationship between the maudsley personality inventory and the course of affective disorders. Br J Psychiatry 116: 11–19

Lewinsohn P (1974) A behavioral approach to depression. In: Friedman R, Katz M (eds) The psychology of depression: contemporary theory and research. Wiley, New York, pp 157–178

Liebowitz MR, Stallone F, Dunner DL, Fieve RF (1979) Personality features of patients with primary affective disorders. Acta Psychiatr Scand 29: 535–544

McGlashan TH (1987) The borderline personality disorder in unipolar affective disorder: long-term effects of comorbidity. J Nerv Ment Dis 175: 467–473

Phfol B, Stangl D, Zimmerman M (1984) The implications of DSM-III personality disorders for patients with major depression. J Effective Disord 7: 309–318

Pfohl B, Coryell W, Zimmerman M, Stangl D (1987) Prognostic validity of self report and interview measures of personality disorder in depressed in patients. J Clin Psychiatry 48: 468–472

Pope HG, Jr, Jonas JM, Hudson JJ, Cohen BM, Gunderson JG (1983) The validity of DSM-III borderline personality disorder: a phenomenologic, family history, treatment response, and long-term follow-up study. Arch Gen Psychiatry 40: 23–30

Reich J (1988) DSM-III personality disorder and family history of mental illness. J Nerv Mental Dis 176: 45–49

Reich J, Noyes R, Hirschfeld R, Coryell W, O'Gorman T (1987) State and personality in depressed and panic patients. Am J Psychiatry 144: 181–187

Shea MT, Glass DR, Pilkonis PA, Watkins J, Docherty JP (1987) Frequency and implications of personality disorders in a sample of depressed outpatients. J Pers Disord 1: 27–42

Shea MT, Pilkonis PA, Beekham E, Collins JF, Elkin I, Sotsky SM (1990) Personality disorders and treatment outcome in the NIMH treatment of depression collaborative research program. Am J Psychiatry (in press)

Zimmerman M, Coryell W, Pfohl B (1986) ECT response of depressed patients with and without a DSM-III personality disorder. Am J Psychiatry 143: 1030–1032

Zimmerman M, Pfohl B, Coryell W, Stangl D, Corenthal C (1988) Diagnosing personality disorder in depressed patients. Arch Gen Psychiatry 45: 733–737

Aggressive Behaviour and Hostility in Depression: Clinical Aspects

P. Castrogiovanni, I. Maremmani, and A. Di Muro

Aggressiveness has been studied chiefly in animals by pharmacologists and ethologists and in man by psychologists and sociologists. Yet, it is also of great interest in psychiatry. Aggressiveness, in terms of violence, has received much attention as has aggressive behaviour in which violent actions are only an aspect.

In depressive disorders aggressiveness has stimulated new interest from a strictly clinical point of view for the following reasons:

1. The growing interest in the serotoninergic system (well-known to be involved both in depression or in aggressive behaviour)
2. The recent availability of substances with a specific action on such a system
3. The constant focus on suicidal behaviour, suggesting some link with the aggressive behaviour
4. The greater sensitivity to problems such as compliance and response predictability, to which the role of aggressiveness cannot be indifferent

At a clinical level various questions arise which are important not only from a theoretical-speculative point of view, but also from a clinical-practical one:

- To what extent is the depressed patient aggressive?
- What kind of aggressiveness prevails (hostility-in or hostility-out; overt-hostility or covert-hostility; direct or indirect)?
- Do different kinds of aggressiveness exist in depression (relating to variables such as diagnosis, age, sex, etc.)?
- What kind of relationship does aggressiveness establish with the symptomatological components of the depressive picture?
- During remission phases, does aggressive behaviour remain unmodified or does it modify itself from a qualitative or quantitative point of view?
- What relation exists between aggressive behaviour and response to antidepressant treatment?
- How does the pharmacological treatment modify aggressive behaviour?

These are the questions we have attempted to answer, even if only partially, utilizing the results of research carried out in recent years at the Psychiatric Clinic of Pisa. We used the Questionario per la Tipizzazione dell'Aggressività by Castrogiovanni et al. (1982) (QTA) which is the Italian version of the Inventory for Assessing Different Kinds of Hostility, by Buss and Durkee (1957). It is made up of 75 items (right/wrong) and provides a global index of aggressiveness and a profile of aggressive behaviour, made up of eight factors: assault (DIR), indirect aggression (IND), irritability (IRR), negativism (NEG), resentment (RES), suspiciousness (SUS), verbal aggression (VER) and guilt (GUI).

Depressive symptomatology has been evaluated in hetero-evaluation by means of the Hamilton Rating Scale for Depression (HRSD) and in self-evaluation by means of the Self-Evaluation Scale for Depression (SAD) by Cassano and Castrogiovanni (1977).

A first study was carried out on 61 patients suffering from depressive disorders, almost globally represented by monopolar depression, treated with tricyclic antidepressants (max. 75 mg/day) and benzodiazepines at a low dosage, or fluoxetine (20–40 mg/day). They were evaluated during the acute phase of the illness and compared with a group of 61 normal subjects homogeneous for sex and age: QTA total mean score shows a slight increase in aggressiveness in depressed patients. The profile is characterized by the relatively high mean values of RES, SUS and GUI, and, to a lesser extent, IRR. A GUI/total score ratio less than 1, shows an inhibition of aggressiveness. Depressed patients' total scores as well as IRR, RES, SUS and GUI, are significantly higher than the controls' scores when using Student's t test (Fig. 1).

In many experimental studies the relationship between the presence and entity of depression with aggressive tendencies less behaviourally expressed, such as RES, SUS and IRR, as well as GUI, has also been repeatedly assessed. This aggressive pattern has been more often defined as "hostility-in" (Busse 1959; Gershon et al. 1968; Friedmann 1970; Schless et al. 1974; Becker and Lesiak 1977; Perris et al. 1983). Our data do not confirm the reduction in verbal aggressiveness (Friedman 1970); reduced in depressed patients, but still always higher than the control group.

In our study, the aggressiveness entity, shown by QTA total score, is not related in a linear way with the depressive state entity, shown either by HRSD

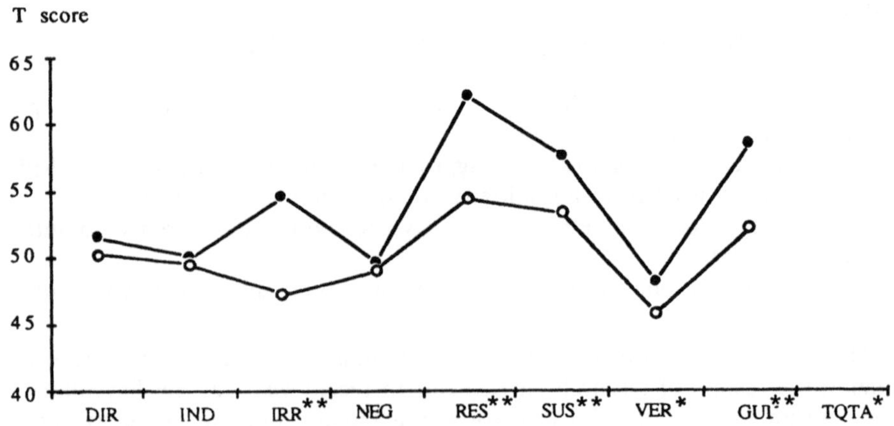

Fig. 1. QTA factors in 61 acute phase depressed patients and 61 controls. ●, depressed; ○, controls; *, $p < 0.05$; **, $p < 0.01$

total or by SAD total (not significant correlation coefficient). Aggressiveness, therefore, is much higher when a depressive disorder is present, but not in proportion to its symptomatological severity (Table 1).

Multiple regression analysis, using QTA scales as predictors and SAD total score as criterion, shows the principal roles of RES, SUS and GUI in predicting the total score in the self-evaluation scale; in this way the prevalent role of inhibited aggressiveness in depression is confirmed (Table 2).

Analogously, the factorial analysis, performed on QTA scales and SAD factors, isolates in the first factor all the aspects that characterize the act of aggression without linking them with any depressed aspect. Only inhibited aggressiveness is linked to some aspects of depression; in the second factor, in fact, we find GUI, RES and NEG (QTA) together with depressed mood, insecurity-sensitivity-guilt, and suicide (SAD) (Table 3).

Table 1. Correlations between QTA scales and HRSD and SAD total scores in 61 depressed patients (acute phase)

	THRSD	TSAD
Direct	n.s.	n.s.
Indirect	n.s.	n,s.
Irritability	n.s.	n.s.
Negativism	n.s.	n.s.
Resentment	n.s.	0.46*
Suspiciousness	n.s.	n.s.
Verbal	n.s.	n.s.
Guilt	n.s.	0.42*
Total score	n.s.	n.s.

*$p < 0.05$.

Table 2. Stepwise regression in 61 depressed patients (acute phase)

	Variables in equation			
Variable	Coefficient	Standard error	Standard coefficient	F to remove
Intercept	40.41			
Resentment	0.56	0.15	0.43	13.02
Suspiciousness	– 0.37	0.12	– 0.35	9.47
Guilt	0.34	0.12	0.33	7.61

	Analysis of variance table			
Source	*df*	Sum squares	Mean square	F test
Regression	3	3083.55	1027.85	11.28
Residual	57	5193.76	91.11	
Total	60	8277.31		

Y1 = TSAD; X = QTA scales

Table 3. QTA-SAD factor analysis in 61 depressed patients (acute phase)

	Factor 1	Factor 2	Factor 3	Factor 4	Factor 5	Factor 6
Direct	0.713					
Indirect	0.84					
Irritability	0.742					
Negativism	0.685	0.405				
Resentment		0.454				0.519
Suspiciousness						0.866
Verbal	0.869					
Guilt		0.782				
Depressed mood		0.623			0.478	
Anxiety			0.856			
Sensitivity-Guilt		0.771				
Somatic symptoms				0.915		
Diurnal variation					0.903	
Suicide		0.612			0.49	
% variance contribution	0.29	0.22	0.11	0.11	0.13	0.11

Orthogonal transformation solution-varimax

This kind of relation is shown more clearly by the analysis of the canonic correlations between QTA scales and SAD factors. In this analysis, along with RES, NEG and GUI, IRR also appears, while, on the depression side, as well as insecurity-sensitivity-guilt, depressed mood, suicide or anxiety also appear (Fig. 2).

The comparison during the remission phase between the QTA profile of the depressed patients and that of 47 patients homogeneous for age, sex and diagnosis, allows one to point out the following (Fig. 3):

1. The remission QTA profile is lower for all the factors than the illness phase profile; this is confirmed by the significant difference in the total scores (Student's *t* test).
2. The more evident differences between the two profiles concern IRR, RES, VER and GUI, whose values during the remission phase are significantly lower (Student's *t* test) than those in the illness phase.
3. In the remission phase, a trend toward a GUI–RES–SUS pattern persists, with a low value particularly for VER but also for DIR, IND, IRR and NEG; this is an expression of hostility-in and therefore of inhibition of aggressiveness, also shown by the relationship between GUI and total score which is, higher than 1 in remission phase patients.

Nevertheless, the comparison between the profile of depressed patients in the remission phase and that of the controls does not point out significant differences. This result shows that the aggressive pattern of the depressed patient is more a state than a trait (Fig. 4).

These analyses allow us to conclude that depression involves a higher level of aggressiveness, which is still not proportional to the symptomatological severity of the clinical picture (showing that aggressiveness is an independent component

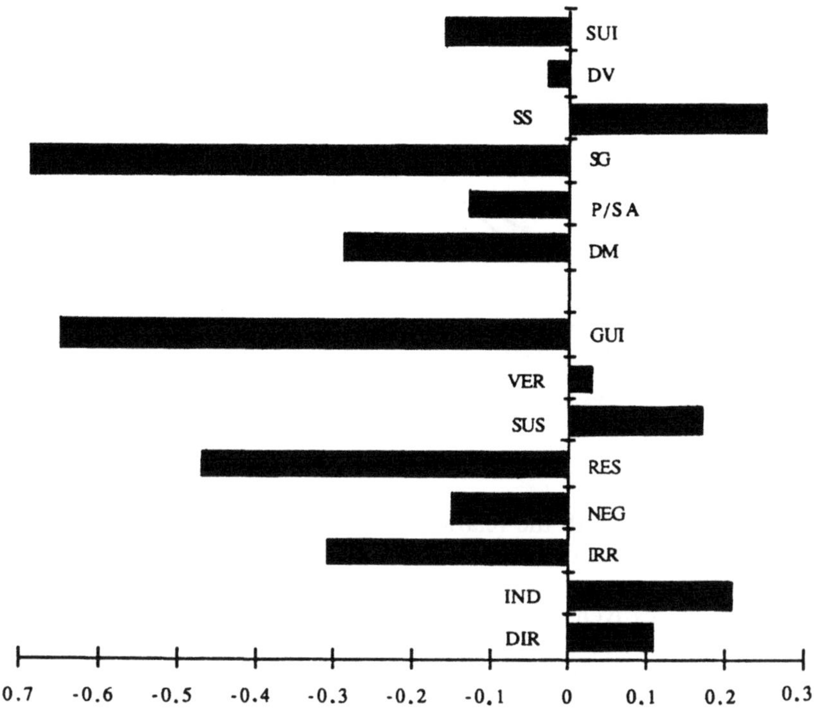

Fig. 2. QTA-SAD canonical variations in 61 acute phase depressed patients. Cancorr = 0.66; Wilks $\lambda = 0.25$; $df = 48$;. $p = 0.01$

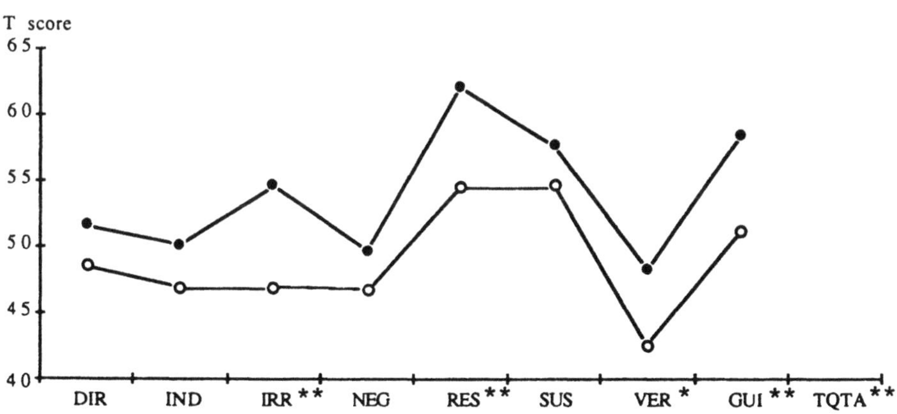

Fig. 3. QTA factors in 61 acute phase and 47 remission phase depressed patients. ●, acute phase; ○, remission; *, $p < 0.05$; **, $p < 0.01$

apart). Aggressiveness is prevalently inhibited, presenting as resentment and suspicious attitudes and feelings, sometimes with negativism, sometimes with irritability, which are linked to depressed mood, but particularly to depressive insecurity and to a lesser extent to suicidal ideas.

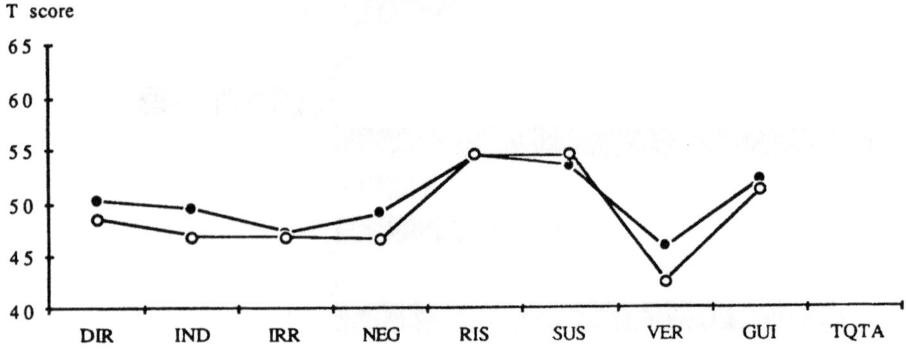

Fig. 4. QTA factors in 47 remission phase depressed patients and 61 controls. ●, controls; ○, remission

Literature that deals with the relation between aggressiveness and suicide, either at a biological level or at a clinical one, is very rich and agrees on a positive correlation between the two. It gives credit to the hypothesis that hetero- and autoaggressiveness are linked together through a common neurochemical basis, represented by a serotoninergic system deficit.

Among depressed patients a higher level of aggressiveness would distinguish subjects with suicidal tendencies from others (Paykel and Dienelt 1971; Weismann et al. 1973; Crook et al. 1975; Yesavage 1983; Farmer and Creed 1986; Farmer 1987), with particular reference to outward hostility (Farmern 1987), so that IND is suggested as a better predictor of suicidal attempts than degree of depression (Yesavage 1983).

In a recent study carried out at the Psychiatric Clinic of Pisa by Conti et al. (1990), 23 attempted suicides were compared with 23 depressed patients without suicide attempts and with 23 healthy controls. The above-described pattern (high values for RES, SUS and GUI and low value for VER was confirmed for attempted suicides and depressed patients: the only statistically significant difference between them concerns GUI, which is higher in attempted suicides. It seems that repressed aggressiveness such as resentment and suspiciousness, and the increase in guilt could cause the move towards self aggressiveness. Therefore behavioural depression is correlated with an activation of aggressive tendencies which:

– Are partially inhibited by guilt, with an increase in hostility-in, covert, hidden and projected hostility, such as resentment and suspiciousness.

– Are partially transferred to a behavioural performance through a hostility-out, or an overt-hostility, which is, however, not openly directed towards other people, but rather indirect or reactive.

– Will partially be directed against self through self-injuring or more particularly suicidal behaviour.

Nevertheless, the stress of aggression during the depressive phase does not seem to be a general rule. In fact, QTA total score of the 61 depressed patients during the acute phase shows high scattering, ranging from a minimum of 38 to a maximum of 70 (Mean 53, 49, standard deviation, SD, ±7.7). The profile, obtained by QTA scales, also shows an analogous high variation in the individual patients.

In fact, the cluster analysis carried out on the 61 depressed patients' QTA profiles allows one to isolate three groups of subjects, each composed of about one third of the examined population (Fig. 5).

A group of 23 patients present a quite normal mean QTA profile (average aggressiveness). Another group of 20 patients show a definitely high mean profile (high aggressiveness group). This shows that in some depressed patients the aggressiveness level is heightened in all its aspects, whether inhibited or expressed.

Finally, the third group (18 patients) shows an aggressiveness not only lower than the depressed sample mean, but lower than the general population mean (low aggressiveness group).

It is interesting to note how, even in this last group, the inhibited aggressiveness aspects (RES, SUS) and GUI maintain high values, even higher than those of the average aggressiveness group.

It is therefore evident that the differences in aggressiveness among depressed patients depend only on the different degrees of hostility-out inhibition: DIR, IND, IRR, NEG and VER are the scales presenting the maximum variation, ranging between the two standard deviations of the standardization sample.

On the contrary, the hostility-in, represented by the couple RES–SUS, always remains high, together with GUI, showing itself as a typical and constant characteristic of the depressed aggressive behaviour during the illness phase.

Therefore, depression, seems to increase, perhaps through guilt hostility-in manifestations; whereas, depression may activate in some people and inhibit in others hostility-out.

What factors are involved in the determination of the different aggressive expressions in depressed patients?

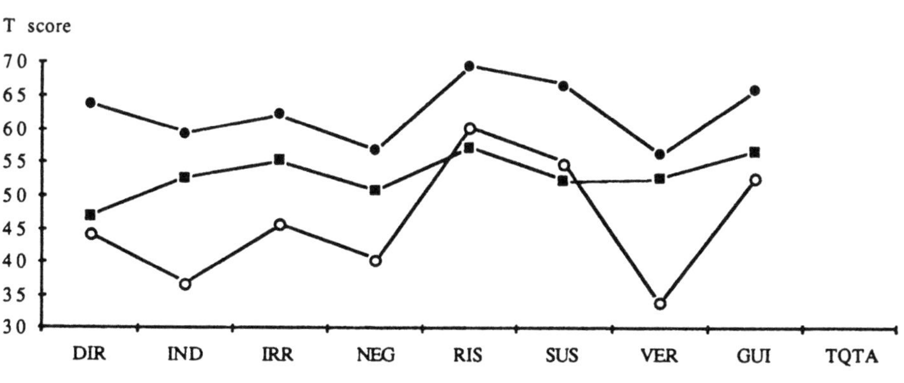

Fig. 5. QTA clustered groups in 61 acute phase depressed patients. ● *HA*, high aggressiveness ($n = 20$); ■ *MA*, medium aggressiveness ($n = 23$); ○ *LA*, low aggressiveness ($n = 18$)

The inhibition of expressed aggressiveness does not depend on guilt. The latter, in fact, is significantly, even if moderately, correlated with total score, IND, NEG, SUS and RES, but always positively. Therefore elevations in hostility-in aspects (RES–SUS) as well as hostility-out aspects (IND, NEG) are proportional to GUI (Table 4).

Previously we have seen that the different aggressiveness entity does not depend on the symptomatological severity of the depressive picture. In fact, QTA total does not correlate significantly with either HRSD total or SAD total (Table 1).

With regard to the diagnosis, too many of our cases are unipolar depressed to allow any comparison. According to literature, we found that the few bipolars were in the lower aggressiveness group.

Finally, as far as sex and age are concerned in the low aggressiveness group, male sex and older age subjects prevail, showing that these characteristics inhibit the expression of aggressiveness. The relation between aggressiveness level and age is significant with chi-squared test (chi-squared = 11.09; $p = 0.02$; Table 5).

Substantially, however, the degree of expressed aggressiveness inhibition, distinguishing the three groups of patients, must now be clarified; it allows one to predict interesting research hypotheses on the neurochemical level as well as on other levels, such as that of personality.

A different involvement of the serotoninergic system in depressed patients with high hostility-out, or a different balance between this neurotransmitter system and the others involved in depression, in particular with the dopaminergic system, could be proposed. We could, in fact, hypothesize that with low

Table 4. Correlations between guilt and QTA factors

QTA factors	GUI	QTA factors	GUI
DIR	0.20	RES	0.45
IND	0.32	SUS	0.32
IRR	0.24	VER	0.13
NEG	0.37	TQTA	0.39

TQTA, QTA total score $r = 0.24$; $p < 0.05$

Table 5. QTA clustered groups (61 depressed patients in acute phase)

		Sex		Age (years)			Diagnosis		
	n	F	M	<40	40–59	60	UD	BD	DYS
High aggression	20	18	2	9	10	1	18		2
Middle aggression	23	18	5	8	11	4	21	1	1
Low aggression	18	11	7	1	10	7	15	2	1

UD, unipolar depressive; BD, bipolar depressive; DYS, dysthymic depressive.

values of serotoninergic activity, the different dopaminergic values could determine the expression or not of aggressive behaviour. In more generic terms, we could hypothesize that the serotonin-dopamine balance has an important role in determining depressed aggressive behaviour. Such a hypothesis has recently been suggested for healthy subjects on the basis of the negative correlation pointed out between serotoninergic and dopaminergic indexes (Castrogiovanni et al. 1989).

However, it must be stressed that the aggressive behaviour variability is typical of the illness phase. In fact, carrying out the cluster analysis in patients in remission phase and also in controls, the average aggressiveness group becomes wider than the high and low ones (Table 6).

Depression, from the aggressive behaviour point of view, would therefore have a dishomogenizing effect, to the same extent as remission would lead to the higher homogeneity of normal people.

This observation is confirmed by the study of variations in aggressive behaviour during antidepressant treatment. In our study the aim was the evaluation of variations in aggression assessed by means of QTA in relation to depression remission. We used as homogeneous a sample as possible, in order to exclude the influence of other variables: all female patients, evaluated during their admission to the clinic, all suffering from major recurrent depression, mean age 47 years, all treated with tricyclic antidepressants, with doses ranging between 75 and 150 mg/day, combined with small doses of benzodiazepines. The 15 patients chosen showed at admission a HRSD total score > 17 and at discharge < 10.

The comparison between the admission QTA total score and the discharge one reveals some variations in the score, but not all in the same direction (Fig. 6): some patients had an increase, while others a decrease. Such a variation explains the lack of statistical significance of the differences; it seems to show that

Table 6. Contingency table of QTA clustered groups in 61 acute phase depressed patients (DEPR) 47 remission phase depressed patients (REM) and 61 controls (CNTR)

Groups	DEPR	REM	CNTR	Totals
HA	47.62	26.19	26.19	100
MA	27.38	27.38	45.24	100
LA	41.86	30.23	27.91	100
Totals	36.09	27.81	36.09	100
HA	32.79	23.40	18.03	24.85
MA	37.70	48.94	62.30	49.70
LA	29.51	27.66	19.67	25.44
Totals	100	100	100	100

All data are percentages

Statistics: *df* 4; total chi square 7.73; G statistic 7.773; contingency coefficient 0.209; Cramer's V 0.151.

HA, high aggression; MA, medium aggression; LA, low aggression

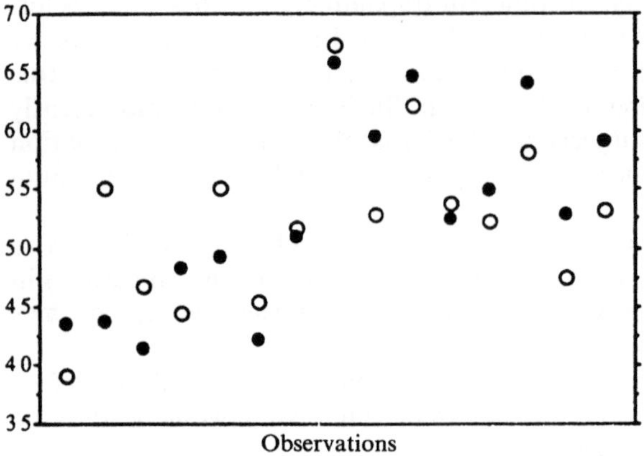

Fig. 6. Baseline (TQTA1) and end of trial (TQTA2) QTA total score differences in 15 inpatients treated with tricyclic antidepressants. ●, TQTA1; ○, TQTA2

variations in aggression, with regard to remission, are accidental; they do not follow a rule. Yet, if we observe the variation in score with respect to the initial level, we notice that the greater the admission score is below 50 (showing poor aggressiveness) the more its variation tends to increase at discharge. On the other hand, there is predominant decrease in aggressiveness in those who start from high levels (Table 7).

In fact, QTA total score variation, during a tricyclic antidepressant treatment, is significantly correlated with QTA total score at the beginning of the treatment; the higher the initial aggressiveness level, the more it will decrease during treatment and vice versa (Fig. 7). Depressive symptomatology remission, achieved with tricyclic antidepressant treatment, would seem therefore to have a "normalizing" effect on the aggressive manifestations of the depressed subject, decreasing, or activating them, according to their high or low entity during the acute phase.

This trend, however, seems to depend on the kind of antidepressant treatment. In fact, a group of 11 patients, suffering for the greater part from major depression, were administered fluoxetine in a single dose of 20–40 mg/day without other antidepressants or tranquillizers for 2 months after wash-out. A different trend in their aggressive behaviour was recorded, but it is awaiting confirmation following the completion of this study on a wider number of cases.

First a significant decrease in QTA total score and a lowering of all the QTA profiles, with significant variations in IRR, occur. Moreover, for this treatment, the relation between entity and direction of aggressive behaviour variation on the one hand, and its initial values on the other, cannot be emphasized (Fig. 8).

If we distinguish between patients with aggressiveness lower than the mean (under-M group) and patients with aggressiveness higher than the mean (over-M group) at the beginning of their antidepressant treatment, the former

Table 7. Baseline-end of trial QTA total score differences in patients treated with tricyclic antidepressants or fluoxetine

Tricyclic antidepressants ($n = 15$)				Fluoxetine ($n = 11$)			
Under-M[a] group ($n = 6$)		Over-M[b] group ($n = 9$)		Under-M group ($n = 6$)		Over-M group ($n = 5$)	
Baseline TQTA	End of trial TQTA	Baseline TQTA	End of trial TQTA	Baseline TQTA	End of trial TQTA	Baseline TQTA	End of trial TQTA
44.59 ± 3.2	47.62 ± 6.3	58.2 ± 5.7*	55.4 ± 6.0	45.1 ± 3.7	44.39 ± 5.2	56.6 ± 3.8**	51.99 ± 5.5

* $T = 2.81$ $p = 0.03$; ** $T = 4.63$ $p = 0.01$.
[a] Patients with baseline TQTA under the means of standard sample.
[b] Patients with baseline TQTA over the means of standard sample.

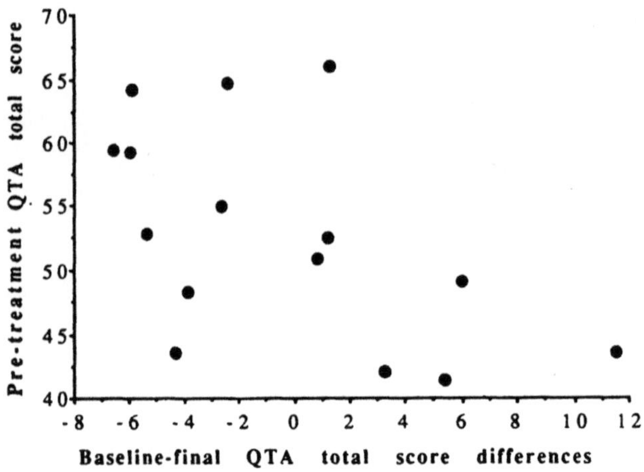

Fig. 7. Correlations between pre-treatment QTA total score and baseline final QTA total score differences. ($r = -.54$)

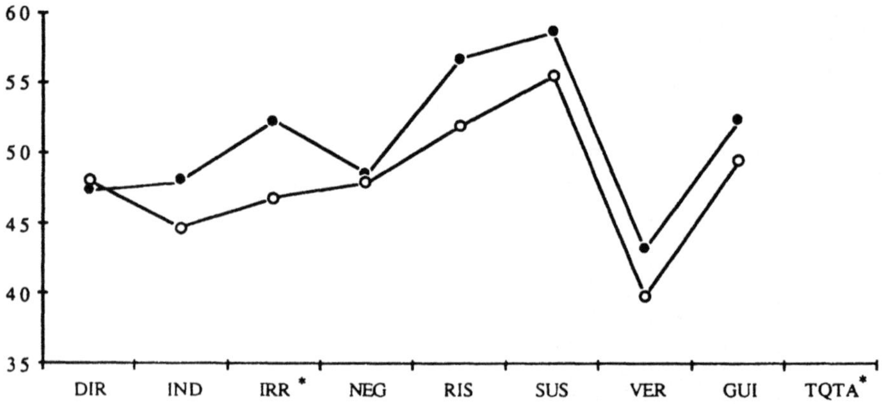

Fig. 8. Pre- and post-treatment (fluoxetine) QTA factors in 11 depressed outpatients. ●, baseline; ○, post-treatment; *, $p < 0.05$

show an increase of aggressiveness and the latter a decrease in the same numerical entity; yet, only the latter is significant, because of the greater number of subjects.

In the group treated with fluoxetine, on the other hand, both patients with high initial aggressiveness and low initial aggressiveness show a QTA total score decrease, even if the variation is only significant with Student's *t* test for the former. The treatment with a drug having an elective action on the serotoninergic system would seem therefore to have a steadier effect on the depressed patient's aggressiveness, causing a decrease; this effect would confirm the implication of this neurotransmitter system in the determination of aggressive behaviour and at the same time testify to the marked and specific serotoninergic action of the substance.

The difference between the treatments is also emphasized by the relation between the effect on aggressiveness (evaluated by means of the difference between the initial and final QTA total scores) and the effect on depressive symptomatology (shown by the final HRSD total score, Fig. 9).

For the 15 patients treated with tricyclic antidepressants and benzodiazepines, variation in aggressiveness does not correlate significantly with improvement in the clinical picture. For the patients treated with fluoxetine, on the contrary, correlation between variation in aggressiveness and improvement in depressive symptomatology is positive and significant ($r = 0.54$). Although the number of cases was small, a trend would seem to exist; those who at the end of the treatment show a worsening of aggressiveness (QTA total score increase) are also those whose HRSD total score does not go below 10, the value traditionally assumed as the threshold for remission.

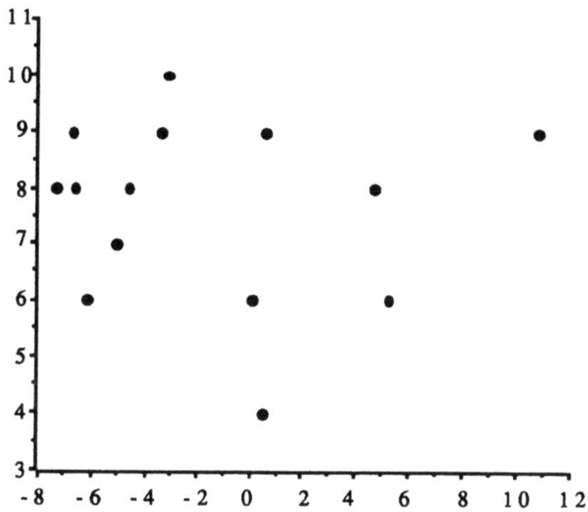

(a)

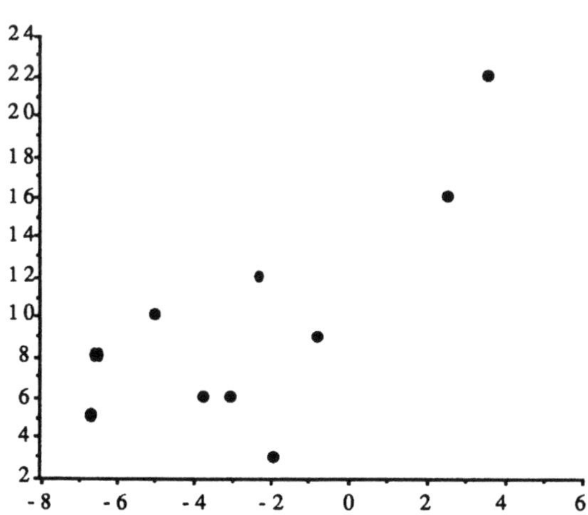

(b)

Fig. 9a, b. Correlations between post-treatment HRSD and baseline end of trial QTA total score differences in (**a**) 15 inpatients treated with tricyclic antidepressants and (**b**) 11 outpatients treated with fluoxetine

If aggressiveness is correlated to a reduction in serotoninergic activity, its variation during treatment could be considered as indicator of the psychotropic substance's agonist effect on such activity. The lack of effect on the aggressive behaviour would therefore show that the patient does not respond to such a drug, showing no significant improvements in the clinical picture on the whole.

In short, the presented results and the developed considerations allow one to suggest various interesting reasons for the study of aggressive behaviour in the field of depressive disorders:

1. To have a psychobiological index of the neurotransmitter systems chiefly involved, as aggressiveness is an expression of biological substratum, perhaps more so than other psychological and psychopathological aspects.
2. Consequently, to develop a typology of depressive disorders, which also considers this psychopathological manifestation; in fact, the latter could reveal itself to be as significant, at least, as other aspects which are more traditionally considered, such as anxiety.
3. To use the entity and kind of depressed patient's aggressive behaviour as a predictor of his/her compliance; in fact, we noticed that the greatest number of drop-outs in the studies mentioned above is in the high aggressiveness group, and in previous studies we observed that the high aggressiveness, depressed patients are those who tend to deny their symptomatology improvement, causing a discrepancy between auto-evaluation (SAD) and hetero-evaluation (HRSD).
4. To isolate within aggressiveness a criterion, extrinsic to the depressive picture in a strict sense, that could be utilized as a more precise indicator for the different antidepressant treatments and as a predictor of therapeutic response.

References

Becker EW, Lesiak WJ (1977) Feelings of hostility and personal control as related to depression. J Clin Psychol 33: 654–657

Buss AH, Durkee A (1957) An inventory for assessing different kinds of hostility. J Consult Psychol 21: 343–349

Busse EW (1959) Psychopathology. In: Birren JE (ed) Handbook of aging and the individual. University of Chicago Press, Chicago

Cassano GB, Castrogiovanni P (1977) SAD, Scala di autovalutazione per la depressione. International Committee for Prevention and Treatment of Depression, Pisa

Castrogiovanni P, Andreani MF, Maremmani I, Nannini-Innocenti MA (1982) Per una valutazione dell'Aggressivita' nell'uomo: contributo alla validazione di un questionario per la tipizzazione del comportamento aggressivo. Riv Psichit 17: 274–282

Castrogiovanni P, Di Muro A, Maremmani I, Perossini M, Marazziti D (1989) Interaction between the serotonin and dopamine systems in humans: preliminary findings. Brain Res 504: 129–131

Conti L, Marazziti D, Toschi D (in press) Aspetti psicopatologici e comportamentali del tentato suicido. The 6th Congress of Proceedings of the Society of Biological Psychiatry

Crook TM, Raskin A, Davis D (1975) Factor associated with attempted suicide among hospitalized depressed patients. Psychol Med 5: 381–388

Farmer R (1987) Hostility and deliberate self-poisoning: the role of depression. Br J Psychiatry 150: 609–614
Farmer R, Creed F (1986) Hostility and deliberate self-poisoning. Br J Med Psychol 59: 311–316
Friedman AS (1970) Hostility factors and clinical improvement in depressed patients. Arch Gen Psychiatry 23: 524–537
Gershon ES, Cromer M, Klerman GL (1968) Hostility and depression. Psychiatry 31: 224–235
Paykel ES, Dienelt MN (1971) Suicide attempts following acute depression. J Nerv Ment Dis 153: 234–243
Perris C, Eisemann M, Ericsson U, von Knorring L, Perris H (1983) Patterns of aggression in the personality structure of depressed patients. Arch Psychiat Nervenkr 233: 89–102
Schless AP, Mendels J, Kipperman A, Cochrane C (1974) Depression and hostility. J Nerv Ment Dis 159: 91–100
Weissman MM, Fox K, Klerman GL (1973) Hostility and depression associated with suicide attempts. Am J Psychiatry 130: 450–455
Yesavage JA (1983) Direct and indirect hostility and self-destructive behavior by hospitalized depressives. Acta Psychiatr Scand 68: 345–350

Course and Outcome

Course as Classifier for Depression*

J. Angst

Introduction

Kahlbaum (1874) proposed the systematic use of the features of the course of a disorder as a classifier, a proposal which was taken up by Kraepelin (1899) later on. In this respect the distinction between single-episode or nonrecurrent and recurrent cases is elementary and seems at first glance to be easy (Table 1).

Recurrence is a prominent characteristic of the course of many depressions. Applying the classification of schizoaffective psychoses of Marneros et al. (1986), recurrent depression can be subdivided into oligophasic (two to three episodes) and polyphasic (more than three episodes) patterns. In addition, a third group consists of continuously recurring cases. They are characterized by multiple brief episodes with short intervals over at least 1 year. They are closely interrelated to the continuous rapid cycling subtype described by Akiskal et al. (1989).

Our definition of continuous rapid cycling requires at least two episodes per month over 1 year, which means only subjects with short cycles. Apart from recurrence, chronicity is an important classifier for depression. Chronicity can develop at any point of time during the course and is defined by nonrecovery over more than 2 years at the last observation.

From a methodological point of view, recurrence depends on the *definition of an episode* and the definition of a subsequent *interval* (interepisodic period). The recurrence observed is also a function of the *length of observation* since onset and

Table 1. Terminology

Phasic course	Number of episodes
Monophasic course	1
Oligophasic course	2–3
Polyphasic course	>3
Continuous recurrent course	Multiple episodes, short intervals over at least 1 year
Chronic course	
Length of episode	>2 years

* Project supported by the Swiss National Science Foundation grant no. 3.873-0.88.

this again may be dependent on *mortality*. Finally, the most important factor is the *selection of the sample* studied. For instance, hospitalized psychiatric patients may differ from cases recruited in community studies and contain many recurrent cases, perhaps resulting in an underestimation of single-episode patients. In studies of hospitalized patients first and readmissions are often not analyzed separately (Zis and Goodwin 1979). Another important variable which has to be taken into consideration is *diagnosis*. It is well-known that bipolar illness is much more recurrent than unipolar depression. This article will concentrate mainly on unipolar depression.

A first question deals with single-episode depression. Does it exist, how frequent is it, and does it differ from recurrent depression? The literature refers to three groups of subjects, psychiatric inpatients, outpatients, and normal subjects.

The *studies of hospitalized depressive patients* have been repeatedly reviewed in this respect (Zis and Goodwin 1979; Bland and Orn 1982; Coryell and Winokur 1982; Fukuda et al. 1983; Angst 1988). The rates of single-episode cases vary between the studies from 13% (Kinkelin 1954) to 61% (Lundquist 1945). The results are highly dependent on the selection of the samples. The highest rates of single-episode patients were observed by Lundquist (1945) and Bland and Orn (1982). The latter followed 102 first-admitted patients over 12–18 years and found 55% single-episode cases. In our own study, Angst and Frey (1976) found 19% single-episode cases in first hospitalized early-onset and 26% in late-onset unipolar depression. The higher rate in the late-onset group was due to a shorter observation period, shorter life, and higher chronicity rate.

Cassano et al. (1989)studied 364 *outpatients* and 41 inpatients, representing consecutive series over an 18-month period in psychiatric facilities. The authors found 23.2% of the patients to have single episodes of depression or hypomania/mania. They mention especially that "single-episode depressions had a later onset, a higher rate of chronicity, a higher prevalence of reported stressors, the lowest family load for mood disorders, and the lowest prevalence of melancholic features."

Up to now, *community studies* did not much focus on the course of affective disorders. In this context the design of the study is highly relevant. Interesting data can be gained from prospective cohort studies. Such a study was carried out in Zurich in a cohort of 591 young adults investigated from age 20 to 30. The methodology of this study has been described earlier (Angst et al. 1984) and some results will be presented here.

Major Depressive Disorder

DSM-III major depressive disorder was tentatively subdivided at each of the four interviews at age 21, 23, 28, and 30 by the number of episodes into monophasic, oligophasic, polyphasic, and more continuously cycling courses. The same was done for recurrent brief depression, considering those with weekly

1–3-day-long episodes as "continuously cycling," the others as polyphasic. The *cross-sectional frequencies* over 1 year are given in Table 2. Among major depressives the rate of single episode cases varies between 33% (1986) and 49% (1988).

Longitudinally, taking into account four interviews (4 years) the single-episode cases drop to 36% ($n = 53$). Two of these subjects were diagnosed as dysthymics and 11 as suffering from recurrent brief depression, and seven others had been treated for depression between the years covered by the interviews. Therefore, we can only be more or less certain in about 22% (33 of 147) of major depressives that they suffered from a single episode only. We shall now compare these 33 single-episode cases with recurrent cases of major depressive disorder in order to validate the distinction and try to reproduce some of the findings described by Cassano et al. (1989).

The comparison is presented between five groups of subjects (Table 3): controls with no depression (219), major depressives with single episodes (28) versus recurrent cases (48), major depressives with comorbidity with recurrent brief depression (46), and finally subjects with recurrent brief depression only (79). The purpose is to show that *single-episode major depressives are much more similar to controls than to recurrent major depressives.*

Table 2. Classification of course based on one interview

	Age 21 (1979)	Age 23 (1981)	Age 28 (1986)	Age 30 (1988)
Major depressive disorder				
Episodes over 12 months				
1 monophasic	20 (43)	22 (49)	16 (33)	23 (49)
2–3 oligophasic	9	5	9	9
>3 polyphasic	9	10	10	2
continuously cycling	8	8	14	13
Recurrent brief depression				
polyphasic	37	27	43	20
continuously cycling	21	13	14	6

Table 3. Marital status, family history

n	No dep. 219	MDD single episodes 28	MDD recurrent episodes 48	MDD +RBD 46	RBD 79	*p*
Married % (age 30)	47	54	33	26	39	0.05
Divorced % (age 30)	3	–	10	13	6	0.05[a]
FH + dep. % (age 28)	37	41	54	78	67	0.001
FH + treated dep. % (age 28)	13	14	23	24	21	0.01[a]

[a] Groups 1+2 vs 3–5

The original marital rate was the same for the five groups, but recurrent depressives have a significantly higher divorce rate, probably as a consequence of the disorder.

A family history for depression was present in all groups but again the single-episode major depressives did not differ from the controls, whereas recurrent depressives showed clearly elevated rates of a positive family history for depression.

Some premorbid (prediagnostic) measures could be taken 1 year prior to the first interview when the subjects underwent a screening procedure with the Symptom Checklist 90-R of Derogatis et al. (1974). At the age of 19/20 years the single-episode depressives did not deviate from the controls prior to the diagnosis of a major depression. It is interesting that we cannot find any difference in any scales measuring depression, anxiety, hostility, phobias, interpersonal sensitivity, or somatization. This is not true for the recurrent depressive cases which showed consistently higher mean values in all scales (Table 4).

At age 30 all subjects interviewed were assessed by the Freiburg Personality Questionnaire (FPI) developed by Fahrenberg et al. (1970). Table 5 shows the results. The depressives did not differ from controls in extraversion and therefore in the primary dimensions sociability and dominance. However, they did differ in all other scales, especially those reflecting emotional lability or neuroticism. Again, the single-episode major depressives did not deviate to a considerable extent from the nondepressed controls. The most deviant group consisted of subjects suffering from both major depressive disorder and recurrent brief depression. This personality measure does not reflect the premorbid but the postmorbid personality.

We could not find significant differences between single-episode and recurrent major depressive patients in symptoms, in precipitating events, or in life events over 12 months assessed by the scale of Tennant and Andrews (1976, 1977).

Table 4. SCL-90-R at age 19/20 (screening) mean values

n	No dep.	MDD single episodes	MDD recurrent episodes	MDD +RBD	RBD
	336	33	61	53	103
Depression	1.9	2.0	2.4	2.7	2.4
Anxiety	1.7	1.8	2.1	2.4	2.1
Hostility	1.7	1.7	2.1	2.1	2.0
Phobia	1.4	1.4	1.6	1.7	1.6
Somatization	1.5	1.6	1.9	1.9	1.8
Interpers. sens.	1.8	2.0	2.3	2.5	2.2
Obsessionality	1.8	1.9	2.1	2.4	2.1
Paranoid	1.8	1.9	2.2	2.5	2.3
Psychoticism	1.6	1.6	1.9	2.0	1.9
Total score	1.7	1.8	2.1	2.2	2.0

The five groups differ significantly in all scales ($p < 0.001$) MDD single episode vs no dep: all comparisons are NS

Table 5. Personality traits (FPI) at age 30

n	No dep. 219	MDD single episodes 28	MDD recurrent episodes 48	MDD +RBD 46	RBD 79	*p*
Nervousness	3.9	4.2	6.0	5.7	5.8	0.001
Aggression	2.4	2.1	2.9	3.7	3.2	0.001
Depression	2.7	3.4	5.1	5.7	5.5	0.001
Irritability	3.8	3.7	4.5	6.0	5.2	0.001
Sociability	7.8	7.3	7.5	8.0	7.2	NS
Frustr. tol.	4.9	4.7	4.6	3.4	3.7	0.001
Dominance	2.7	2.6	2.7	3.1	3.3	NS
Inhibition	3.6	4.2	4.8	4.7	5.3	0.001
Frankness	4.4	4.3	4.7	5.1	5.0	0.003
Extraversion	5.5	5.1	5.3	5.7	5.1	NS
Neuroticism	3.7	4.1	5.6	6.3	6.1	0.001

MDD single episode vs no dep: all comparisons are NS

Dysthymic Disorder

Dysthymic disorder was defined by DSM-III-R criteria. At age 28 we found a 1-year prevalence rate of 3.4%. Within the same year, 16 of 25 cases were associated with recurrent brief (5) or major depression (11). Two years later we identified only 11 cases of dysthymia, 9 of them overlapping with major depression and two with recurrent brief depression. For this and other reasons the diagnostic category of dysthymia has been questioned.

Kocsis and Frances (1987) described that 95% of DSM-III dysthymic patients met the symptomatic criteria for major depressive disorder. They studied a psychiatric outpatient sample of 39 cases. Our study confirms in an impressive way their findings (Table 6).

Table 6. Dysthymia and number of criterial symptoms

Dysthymia	No. of criterial symptoms for major depression DSM-III			
	n	<4	⩾4	%
Kocsis and Frances 1987				
DSM-III	39	2	37	95
Our study:				
DSM-III 1986	19	0	19	100
1988	6	0	6	100
DSM-III-R 1986	25	1	24	96
1988	10	0	10	100

In our community study, all 25 cases of DSM-III dysthymic disorder met the symptomatic criteria for major depression, which means four or more of the eight criterial symptoms. DSM-III-R criteria are softer, which results in an increase from 25 to 35 cases (+36%). It is remarkable that only 1 of our 35 DSM-III-R cases of dysthymia was under the symptomatic threshold of major depression. The two studies (Kocsis and Frances 1987 and ours) suggest the existence of a uniform broad major depressive syndrome independent of its course. Chronic dysthymia, recurrent brief depression, and major depression would then be interrelated and represent only subgroups defined by different course patterns.

Recurrent Brief Depression

In the community we found that only about 50% of all subjects treated for depression met diagnostic criteria for major depressive disorder or dysthymia. Analyzing the other 50% of treated depressives we came up with the definition of a new group of depressives characterized by brief episodes but high recurrence. This group was called recurrent brief depressives (Angst et al. 1990).

The definition of recurrent brief depression, compared with DSM-III major depressive disorder, is described in Table 7. Subjects with recurrent brief depression suffer from the full depressive syndrome and meet all the symptomatic criteria of major depression. But the episodes of recurrent brief depression are brief, usually lasting only 1–3 days and show a high recurrence. Half of the cases suffer from one or two episodes per month, the other half from weekly spells of depression over 1 year. In community studies it is recommendable to diagnose recurrent brief depressives only when the subjects have a subjective work impairment.

Patients with recurrent brief depression do not differ from those with major depression in common validators, for instance, number and quality of symptoms, lifetime treatment rates, rates of suicide attempts, course studied prospectively, and a family history in first-degree relatives of treated depression.

Table 7. Criteria for DSM-III-major depression (MDD) and recurrent brief depression (RBD)

	DSM-III MDD	DSM-III-R MDD	RBD
Dysphoric mood	+	+	+
Duration (weeks)	2	2	<2
Symptoms	4/8	5/9	4/8
Impairment	No	No	Yes
Recurrence	No	No	Yes
Structured instrument	DIS	SCID	SPIKE

Table 8. One-year prevalence rates

	Age 28 1986	Age 30 1986
Major dep. dis. (DSM-III)		
Males	4.6	7.1
Females	10.0	11.6
M + F	7.3	9.4
Dysthymia (DSM-III-R)		
Males	3.4	0.8
Females	3.5	0.4
M + F	3.4	0.6
Recurrent brief dep.		
Males	4.4	3.8
Females	14.3	3.6
M + F	9.4	3.7

The diagnostic categories are not mutually exclusive

Table 8 gives the prevalence rates of recurrent brief depression and major depressive disorders in the Zurich cohort study separated by sex at ages 28 and 30. Recurrent brief depression and major depression show prevalence rates of between 4% and 9%. If we consider unweighted rates, females outweigh males more among patients with major depressives than among those with recurrent brief depression.

Therefore, in the general population we can identify a highly prevalent form of brief and highly recurrent depressives. Longitudinally, the major depression and recurrent brief depression show considerable interchange, and we do not consider recurrent brief depression to be a new illness. It is a subtype of the course of major depressive syndromes as long as we define this by symptoms and not by duration.

Conclusions

Using the course pattern as a classifier for depression, we started our analysis with the definition of a depressive syndrome identical to a major depressive episode according to DSM-III requiring at least four of eight criterial symptoms. Subjects with less than four symptoms are considered to suffer from a minor depressive syndrome. Characteristics of the course patterns of episodes can be applied to both, to minor or to major depressive syndromes in an identical way (Fig. 1).

Two criteria can be applied: (a) length in days, weeks or years and (b) recurrence defined by the number of episodes. With the length of the episodes one can distinguish brief spells of depression (lasting days), major episodes (lasting at least 2 weeks), a dysthymic course (with at least 50% of the

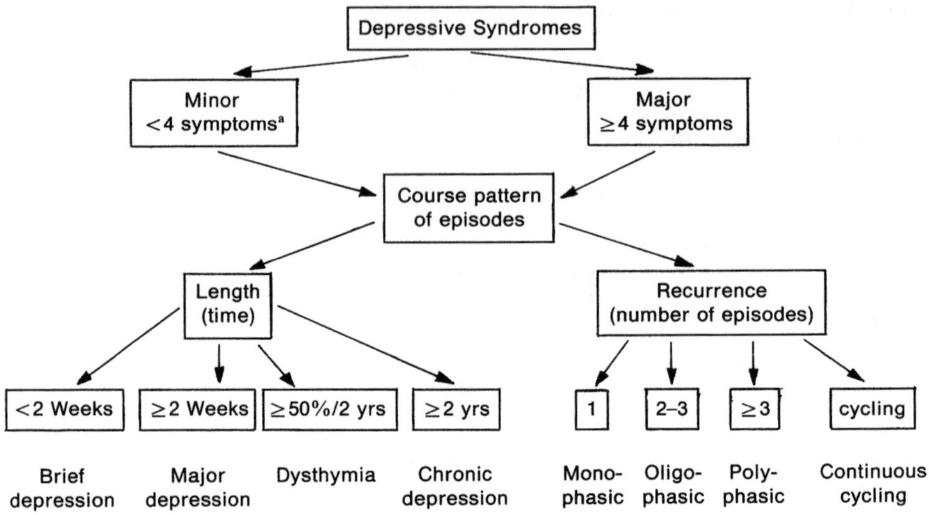

Fig. 1. Course as classifier. [a] Criterial symptoms DSM-III

time over 2 years spent in depression), and finally chronic depression (defined as nonrecovery from an episode over at least 2 years). Based on the recurrence of depressive episodes one can distinguish monophasic, oligophasic, polyphasic, and continuous cycling course patterns.

On the syndrome level there is a spectrum of four diagnostic groups: recurrent brief depression, major depression, major dysthymia, and chronic major depression. The same subdivision can be applied to minor depressive syndromes (Fig. 2).

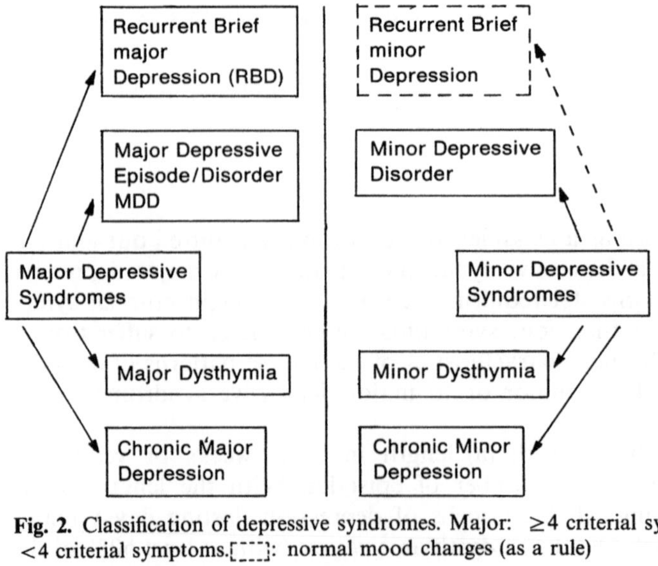

Fig. 2. Classification of depressive syndromes. Major: ≥4 criterial symptoms (DSM-III). Minor <4 criterial symptoms. [dashed box]: normal mood changes (as a rule)

The main conclusion is that we can identify in the community a broad depressive syndrome defined operationally by the number of criterial symptoms. Subdividing the syndrome by length and periodicity we can obtain subgroups, but they share many features and belong more or less to the same depressive disorder. This is especially true for major depression, dysthymia, and recurrent brief depression. Up to now an exception can only be postulated for monophasic (single-episode) major depression which may occur in premorbid normal persons with no hereditary load. Further research on single-episode major depressive patients validated by a longer follow-up might be very interesting.

References

Akiskal HS, Cassano GB, Musetti L, Perugi G, Tundo A, Mignani V (1989) Psychopathology, temperament, and past course in primary major depressions. I. Review of evidence for a bipolar spectrum. Psychopathology 22: 268–277

Angst J (1988) Clinical course of affective disorders. In: Helgason T, Daly RJ (eds) Depressive illness: prediction of course and outcome. Springer, Berlin Heidelberg New York, pp 1–48

Angst J, Frey R (1976) Endogene Früh- und Spät-Depressionen zeigen mehr Gemeinsamkeiten als Unterschiede. Med Tribune 39: 5

Angst J, Dobler-Mikola A, Binder J (1984) The Zurich Study. A prospective epidemiological study of depressive, neurotic and psychosomatic syndromes. I. Problem, methodology. Eur Arch Psychiatry Neurol Sci 234: 13–20

Angst J, Merikangas K, Scheidegger P, Wicki W (1990) Recurrent brief depression. A new subtype of affective disorder. J Affective Disord 19: 87–98

Bland RC, Orn H (1982) Course and outcome in affective disorders. Can J Psychiatry 27: 573–578

Cassano GB, Akiskal HS, Musetti L, Perugi G, Soriani A, Mignani V (1989) Psychopathology, temperament, and past course in primary major depressions. 2. Toward a redefinition of bipolarity with a semistructured Interview for depression. Psychopharmacology 22: 278–288

Coryell W, Winokur G (1982) Course and outcome. In: Paykel ES (ed) Handbook of affective disorders. Churchill Livingstone, Edinburgh, pp 93–106

Derogatis LR, Lipman RS, Rickels K, Uhlenhuth EH, Covi L (1974) The Hopkins Symptom Checklist (HSCL): a measure of primary symptom dimensions. In: Pichot P (ed) Psychological measurements in psychopharmacology. Karger, Basel, pp 1–15 (Modern problems in pharmacopsychiatry, vol 7)

Fahrenberg J, Selg H, Hampel R (1970) Das Freiburger Persönlichkeitsinventar (FPI), 3rd edn. Hogrefe, Göttingen

Fukuda K, Etoh T, Iwadate T, Ishii A (1983) The course and prognosis of manic-depressive psychosis: a quantitative analysis of episodes and intervals. Tohoku J Exp Med 139: 299–307

Kahlbaum J (1874) Die Katatonie oder das Spannungsirresein. Eine klinische Form psychischer Krankheiten. Hirschwald, Berlin

Kinkelin M (1954) Verlauf und Prognose des manisch-depressiven Irreseins. Schweiz Arch Neurol Neurochir Psychiatr 73: 100–146

Kocsis JH, Frances AJ (1987) A critical discussion of DSM-III dysthymic disorder. Am J Psychiatry 144: 1534–1542

Kraepelin E (1899) Psychiatrie. Ein Lehrbuch für Studierende und Aerzte, 6th edn. Barth, Leipzig

Lundquist G (1945) Prognosis and course in manic-depressive psychoses: a follow-up study of 319 first admissions. Acta Psychiatr Scand [Suppl] 35: 1–96

Marneros A, Rohde A, Deister A, Risse A (1986) Features of schizoaffective disorders: the cases in between. In: Marneros A, Tsuang MT (eds) Schizoaffective psychoses. Springer, Berlin Heidelberg New York

Tennant C, Andrews G (1976) A scale to measure the stress of life events. Aust NZ J Psychiatry 10: 27–32
Tennant C, Andrews G (1977) A scale to measure the stress of life events. Aust NZ J Psychiatry 11: 163–167
Zis AP, Goodwin FK (1979) Major affective disorder as a recurrent illness. A critical review. Arch Gen Psychiatry 36: 835–839

Course and Outcome: Definitional Dilemmas*

D.J. Kupfer and E. Frank

Introduction

Effective pharmacological and psychotherapeutic treatments for affective disorders have been developed. Despite their extensive testing in clinical trials, our understanding of the differential effectiveness of various treatment approaches is very limited. More treatment research and novel treatment modalities are needed.

In discussing potential contributions to the area of treatment research, it was concluded early in the planning process of a program sponsored by the John D. and Catherine T. MacArthur Foundation (the Network on the Psychobiology of Depression and Related Disorders) that while treatment research per se is sufficiently well funded by governmental agencies and the pharmaceutical industry, none of the many sponsors have found room to support work on a vital and basic problem impeding research in this area which limits the generalizability of reports on treatment outcome and the efficacy of various treatment modalities. This problem is that the enormous variability in the use of labels to identify change points in the course of illness (such as "response," "recovery," "recurrence," and "relapse") has created "Tower-of-Babel" conditions in the field which have rendered comparison of results across treatment studies virtually impossible.

Even one example will suffice to make this point. If one study defines "recovery" from depression as a 50% symptom reduction at the 8-week point (irrespective of whether or not the patient still meets criteria for the disorder), while another study considers "recovery" as being symptom-free for a period of 8 months (the presumptive end of the "episode" of depression), while yet a third study considers the former a "response" and the latter a "remission" and defines "recovery" as something in between, it is clear that one cannot compare these "recoveries" and easily evaluate which of the treatment procedures described in these three studies was more "effective." Moreover, many study reports fail to specify how exactly they defined the terms employed to label change points in course. In summary, while treatment studies are well supported and there is a large body of treatment literature, its findings are less conclusive than is

* Supported in part by a grant from the John D. and Catherine T. MacArthur Foundation Research Network on the Psychobiology of Depression. The authors wish to thank Ms. Herma Rojahn.

generally assumed. This fact has major public health implications in that it not only affects research progress, but constitutes a major impediment to optimizing clinical care.

It was on this background that our group of scientists concluded that conceptual work in this area might well constitute a unique network contribution to the area of treatment research which might have a major impact on research and clinical practice. As stated earlier, the major goal was to formulate empirically derived operational criteria for change points in the course of major depressive disorder. Such criteria are desirable for the improved design, interpretation, and comparison of studies of the natural course of the disease and clinical trials; for the clarification of relationships between biologic and psychological correlates of illness; for more rational drug development planning by individual investigators and the pharmaceutical industry; for improved guidelines for the evaluation of clinical efficacy and other treatment criteria of regulatory agencies; and finally, for the development of improved treatment guidelines for clinical practice.

Following these recommendations, a task force was formed, chaired by Dr. Robert Prien of the National Institute of Mental Health and consisting of leading treatment researchers with access to large data sets and an expert biostatistician, to begin work on these issues. The task force conceptualized its work as consisting of three related endeavors: (1) arriving at consensus definitions of the relevant terms, (2) proposing tentative operational criteria for each of the definitions, and (3) testing these operational criteria for validity. As a first step, the task force worked on the development of preliminary consensus definitions of terms relating to course of affective illness (the "R" terms, thus "RRR" Task Force). Great care was given to base the definitions exclusively on observable symptomatology rather than any given theoretical model of the disease, since models are based on assumptions about the nature of the underlying, but inherently unobservable, course of the illness and tend to differ between treatment researchers of different backgrounds and scientific persuasion. In an iterative process, preliminary consensus definitions were developed, and methods for testing these definitions in existing data sets were devised. Five terms were found necessary to describe the course of major depression: episode, remission, recovery, relapse, and recurrence. As shown in Fig. 1, a prototype of an episode of major depression can be portrayed. Such an example provides one strategy based on the definition of "episode" to indicate discriminating points for response, remission, relapse, recovery, and recurrence.

Simultaneously, an extensive literature review was conducted to document the variability of the terms relating to course applied in recent publications of treatment research in five leading journals. The results of this review confirmed the very serious nature and extent of the problem. In the articles reviewed, an even greater than expected variety of terms labeling change points in course were found, several of them "word creations" appearing in only one report. One-hundred twenty-one studies were reviewed, and 28 different labels were found. Including frequently used modifiers (e.g., complete, partial, marked, moderate), the number of different labels applied in these studies was 64. As expected, it was also found that commonly used terms to describe improvement of symptoms

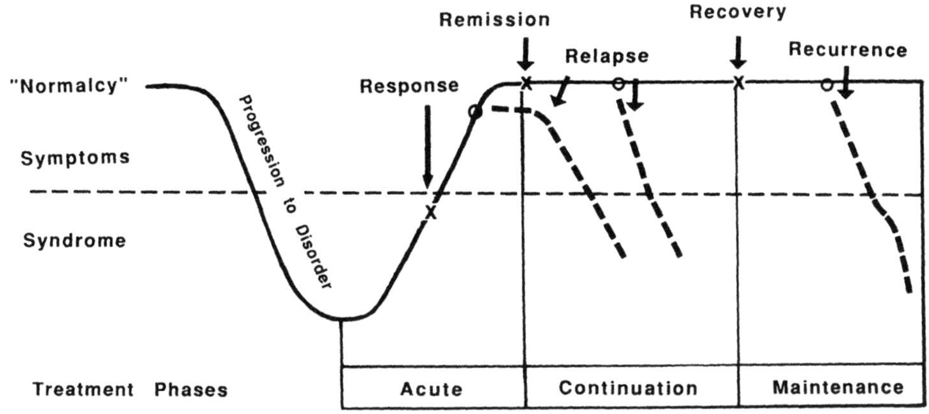

Fig. 1. Response, remission, recovery, relapse, recurrence. (Reprinted from the *Journal of Clinical Psychiatry* 1991, 52 (Suppl. 2), 12–16. Physicians Postgraduate Press.)

(such as "recovery" and "remission") were used interchangeably. These results reinforced the notion that the existing treatment literature is inconclusive and that the operationalization of the terms relating to change points in course is of vital importance to both research and clinical practice (Prien et al. 1991).

The task force jointly prepared several manuscripts which have been published and communicate the task force's activities to the wider research community. A first paper communicates the results of the literature review and documents the extent of the "semantic" problem in the field (Prien et al. 1991). A second paper proposes the preliminary consensus definitions and seeks feedback and dialogue in the process of further refining these definitions (Frank et al. 1991).

In this consensus document, Frank et al. (1991) have proposed definitions and operational criteria for major depressive disorder. They utilized the following three principles to construct the definitional scheme: (a) the definitional scheme is based on observable, measurable phenomena; (b) the initiation or withdrawal of any form of treatment may change the meaning of remission, recovery, relapse, and recurrence, but not their phenomenological expression (i. e., observable events); and (c) the temporal focus of the definitional scheme is lifelong rather than episode specific. They concluded that only five terms (six, if response and partial remission are considered separately) were required to designate the relevant change points in the course of unipolar depressive illness. They also realized that a coherent definitional scheme for these terms leads to a definition of what constitutes an "episode" of illness (and vice versa). Two types of variations were fundamental to their definitions: (a) *severity* (number of intensity of symptoms) and (b) *duration* (of symptomatic deterioration or *improvement*). By this simplification they hoped to isolate the part of the problem of definition that depends on the description of the number and intensity of symptoms from the part that is tied to the timing of changes in symptoms.

Episode

Conceptualization of Episode

An episode is a period of time, lasting longer than D days, during which the patient is consistently within the fully symptomatic range on a sufficient number of symptoms to meet syndromal criteria for the disorder. Syndromal criteria are defined by any of several criterion-based assessment systems such as the Research Diagnostic Criteria or the Diagnostic and Statistical Manual of Mental Disorders. It should be noted that some of these assessment systems specify a pattern as well as number, severity, and duration of symptoms.

Any time period prior to the patient's first episode, during which the patient is in the asymptomatic range except for short periods (<D days), is said to be disorder-free. A short (<D days) time period during which the patient is outside the asymptomatic range is called a "flurry." A flurry can occur either prior to onset or after the resolution of an episode. An episode does not end until a patient reaches recovery (see below).

Rationale for the Conceptualization of Episode

Both clinicians and researchers must decide when a patient is clearly ill. For the clinician, this typically triggers a decision to treat; for the researcher, this designation signals the appropriateness of including the patient in a group of individuals with the same illness.

Response and Partial Remission

Conceptualization of Partial Remission

"Partial remission" is a period of time during which an improvement of sufficient magnitude is observed such that the individual is no longer fully symptomatic (i.e., no longer meets syndromal criteria for the disorder), but continues to evidence more than minimal symptoms. Treatment is not a requirement of the definition; partial remission can be spontaneous.

A "response" can be thought of as the point at which a partial remission begins. Theoretically, a response, unlike a partial remission *does* require treatment and, thus, implies that the cause of the change in the patient's condition is known, which may or may not be a valid assumption.

Rationale for the Conceptualization of Partial Remission

In deciding when and how to intervene, the clinician usually chooses to intervene when the patient suffers from the disorder. If the disorder is in partial remission (either by natural course or in association with treatment), the clinician may choose to observe rather than alter the patient's regimen. If a partial remission fails to become a full remission after a reasonable period of time, the clinician will typically alter treatment, either by increasing the intensity (through a higher dose of medication or more frequent therapy sessions) of the current treatment, adding additional treatments to the one associated with the partial remission, or by switching to a new treatment. If the disorder is not being treated and partial remission fails to become a full remission after a reasonable period of time, the clinician will typically initiate treatment. For the researcher, the failure to proceed from partial to full remission in a naturalistic study may imply the need for placing the subject in a separate category of patients. In a treatment study with a specified treatment protocol, it may imply the need to drop the subject from the study.

Full Remission

Conceptualization of Full Remission

A "full remission" is a relatively brief ($>$E days, but $<$F days) period of time during which an improvement of sufficient magnitude is observed such that the individual is asymptomatic (i.e., no longer meets syndromal criteria for the disorder and has no more than minimal symptoms). Again, treatment is not a requirement; full remission can be spontaneous.

Rationale for the Conceptualization of Full Remission

A declaration of remission implies that no increase in the intensity of the treatment regimen is required. Depending upon the treatment and assumptions about its mechanisms of action, a full remission might imply that a decrease in the intensity of treatment could be attempted.

Recovery

Conceptualization of Recovery

A remission which lasts $\geq$F days is a "recovery." Recovery can be spontaneous and can last for an indefinite period. The term is used to designate recovery from the episode, not from the illness per se.

Rationale for the Conceptualization of Recovery

In a clinical setting, a declaration of recovery raises the possibility that: (a) treatment can be discontinued or (b) if continued, the aim is prevention of a subsequent episode. In a research setting, it might mean that treatment efforts can now be focused on maintenance of the well state or that the subject moves on into a no-treatment follow-up phase in which the focus is the extent to which treatment-associated improvement is maintained.

Relapse

Conceptualization of Relapse

"Relapse" is a return of symptoms satisfying the full syndrome criteria for an episode which occurs during the period of remission, but prior to recovery as defined above. Relapse can represent a change from either partial or full remission to full syndrome criteria for the disorder.

Rationale for the Conceptualization of Relapse

A relapse signals a need for treatment intervention or modification of ongoing treatment since the disorder has returned. In a study of acute or continuation treatment, it may represent one outcome of interest.

Implicit in the distinction between a relapse and a recurrence (see below) is the hypothesis that relapse represents the return of the symptoms of a still ongoing, but symptomatically suppressed episode, while a recurrence represents an entirely new episode; however, in a definitional scheme based exclusively on observable events, this distinction must be made in probablistic terms.

Recurrence

Conceptualization of Recurrence

A recurrence implies: (a) need for treatment and (b) a revision in the history of the course of illness (i.e., a new episode has occurred). The latter may have prognostic and treatment implications. In studies of maintenance therapy, recurrence is typically the outcome of primary interest.

After describing the conceptualization and rationale for each of the terms, they discussed proposed operational criteria and strategies for testing the definitional scheme. Such a strategy would involve finding valid specifications for the severity and duration parameters in our definitional scheme involves

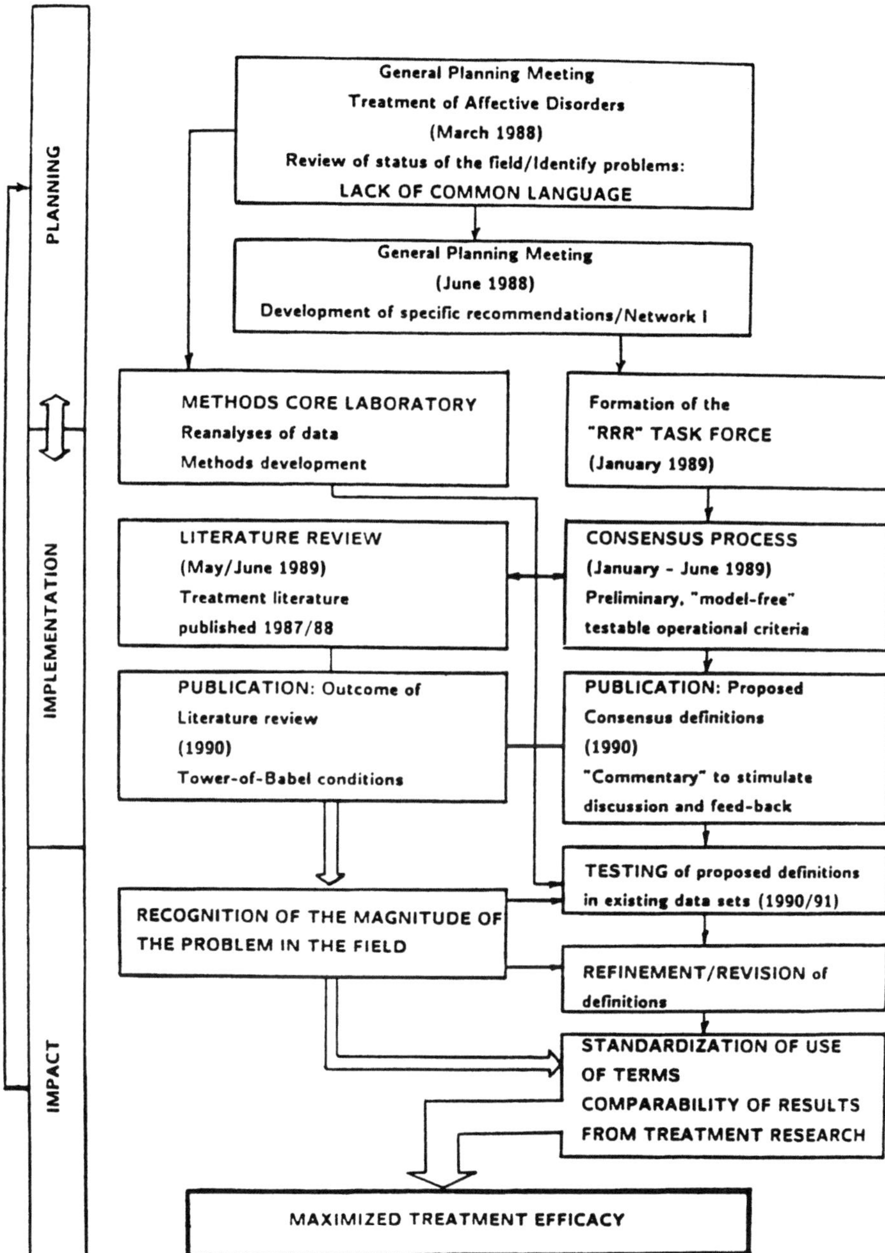

Fig. 2. Network I initiative. Change points in the course of depression: response, recovery, relapse, recurrence, and remission

analysis of longitudinal data sets on patients in long-term treatment and follow-up studies or on patients in naturalistic follow-up studies.

A series of subsequent papers will report results of testing the preliminary definitions in existing data sets. It is hoped that refined and tested consensus definitions will ultimately be adopted widely in the field.

The testing of definitions in existing data sets and further work of this task force will be supported by the establishment of a core laboratory for longitudinal studies which will serve as a service, training, and research resource for longitudinal studies throughout the network. This cluster of activities represents an excellent example for the type of methods development and conceptual work which we believe a research network is uniquely suited to pursue. Figure 2 is a graphic presentation of the network's integrated strategy of activities in this area. It depicts activities undertaken since 1988 up to the present time.

References

Frank E, Prien R, Jarrett RB, Keller MB, Kupfer DJ, Lavori P, Rush AJ, Weissman MM (1991) Conceptualization and rationale for consensus definitions of terms in major depressive disorder: remission, recovery, relapse, and recurrence. Arch Gen Psychiatry 48: 851–855

Prien RF, Carpenter LL, Kupfer DJ (1991) The definition and operational criteria for treatment outcome of major depressive disorder: a review of the current research literature. Arch Gen Psychiatry 48: 796–800

Bipolar Disorders in Prepubertal Children

E.B. Weller and R.A. Weller

Introduction

Historically, mood disorders in the United States have received little attention as it was felt that children's immature superegos would protect them from experiencing and expressing depression. Childhood was seen as a time of growth and development, and the unfolding of the young life would make it impossible to give up hope and succumb to depression. Furthermore, it was felt that children's behavior which is typically full of energy and enthusiasm made it harder to diagnose mania.

Esquirol (1845) described mania in children in the middle of the nineteenth century. Other authors have also discussed childhood mania, the most prominent being Kraepelin (1921) who felt the condition was rare in children but that there was a surge in cases with adolescence. Approximately 0.4% of his 800 adult manics had their first episode below age 10. Loranger and Levine (1978) reported 0.5% of patients with mania had their first episode between the ages of 5 and 9 while 7.5% had an onset between 10 and 14 years of age. Other prominent child psychiatrists such as Kanner (1946) have doubted the existence of mania in children. Anthony and Scott (1960) reviewed 60 previously reported cases and reported that only 3 of 60 satisfied their very stringent criteria to diagnose mania. They also reported a case of their own, a 12-year-old who exhibited full-blown mania similar to that observed in adults. The criteria Anthony and Scott presented included the following:

1. An abnormal psychiatric state approximating descriptions by Kraepelin, Bleuler, Meyer and others
2. Positive family history for mania
3. Early indicators including cyclothymia and sporadic manic or depressive outbursts
4. Two or more similar episodes
5. Diphasic presentation, i.e., elation and depression
6. The condition should be endogenous, i.e., minimally affected by the environment
7. If treated, treatment should be on an inpatient basis, with heavy sedation or ECT
8. There should be an abnormal underlying personality

9. There should be an absence of schizophrenia or organic states
10. The assessment should be current and not retrospective

Subsequently, Weinberg and Brumback (1976) adjusted the criteria presented by Feighner et al. (1972) for diagnosing mania in adults to be applicable to children. Their criteria included the following:

1. Euphoric, irritable, or agitated mood
2. The presence of three or more of the following symptoms which should be a distinct change from the child's normal behavior:

   a) Hyperactive or intrusive behavior
   b) Push of speech
   c) Flight of ideas
   d) Grandiosity
   e) Disturbed sleep, including decreased amount or unusual pattern
   f) Distractibility

3. Duration of at least 1 month.

In 1979 Davis described "the manic depressive variant syndrome." According to Davis, for a child to have this syndrome he should satisfy *all* of the following primary criteria: (a) affective storms which are irregular and transient, (b) family history of mania, (c) hyperactive behavior, (d) chronically disturbed personal relationships, and (e) no psychotic thought disorder.

Furthermore, at least one of the following should be present from the secondary criteria: (a) soft neurological signs, (b) sleep disturbance, (c) abnormal EEG, (d) evidence of minimal brain dysfunction, and (e) enuresis.

More recently several researchers have suggested mania could be diagnosed in children and adolescents using the same criteria as adults with only minor modifications to adjust for the different developmental stages of children (Carlson 1983; Weller et al. 1986a). Weller et al. (1986a) did a detailed review of cases of psychotic and severely disturbed children from 1809 to 1984. Over 200 articles were reviewed where cases diagnosed as schizophrenic, atypically manic, or "severely disturbed" and psychotic children were described. The following diagnoses were excluded from consideration: (a) mental retardation, (b) organic brain disease, (c) attention deficit disorder with hyperactivity, (d) drug or alcohol abuse, and (e) pervasive developmental disorder; 157 cases remained. These were blinded and rediagnosed independently by two child and adolescent psychiatrists using DSM-III criteria. There was full agreement in diagnosis in all but four cases. In three cases the disagreement was whether the mania was possible or probable. In one case one child psychiatrist diagnosed mania while the other diagnosed attention deficit hyperactivity disorder. A third psychiatrist blindly reviewed the cases to make a final determination in these cases. Although DSM-III criteria were used to rediagnose these cases, the criteria as they were applied were somewhat more restrictive. For example, one criterion requiring excessive involvement in activities with a high potential for painful consequences was excluded as this symptom was common in conduct disorder and attention deficit disorder. Also, four symptoms were required to make the diagnosis regardless whether the mood was irritable or euphoric.

Thus, four of six possible criteria (excluding the painful consequences criterion) were needed to make the diagnosis of definite mania. Three criteria made the diagnosis of probable mania, and possible mania was diagnosed when three criteria were met and there was no specification of mood or duration of symptoms. As a result of this extensive review, 33 children were diagnosed as manic, of these 17 (52%) had been previously diagnosed as having schizophrenia, obsessive complusive disorder, psychosis, loss reaction, "chronic personality change," "psychopathic personality," or as being borderline, immature, or neurotic. Thus, 50% of manic children who appeared to have met stringent DSM-III criteria for mania had previously received another diagnosis.

Etiology

Psychodynamic

In this theory, mania is considered as a reaction formation to depression. The manic focuses on other's weaknesses to avoid looking at his own weaknesses.

Genetics

There are three different approaches to studying the effects of genetics in prepubertal mania: (a) twin studies, (b) adoption studies, and (c) family studies. To date there are no twin or adoption studies in prepubertal children.

Family Studies

In regard to studies of *relatives of bipolar prepubertal children*, Varanka et al. (1988) reported on ten hospitalized prepubertal 6 to 12-year-old children who had mania with psychotic features. All ten had a positive family history of psychiatric disorders: 20% had mania, 50% had depression, and 60% had alcoholism in the family history; 80% had depression, mania, or alcoholism in their families. Other diagnoses included drug abuse, antisocial personality, and paranoid disorder. This history was collected by the family history method; hence, it is a conservative estimate.

Strober et al. (1988) reported on the family histories of adolescents with mania. When they stratified their sample into those with prepubertal onset of psychiatric problems vs those with adolescent onset, the prepubertal onset group had three times the familial psychopathology of that of the adolescent onset group.

Children of Bipolars

Although suggestive, these studies cannot be considered definitive due to inadequate attention to: (a) polarity of parent, (b) small samples sizes, and (c) lack of control group. Mayo et al. (1979) studied 25 children (5–17) from 12 families with a bipolar parent. The diagnoses of the children included depression 2/25 (8%) behavioral disorder 9/25 (36%), paranoia (4%), and learning disabilities with depression (4%). Others such as LaRoche et al. (1981) and Decina et al. (1983) reported an increased incidence of depression and dysthymia in children of bipolars compared with children of controls.

Cytryn et al. (1982) reported on 13 bipolar depressed parents with 19 children. In 85% of these families there was at least one depressed child compared with 23% of the families of normal controls.

Akiskal et al. (1985) reported increased mood disorders in offspring and siblings of bipolar patients. These included 35% major depression, 18% dysthymia, 16% mania, 15% cyclothymia, and 16% substance abuse. There was also a high rate of fall and winter episodes for all bipolar patients.

Using sophisticated research techniques, Gaensbauer et al. (1984) studied the infant children of seven manic-depressive couples at 12, 15, and 18 months. They found a disturbance in the quality of attachment to mother, disturbance in regulation of emotions of the infants, and an increase in disturbance on follow-up.

Parent-Child Interaction Model

Prepùbertal children are dependent on their parents more than adolescents who are in the process of separation, individualization, and emancipation. Infants and toddlers are at increased risk as they do not attend school and may be constantly around their parents. Davenport et al. (1984) studied seven couples where one of the partners had a bipolar illness. Their children were evaluated at 12, 15, and 18 months and compared with age-, sex-, and socioeconomic-status-matched controls. Mothers in the bipolar families were less attentive to their children's health needs, overemphasized performance, were more overprotective, and reported more negative affect toward their children. They were more disorganized, less active, more unhappy, more tense, ineffective, and had more problems with family interactions and social adjustment. They were less likely to encourage curiosity and exploratory behavior and less likely to joke and play with their children. They were more likely to encourage isolation than the control parents.

Cohort Effect

Klerman et al. (1985) and Gershon et al. (1987) have reported progressive increase in the lifetime rates of major depression, schizoaffective disorder, and bipolar disorder in subsequent generations over the last 70 years. They report higher rates of affective disorder among relatives of probands with a younger age of onset. The age of onset appears to be decreasing in successive generations. If this observation holds true and continues, bipolar disorder in children may be seen with increased frequency. It has been postulated that an interaction between genes and environment may account for this effect.

Epidemiology

As of this date there are no published studies on the epidemiology of mania in prepubertal children.

Clinical Presentation

Carlson (1983) has done an analysis of symptom patterns of younger manic children (less than 9) compared with older children. She concluded that younger children present with irritability and emotional lability, while older children present with euphoria, elation, paranoia, and grandiose delusions. Hyperactivity, push of speech, and distractibility were equally present in both age groups. Similarly, DeLong and Aldershof (1987) suggest prepubertal bipolar children have cycles where dysphoria, hypomania, and agitation are commonly intermixed and extremes of manic excitement become more apparent with onset of puberty.

Varanka et al. (1988) reported on the clinical symptoms of ten psychotic manic hospitalized children (6-12 years old). Half presented with elation while the other half had an irritable mood. All were restless; 60% had increased sexual activity or interest, 50% had increased talkativeness, 60% had push of speech, 50% flight of ideas, 60% had racing thoughts, 90% reported decreased sleep, and 50% were distractible. All reported psychotic symptoms. These included visual hallucinations (70%), auditory hallucinations (50%), persecutory delusions (70%), and grandiose delusions (20%). The psychotic symptoms reported by the children included: "the devil and the angel talk to me," "voices are calling me dirty names," "I can see the devil," "I see people with purple eyes," "I see people's heads glaring at me from the window," "the Wolfman is after me," "I am the President of the United States of America."

Differential Diagnosis

Several medical and psychiatric conditions may mimic mania (Weller and Weller 1990a). Medical conditions include: (a) medications, e.g., steroids and amphetamines, (b) endocrine disorders, e.g., hyperthyroidism, and

(c) neurological conditions such as multiple sclerosis, head trauma, seizure disorders, and brain tumors.

Psychiatric conditions that should be ruled out in manic children include the following:

1. Attention Deficit Hyperactivity Disorder (ADHD). There are similarities and differences between manic and ADHD children. Both may be distractible and may have psychomotor agitation, increased talkativeness, and excessive involvement in activities with painful consequences. However, age of onset in mania is usually after 7. The self-esteem of manic children is often grandiose. They have hallucinations, delusions, and flight of ideas. By comparison, children with ADHD have onset prior to 7, usually have poor self-esteem, and do not have psychotic symptoms.

2. Conduct Disorder. This is often a comorbid condition in bipolar children. However, children with pure conduct disorder do not have push of speech, flight of ideas, delusions, or hallucinations.

Comorbid Conditions

Prepuberal children with mania very often have the following comorbid conditions:

1. ADHD. Usually this is a very common misdiagnosis prior to establishing a definitive diagnosis of mania because of the increased motor activity present.

2. Conduct Disorder. This is usually a coexisting diagnosis as manic children often have been involved in activities that got them in trouble.

Assessment

Psychometric tests can sometimes be helpful in diagnosing mania. These include the diagnostic interview for children and adolescents (DICA-R) by W. Reich and Z. Welner (1988, The Diagnostic Interview for children and Adolescents-Revised, unpublished manuscript, Washington University, St. Louis) as well as the Semi-structured Interview (K-SADS) by chambers et al. (1985).

Currently there is at least one study in progress to develop a Mania Rating Scale for Prepubertal Children to assess the severity of mania by Fristad and coworkers (1989). The Mania Rating Scale (MRS) (Young et al. 1978) was modified so it could be used in prepubertal children. This 11-item instrument rates elevated mood, increased sexual activity, increased irritability, language thought disorder, appearance, insight, increased motor activity, decreased sleep, increased speech, content of thought, and disruptive/aggressive behavior. Preliminary results suggest this instrument differentiates bipolar children from attention deficit hyperactive children on all but two individual items as well as overall score.

Treatment

A manic child is at best treated in an inpatient setting where a well-controlled environment will provide an opportunity of observation around the clock as well as keep the child from harming himself or others (Weller and Weller 1990b).

It is important for the physician to educate the parents and the child about the disorder. Often strict behavior modification accompanied by individual group and family therapy with educational and social intervention is helpful. Support groups organized through the Association of the Mentally Ill (AMI) or similar groups may be available in some communities.

Before giving any psychotropic medications to children below the age of 12, consent from parent and assent from children should be obtained and the known side effects should be explained. To date lithium has been the most commonly prescribed medication for mania. Common side effects of lithium include nausea, hyperphagia, weight gain, polyuria, polydypsia, and hand tremor. An increase in enuresis in children with a preexisting history of bedwetting is common. A thorough medical work-up including complete blood cell count (CBC) with differential, blood urea nitrogen (BUN), creatinine, creatinine clearance, urine osmolality, electrolytes, and thyroid function tests are necessary. Lithium can be started in a safe manner according to the protocol reported by Weller et al. (1986b). Lithium levels as high as 1.4 mEq/liter can be used. In general, children tolerate lithium better than adults due to their increased glomerular filtration rate.

As lithium treatment needs close monitoring, frequent serum samples by venipuncture are needed. However, children often resent this and may resist giving blood samples. In an attempt to help overcome this problem, Weller et al. (1987) examined the possibility of using saliva lithium levels to monitor treatment by determining the correlations between saliva and serum levels. The concentration of lithium in saliva was almost two times that in the serum, and there was more variability of saliva levels than serum levels. It was possible to predict serum levels from saliva levels using regression analysis.

Other medications have been less well studied in children. Some have used carbamazepine (Tegretol) either separately or in combination with lithium to augment its effects. However, there are no well-designed studies of carbamazepine (Tegretol) in manic children. Valproic acid and clonazepam have been used in children, but well-designed studies are advised before these medications can be recommended for children.

Outcome and Follow-up Data

There are no published data on the follow-up of mania in prepubertal children. In our clinical experience we have encountered some children who have not been able to function without lithium carbonate maintenance. The most fortunate children are those who do not experience recurrent episodes.

Research Directions

Diagnostic instruments should be refined so that mania is not overdiagnosed. Also, double-blind, placebo-controlled studies are needed to demonstrate the importance of the medication management in these children. Studies of children at high risk for bipolar disorder such as children of bipolar parents, children with a family history of bipolarity, and depressed or dysthymic children may also yield valuable information regarding the disorder.

References

Akiskal HS, Weller EB (1989) Mood disorders and suicide in children and adolescents. In: Kaplan, Sadock (eds) Comprehensive textbook of psychiatry, vol 2, 5th edn. Williams and Wilkins Baltimore

Akiskal HS, Downs J, Jordan P, Watson S, Daugherty D, Pruitt DB (1985) Affective disorders in referred children and younger siblings of manic- depressives. Arch Gen Psychiatry 42: 996–1004

American Psychiatric Association (1987) Diagnostic and statistical manual of mental disorders, 3rd edn, revised. American Psychiatric Association, Washington DC

Anthony J, Scott P (1960) Manic-depressive psychosis in childhood. Child Psychol Psychiatry 4: 53–72

Carlson GA (1983) Bipolar affective disorders in childhood and adolescence. In: Cantwell DP, Carlson GA (eds) Affective disorders in childhood and adolescence – an update. Spectrum, New York pp 61–84

Chambers WJ, Puig-Antich J, Hirsch M, Paez P, Ambrosini PJ, Tabrizi MA, Davies M (1985) The assessment of affective disorders in children and adolescents by semistructured interview. Arch Gen Psychiatry 42: 696–702

Cytryn L, McKnew DH, Zahn-Waxler C, Gershon ES (1986) Developmental issues in risk research: the offspring of affectively ill parents. In: Rutter M, Izard CE, Read PB (eds) Depression in young people: clinical and developmental perspectives. Guilford, New York

Davenport YB, Zahn-Waxler C, Adland ML, Mayfield A (1984) Early child-rearing practices in families with a manic-depressive parent. Am J Psychiatry 141(2): 223–229

Davis RE (1979) Manic-depressive variant syndrome in childhood: a preliminary report. Am J Psychiatry 136(5): 702–706

Decina P, Kestenbaum CJ, Farber S, Kron L, Gargan M, Sackeim HA, Fieve RR (1983) Clinical and psychological assessment of children of bipolar probands. Am J Psychiatry 140: 548–553

DeLong GR, Aldershof AL (1987) Long-term experience with lithium treatment in childhood: correlation with clinical diagnoses. J Am Acad Child Adolesc Psychiatry 26: 389–394

Dwyer JT, DeLong GR (1987) A family history study of twenty probands with childhood manic-depressive illness. J Am Acad Child Adolesc Psychiatry 26(2): 176–180

Esquirol E (1845) Mental maladies. Lea and Blanchard, Philadelphia, 33

Feighner J, Robins E, Guze S, Woodruff R, Winokur G, Munoz R (1972) Diagnosing criteria for use in psychiatric research. Arch Gen Psychiatry 26: 57–63
Fristad MA, Weller EB, Weller RA, McCormick L (1989) Assessing mania in prepubertal children. Presented at Poster Session at the 36th annual meeting of the American Academy of Child and Adolescent Psychiatry, New York, 11–15 Oct 1989
Gaensbauer TJ, Harmon RJ, Cytryn L, McKnew DH (1984) Social and affective development in infants with a manic-depressive parent. Am J Psychiatry 141: 223–229
Gershon ES, Hamovit JH, Guroff JJ, Nurnberger JI (1987) Birth cohort changes in manic and depressive disorders in relatives of bipolar and schizoaffective patients. Arch Gen Psychiatry 44: 314–319
Kanner L (1960) Do behavioral symptoms always indicate psychopathology? J Child Psychol Psychiatry 1: 17–25
Klerman GL, Lavori PW, Rice J et al. (1985) Birth-cohort trends in rates of major depressive disorder among relatives of patients with affective disorder. Arch Gen Psychiatry 42: 689–693
Kraepelin E (1921) Manic depressive insanity and paranoia. Livingstone, Edinburgh
LaRoche C, Cheifetz P, Schibuk L, DiTomasso E, Englesman F (1985) Psychopathology in the offspring of parents with bipolar affective disorders. Can J Psychiatry 30: 337–343
Loranger AW, Levine PM (1978) Age of onset of bipolar affective illness. Arch Gen Psychiatry 35: 1345–1348
Mayo JA, O'Connell RA, O'Brien JD (1979) Families of manic-depressive patients: Effects of treatment. Am J Psychiatry 136: 1535–1539
Mendelwicz J, Fieve RR, Rainer JD, Fleiss JL (1972) Manic depressive illness: a comparative study of patients with and without a family history. Br J Psychiatry 120: 523–530
Strober M, Morrell W, Burroughs J, Lampert C, Danforth H, Freeman R (1988) A family study of bipolar I in adolescence: early onset of symptoms linked to increased familial loading and lithium resistance. J Affective Disord 15: 255–268
Varanka TM, Weller RA, Weller EB, Fristad MA (1988) Lithium treatment of manic episodes with psychotic features in prepubertal children. Am J Psychiatry 145: 1557–1559
Weinberg WA, Brumback RP (1976) Mania in childhood. Am J Dis Child 130: 380–385
Weller EB, Weller RA (1990a) Mood disorders in children and adolescents. In: Lewis M (ed) Child and adolescent psychiatry: a comprehensive textbook. Williams and Wilkins, Baltimore (in Press)
Weller EB, Weller RA (1990b) Mood disorders in prepubertal children. In: Weiner J (ed) The comprehensive textbook of child and adolescent psychiatry. American Psychiatric Press, Washington DC (in press)
Weller RA, Weller EB, Tucker SG, Fristad MA (1986a) Mania in prepubertal children: has it been underdiagnosed? J Affective Disord 11: 151–154
Weller EB, Weller RA, Fristad MA (1986b) Lithium dosage guide for prepubertal children: a preliminary report. J Am Acad Child Psychiatry (25)1: 92–95
Weller EB, Weller RA, Fristad MA, Cantwell M, Tucker S (1987) Saliva lithium monitoring in prepubertal children. J Am Acad Child Adolesc Psychiatry 26(2): 173–175
Young RC, Biggs JT, Ziegler VE, Meyer DA (1978) A rating scale for mania: reliability, validity and sensitivity. Br J Psychiatry 133: 429–435
Zahn-Waxler C, McKnew DH, Cummings EM, Davenport YB, Radke-Yarrow M (1984) Problem behaviors and peer interactions of young children with a manic-depressive parent. Am J Psychiatry 141: 236–240

Bipolar Disorder in Adolescence

G.A. Carlson

Introduction

Manic depressive illness, or bipolar disorder as it is now labeled in the United States (DSM-III/III-R, American Psychiatric Association 1980, 1987) not infrequently has its onset in adolescence. Up to 25% of patients will report episodes of depression, hypomania, or mania beginning before age 19 (Carlson et al. 1977; Loranger and Levine 1978; Joyce 1984). In spite of this ubiquitous observation, recognition of the disorder at its onset has been slow in coming. Although there have been flurries of reports and descriptions periodically in the English-language literature at least, concerted interest in adolescent bipolar disorder has occurred only in the past 20 years (Carlson 1990a, for review).

In this brief talk, I will address three specific issues pertinent to the topic of adolescent onset bipolar disorder:

1. Do episodes of depression or mania which begin in adolescence continue into adulthood?
2. Does adolescence change the phenomenology of mania or depression?
3. Does early age of onset predict a more serious disorder in terms of natural history, rates of affective disorders in families, or treatment resistance?

Is There Continuity into Adulthood?

This issue is much less compelling than it was when diagnoses were formulated on the basis of ego structure. The rationale for being oblivious to depression and mania in adolescents had been that the superego was not sufficiently formed until late adolescence to produce depression and its defense, mania (Anthony 1975). As I mentioned above, however, there are many reports from articulate adults who describe episodes beginning in adolescence and occasionally even prepubertally.

On the other hand, there are fewer prospective studies in which adolescents with depression and/or mania are followed into adulthood. In one study, 60 adolescents hospitalized with major depression which met RDC criteria (Spitzer et al. 1978) were followed up 4 years later (at which time they were between ages 17 and 21) (Strober and Carlson 1982): 20% of these adolescents developed manic episodes. This subsample was characterized by depressive episodes with an acute onset, psychomotor retardation, and psychosis. Family histories of major depression and/or bipolar disorder (often going back for three successive generations) and a hypomanic response to antidepressant medication were also prominent in this sample.

In a 3-year prospective follow-up study of clinically referred 6- to 24-year-old siblings and offspring of bipolar probands, Akiskal et al. (1985) also found high rates of recurrence of affective episodes (71%). Half of these cases evidenced signs of bipolarity.

Recently, Harrington and his colleagues in England (Harrington et al. 1990) accomplished a follow-up study of 52 depressed children and adolescents and 52 case controls who had been evaluated and treated at the Mandsley Hospital in London from 1968 to 1969. Although the 52 depressed subjects had been selected using an earlier delineation of depression, of the 30 adolescents, 80% met RDC criteria (as accomplished by chart review) for major depression. In the intervening years since age 17, five have met criteria for bipolar disorder as assessed by SADS-L interviews. None of the prepubertal depressives or case controls had developed manic episodes.

There is, therefore, not only clear evidence from a significant number of adults that their disorder began in adolescence, there are also data that a substantial minority of adolescents psychiatrically referred for major depression will have a bipolar course.

What Kind of Impact, if Any, Does Adolescence Have on the Phenomenology of Bipolar Disorder?

First, even determining how frequently bipolar disorder occurs in an adolescent population depends on how strictly one defines mania and hypomania. While boundary issues distinguishing hypomania from mood lability at the mild extreme and mood incongruent affective psychosis from schizophrenia at the other are important in any age group, they are particularly complicated in adolescence (Carlson 1990a, for review).

A brief review of what little epidemiologic data there are bears this out. In a study of a community sample of adolescents from a university town in the midwest of the United States (Carlson and Kashani 1988), the following lifetime rates of mania and depression were ascertained by structured interviews of parents and adolescents. Using RDC criteria (1 week of manic symptoms producing impairment), 0.6% of the sample had had a manic episode and at least one major depressive episode. This is comparable to the rates found in the ECA adult studies (0.6%–1.0% depending on the cite) (Robins et al. 1984). If impairment was not felt to be present or was equivocal, downgrading the severity of hypomania, lifetime rates increased to 7.3%. If neither duration nor severity are defined (DSM-III-R) rates of at least bipolar NOS increase to 13.3%.

The reasons why adolescence complicates the identification of bipolar disorder are several (Carlson 1990a). The first is obvious and not exclusive to adolescence, though more likely to be an issue here. That is, if bipolar disorder is recurrent and this is a first episode, one does not have pattern recognition to help with the identification of the disorder. Another problem has, in part, to do with biases that clinicians have about adolescent psychopathological conditions. I shall elaborate on this more in a moment. The final complication is that there may be something developmental that alters the phenomenology of depression and/or mania somewhat, at least initially.

The clinical biases which affect adolescents are twofold. On one hand, even when an adolescent has an episode of disorder which clearly meets criteria for major depression or mania, if it is preceded by any kind of crisis (and it is difficult for adolescents not to be experiencing some kind of interpersonal, family, scholastic, or existential stressor), it tends to be dismissed as an adjustment reaction. In relatively well-adjusted youngsters for whom the manic or depressive symptoms are a clear change from their premorbid level of functioning, there is, frankly, little excuse for this kind of diagnostic error. There are, however, a substantial minority of adolescents with long-standing psychiatric (usually behavioral) problems which often begin in early childhood (Carlson 1990b). When these young people develop mania and/or depression, the affective disorder is often harder to distinguish from their premorbid personalities and otherwise stormy life styles, and, as I will discuss shortly, are more difficult to treat. Many of these adolescents are described as having concurrent personality disorders and they are frequently substance abusing and suicidal. This kind of comorbidity has been called "complicated mania" (Black et al. 1988). Whether it occurs more frequently among adolescent onset vs young adult bipolars has not been studied.

The other bias, which is not as pervasive as it once was, is that psychosis in adolescence is invariably a sign of schizophrenia. In fact, psychotic symptoms in a previously well-functioning adolescent with clear-cut affective symptoms are more likely to be a sign of bipolar disorder (either mania or depression) providing the hallucinations are not pervasive and constant, the premorbid personality is indeed intact, and the affective symptoms are clear and prominent (Carlson 1990a). Among the legitimate reasons for confusing bipolar disorder and schizophrenia is the fact that, as mentioned earlier, a history of cycles may not yet be present, family history may not add helpful information because members are not themselves through the age of risk, and finally, the affective and psychomotor features of both disorders are easy to confuse. Distinguishing the difference between flat vs depressive affect, severe psychomotor retardation vs catatonia, anhedonia and social withdrawal vs autistic withdrawal, and the thought disorder of severe mania vs the thought disorder of an excited schizophrenic may require good clinical acumen and experience. The final question, which has not really been addressed (though it is not exclusive to adolescents), is how mood incongruent can psychotic symptoms be before they are too incongruent to have any predictive validity for treatment or course of illness.

Is There Evidence that Adolescence or Even Childhood Alters the Phenomenology of Bipolar Disorder?

The diagnoses which occur not infrequently in the histories of early onset bipolar disorders are "school phobia," "anorexia nervosa," and "externalizing disorders" (Carlson 1990a). In the first two diagnoses it is clear that a depressive disorder was at least co-occurring, though the separation anxiety and bizarre weight and food preoccupations were prominent as well. The relationship between these disorders may only occur in young people at risk for bipolar disorder since family and follow-up studies of 'school phobias' and people with anorexia nervosa do not show a relationship to bipolar disorder. A similar phenomenon can be found with externalizing disorders (attention deficit hyperactivity disorder and/or conduct disorder) in that a significant number of adolescent onset bipolar patients will have histories of externalizing disorders though follow-up and family history studies of children with externalizing disorders do not show a relationship to bipolar disorder (Carlson 1990b). It is interesting that even mild behavior disorders do occur significantly more often in nonreferred children at risk for bipolar disorders vs nonreferred psychiatric controls, and in a blind follow-up study, these behavior-disordered children had higher rates of bipolar disorder but also of alcohol/substance abuse problems than bipolar risk children without such histories (G.A Carlson and S. Weintraub, in press).

The confusion between schizophrenia and bipolar disorder has been demonstrated all over the world (Joyce 1984). In addition to the reasons I discussed earlier, there is also suggestive evidence from a comparison of adolescent episodes and those occurring over age 30 as well as retrospective recollection of symptoms that adolescents may be more psychotic during their episodes than people whose disorders start later (Ballenger et al. 1982; Rosen et al. 1983). Whether all of these phenomena are explained by the observation that illnesses of all kinds are more diffuse in their earlier stages or that there is a specific impact of the neuroendocrine changes occurring during this age span should be a focus of future research.

Does Early Age of Onset Predict a More Serious Disorder in Terms of Natural History, Greater Prevalence of Disorder in Families, or Treatment Resistance?

In patients with uncomplicated mania, adolescent onset of bipolar disorder confers no worse a prognosis than bipolar disorder beginning later, that is, even though there may be recurrences, about half are able to maintain an IQ- and SES-appropriate educational, interpersonal, and occupational standard of function (Carlson et al. 1977; McGlashan 1988). Twenty percent are so incapacitated by chronic affective disorder (e.g., depression, rapid cycling) that they function poorly. Moreover, lithium response is about the same as one finds in adult studies (Youngerman and Canino 1978; DeLong and Aldershof 1987; Strober et al. 1988). On the other hand, although specific follow-up studies on adolescents with complicated mania have not been done, data from a variety of small studies suggest poor treatment compliance, poor treatment response, and high lethality (Welner et al. 1979; Kutcher et al., personal communication). In a follow-up of 12 bipolar onset adolescents with comorbid personality and substance abuse problems, 25% had committed suicide. These data are consistent with adult complicated manics in whom Black and colleagues (1988) found higher rates of suicide attempts (26% vs 12%), lower rates of recovery (44% vs 68%), and more inadequate lithium treatment (53% vs 28%).

Family studies (Dwyer and DeLong 1987; Strober et al. 1988) consistently show higher rates of bipolar disorder among relatives of adolescent onset bipolar patients (13.6%) (Strober et al. 1988) than among adult bipolars (though these may have included some with adolescent onsets) (5.8%) (Andreason et al. 1987). In the one study examining first- and second-degree relatives of adolescent bipolar patients with prepubertal psychopathology, rates of 36.5% were found for bipolar disorder (Strober et al. 1988). One can hypothesize a number of explanations for this finding such as increased family loading lowers age of onset in those at risk either by genetic mechanisms or by environmental ones, i.e., the stress of living in the chaos induced by parental psychopathology advances or unmasks expression of the disorder.

In summary, the major modifying effects adolescence per se has on bipolar disorder are in phenomenology. Even those effects are inconsistent and may have more to do with diagnostic practice. Unless it can be shown that complicated mania occurs more frequently in adolescence, it is unlikely that onset of disorder after puberty in itself confers a different clinical course, even though family genetic loading appears to be greater.

References

Akiskal HS, Downs J, Jordan P, Watson S, Daugherty D, Pruitt DB (1985) Affective disorders in referred children and younger siblings of manic depressives. Arch Gen Psychiatry 42: 996–1004

American Psychiatric Association (1980) Diagnostic and statistical manual of mental disorders (DSM III), 3rd edn. American Psychiatric Association, Washington DC

American Psychiatric Association (1987) Diagnostic and statistical manual of mental disorders (DSM III-R), 3rd edn, revised. American Psychiatric Association, Washington DC

Andreasen NC, Rice J, Endicott J, Coryell W, Grove WM, Reich T (1987) Familial rates of affective disorder. Arch Gen Psychiatry 44: 461–469

Anthony EJ (1975) Childhood depression. In: Anthony EJ, Benedek T (eds) Depression and human existence, Little and Brown, Boston, pp 253–254

Ballenger JC, Reus VI, Post RM (1982) The "atypical" presentation of adolescent mania. Am J Psychiatry 139: 602–606

Black DW, Winokur G, Bell S, Nasrallah A, Hulbert J (1988) Complicated mania – comorbidity and immediate outcome in the treatment of mania. Arch Gen Psychiatry 45: 232–236

Carlson GA (1990a) Bipolar disorder in children and adolescents in psychiatric disorders. In: Garfinkel B, Carlson GA, Weller EB (eds) Psychiatric disorders in children and adolescence Saunders, Philadelphia

Carlson GA (1990b) Annotation: child and adolescent mania – diagnostic considerations. J Child Psychol Psychiatry (in press)

Carlson GA, Kashani JH (1988) Manic symptoms in a nonreferred adolescent population. J Affective Disord 15: 219–226

Carlson GA, Strober M (1978) Manic depressive illness in early adolescence: a study of clinical and diagnostic characteristics in six cases. J Am Acad Child Psychiatry 17: 138–153

Carlson GA, Davenport YB, Januson K (1977) A comparison of outcome in adolescent and late onset bipolar manic depressive illness. Am J Psychiatry 134: 919–922

Carlson GA, Weintraub S (in press) Childhood Behavior Problems and bipolar disorder – relationship or coincidence. J Affective Disorders

DeLong GR, Aldershof AL (1987) Long-term experience with lithium treatment in childhood: correlation with clinical diagnoses. J Am Acad Child Adolesc Psychiatry 26: 389–394

Dwyer JT, DeLong GR (1987) A family history study of twenty probands with childhood manic depressive illness. J Am Acad Child Adolesc Psychiatry 26: 176–180

Harrington R, Fudge H, Rutter M, Pickles A, Hill J (1990) Adult outcome of childhood and adolescent depression. Arch Gen Psychiatry (in press)

Joyce PR (1984) Age of onset in bipolar affective disorder and misdiagnosis as schizophrenia. Psychol Med 14: 145–149

Loranger AW, Levine PM (1978) Age of onset of bipolar affective illness. Arch Gen Psychiatry 35: 1345–1348

McGlashan TH (1988) Adolescent versus adult onset of mania. Am J Psychiatry 145: 221–224

Robins LN, Helzer JE, Weissman MM, Orvaschel H, Gruenberg E, Burke JD, Regier DA (1984) Lifetime prevalence of specific psychiatric disorders in three sites. Arch Gen Psychiatry 41: 949–958

Rosen LN, Rosenthel NE, VanDosen PH, Dunner DL, Fieve RR (1983) Age at onset and number of psychotic symptoms in bipolar I and schizoaffective disorder. Am J Psychiatry 140: 1523–1524

Spitzer RL, Endicott J, Robins E (1978) Research diagnostic criteria rationale and reliability. Arch Gen Psychiatry 35: 773–782

Strober M, Carlson GA (1982) Bipolar illness in adolescents with major depression: clinical, genetic, and psychopharmacologic predictors in a 3 to 4 year prospective follow-up investigation. Arch Gen Psychiatry 39: 549–555

Strober M, Morrell W, Burroughs J, Lampert C, Danforth H, Freeman R (1988) A family study of bipolar I in adolescence: early onset of symptoms linked to increased familial loading and lithium resistance. J Affective Disord 15: 255–268

Welner A, Welner Z, Fishman R (1979) Psychiatric adolescent inpatients – 8–10 year follow-up. Arch Gen Psychiatry 36: 698–705

Youngerman J, Canino I (1978) Lithium carbonate use in children and adolescents: a survey of the literature. Arch Gen Psychiatry 35: 216–224

Diagnosis, Clinical Assessment, and Treatment of Late-Life Depression

A.C. Altamura, G. Invernizzi, S. Gianetti, and M.C. Mauri

Introduction

In the elderly, the term "depression" is used to describe highly heterogeneous nosographic entities. In fact, it refers to subclinical problems such as general feelings of sadness and demoralization, but also to acute or chronic clear-cut psychopathological pictures, such as dysthymia and major depression.

Concerning epidemiologic data on major depression, the most defined and severe syndrome, some authors believe that its incidence in the elderly is overestimated. Actually, some data seem to indicate that rates for major depression are somewhat lower in the elderly (about 2%) compared with younger subjects (3%–5%) (Blazer et al. 1987; Blazer and Williams 1980; Klerman et al. 1985; Myers et al. 1984).

This is in part contradicted by data on suicide and use of antidepressants in the aged population: in the United States, the suicide rate is higher (35 per 100 000) in the elderly than in any other age group, irrespective of underlying diagnoses (Rich et al. 1986), and use of antidepressants seems to be more common over 60 years of age (Grimmson et al. 1977).

However, when the entire depressive spectrum, according to DSM-III-R, is considered, up to 20% of the elderly meet criteria for dysthymia in epidemiologic surveys (Blazer and Williams 1980; Dovenmuehle et al. 1970; Gurland et al. 1980), and this figure increases to 31% for patients in geriatric evaluation units (Borson et al. 1986; Cheah and Beard 1980).

On the other hand, many medical conditions particularly significant in older patients such as coronary artery disease, endocrinologic abnormalities, neurological disorders, metabolic disturbances, and cancer have been associated with some depressive features. In particular, approximately one-third of medically ill subjects were found to have depressive symptoms and up to one-fourth met criteria for a depressive syndrome (Clark et al. 1983; Moffic and Paykel 1975; Nielsen and Williams 1980).

These epidemiologic discrepancies may reflect the use of different diagnostic and measurement instruments, the higher incidence of atypical depressive pictures in the elderly, masked by medical disorders, and socioeconomic stressors.

In fact, in late life, depressive syndromes are characterized by a higher etiopathogenetic heterogeneity, but also by a more evident complexity in semeiologic, diagnostic, nosographic, and accordingly therapeutic terms as will be discussed below.

Diagnosis

From an etiopathogenetic point of view, depression in the elderly generally arises from a mixture of sociogenetic, psychogenetic, and biologic factors, whose weight is difficult to elucidate (Fig. 1).

First, it is important to stress the interrelationship between depression and cognitive impairment in the sense that they have a reciprocal influence, and it is often very difficult to discriminate how primary or secondary they are.

Therefore, any attempt to perform a nosographic subdivision in the two major syndromes, endogenous vs reactive ones, using for instance the Newcastle Inventory Scale can be frustrating, since there is a huge imbalance due to the burden of sociogenetic and environmental factors (Post 1976).

Recently, a possible reconsideration of an obsolete kraepelinian nosographic entity, "involutional melancholia" (Kraepelin 1907), completely forgotten by DSM-III, has been proposed (Brown et al. 1983). Despite poor evidence for considering involutional melancholia a definite clinical entity, genetic and biochemical data, besides clinical and therapeutic considerations, support the idea that depression in the elderly could be, possibly, a diagnostic subtype among depressive disorders (Brown et al. 1983).

On the other hand, the occurrence of atypical symptoms such as somatic complaints (abdominal problems, constipation), agitation, insomnia, hypochondriasis, obsessional thoughts, and lack of periodicity make problematic to achieve a reliable diagnosis (Sunderland et al. 1988).

Therefore, cognitive impairments make an early detection of the disorder difficult which can often be confounded by organic deterioration and diagnosed as dementia (see differential diagnosis between depressive pseudodementia and dementia with depressive features). In this case, an instrumental approach with

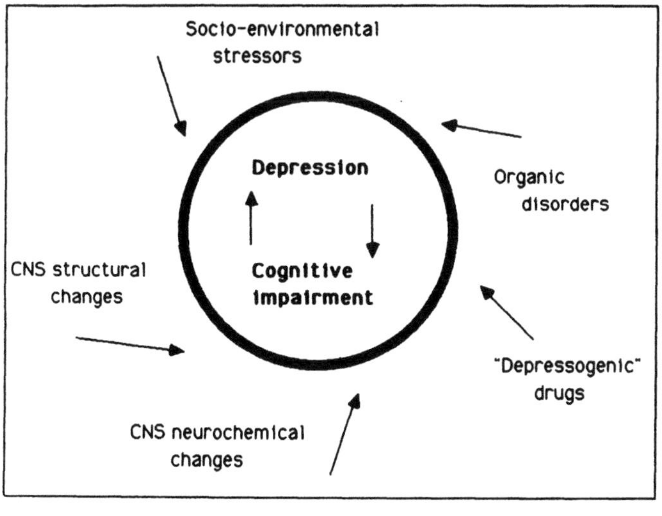

Fig. 1. Different factors contribute to cause depression but also cognitive impairment and they influence each other reciprocally.

CAT or NMR could be highly helpful in formulating a reliable diagnosis although the absence of any pathological pathway does not exclude the diagnosis of dementia (and vice versa), whose assessment should be based merely on the clinical picture (Altamura et al. 1990; Riege and Metter 1988).

In other words, from the semeiologic point of view, the symptoms of depressive series are variable, often more or less partially masked, generally anomalous vs those observed in adults, generally not dealing with clear-cut depressive states, but mostly with masked ones (Fassler and Gaviria 1978). On the other hand, there are recent literature data that do not agree on considering the depressive symptomatology atypical in the elderly (Musetti et al. 1989).

When trying to classify depressions in the elderly, the role played by four main variables should be considered: concomitant CNS or extra-CNS organic disorders vs environmental factors and endogenous vs psychogenic features. To relate these variables to the antidepressant response, a classification "ex iuvantibus" of elderly depressions can be tentatively proposed, leading to recognition of the following nosographic forms.

1. Organogenetic. These forms are secondary to a pathological organic condition (both in SNC or extracerebral). These disorders are described in DSM-III as organic affective syndromes, characterized by the prevalence of mnestic and cognitive impairment, often with symptoms of anxiety, with poor response to the treatment, high sensitivity to antidepressant side effects.

2. Non-Organogenetic. These forms include major depression, dysthymia, and adjustment disorders with depressive mood (DSM-III-R). The first one is characterized by a biologic depressive core, with a clinical picture which includes suicidal ideas, loss of weight, sleep disturbances, often accompanied by anxious features. Among these forms, subtypes can be recognized as "reactive" and "endogenous." The former are characterized by anxiety, psychomotor activation, somatizations, sleep disturbances, and the drug response is partial. On the other hand, "endogenous" ones respond better to antidepressants but less efficiently compared with adults because of the possible negative impact of psychological, environmental, or antidepressant side effects which can "mask" or counteract therapeutic response.

3. Intermediate. In our experience, these are the most common pathological forms in the elderly. These forms are characterized by a mixture of clinical symptoms of endogenous, reactive, and organic (cognitive disturbances) types and the drug response is unpredictable, depending on the prevalence of different symptoms in the individual patient.

Clinical Assessment

On these bases the assessment of depression in the elderly is more difficult than in adults, and the rating scales used as dependent variables in psychopharmacological studies may need to be adjusted accordingly (McGarvey et al. 1982).

For example, the use of the HRS-D scale could be problematic for assessing the severity of depression in the elderly because it is heavily weighted toward somatic symptoms (9 of the basic 17 depression items involve ratings of somatic complaints). In light of the assumed higher prevalence of physical impairment in normal aging, the HRS-D may tend to overestimate depression. Moreover, despite its wide use, the psychometric properties of the HRS-D are not well established in elderly (Thompson et al. 1988). On the other hand, the GDS has been shown to be reliable and valid for older persons (Yesavage 1986; Yesavage et al. 1983), and scores on the GDS were highly correlated with severity of depression. In addition, using designated cutoff scores, the GDS was shown to have high sensitivity (>78), high specificity, and to correctly diagnose at least 77% of older depressed patients (Norris et al. 1987).

In a multicenter controlled study comparing the effect of trazodone vs mianserin and amitriptyline on 106 elderly inpatients with major depression, the discrepancy in the onset of amelioration of the clinical picture observed at the HRS-D (from the 1st week of treatment) as compared with that observed at the

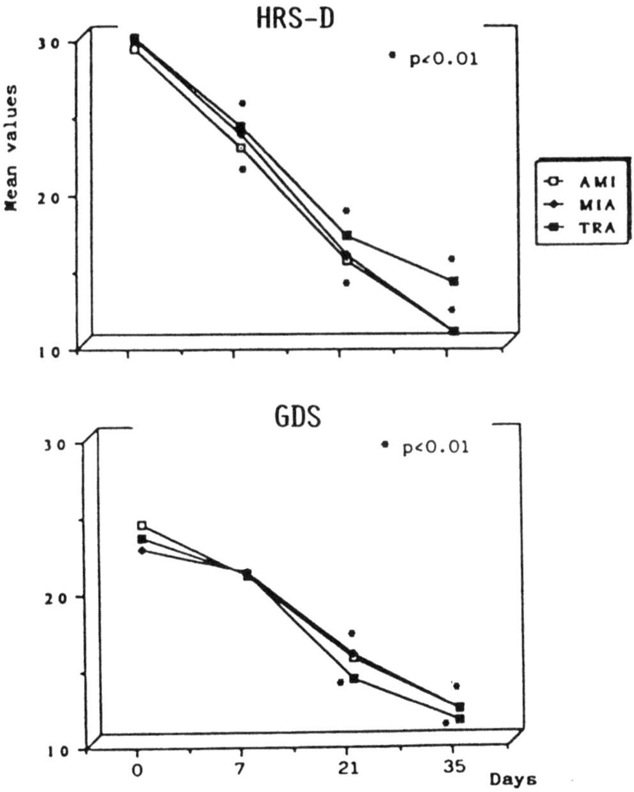

Fig. 2. Patterns of the total HRS-D and GDS scores (mean values) recorded in the course of the study on elderly depressed patients treated with trazodone, mianserin, or amitriptyline, indicating a significant decrease ($P < 0.01$ vs time 0) from the 7th day at the HRS-D and from the 21st day at the GDS. (Altamura et al. 1989)

GDS (from the 3rd week) was explained considering the higher degree of specificity of the latter (Altamura et al. 1989) (Fig. 2). Actually, "specific" symptoms for major depression, such as retardation, guilt, and loss of libido, showed an improvement after the 3rd week of treatment. In contrast, anxiety, which is almost invariably coupled or combined with depression in the elderly (Altamura 1987), ameliorated after the 1st week, possibly due to the anxiolytic properties of the antidepressant. In other words, the GDS was confirmed to reflect changes occurring in the specific biologic symptoms of depression, whereas the HRS-D reflected both specific and nonspecific symptoms (Altamura et al. 1989).

In any case, it does not seem correct, when *dealing with depressive disorders, to extrapolate from diagnostic and assessment patterns used in adults those concerning the elderly.*

Treatment

Also from the therapeutic point of view the use of antidepressants is particularly complex in the elderly. We must consider a number of problems: alterations in drug sensitivity, pharmacokinetic pattern modifications, a more pronounced susceptibility to side effects, poor compliance, the influence of therapeutic "milieu", and interaction with concurrent medication.

The rate of response to antidepressants is often unsatisfactory in late life due to pharmacodynamic and pharmacokinetic factors. Concerning pharmacodynamic factors, there is functional impairment of the main neurotransmitter pathways including cholinergic, dopaminergic, and noradrenergic systems (Carlsson 1986; Gibson 1981). This is clearly shown, for example, by the acute administration of an atypical antidepressant, mianserin, blocking α_2-presynaptic receptors that activated GH secretion in adults but elicited a blunted response in the elderly. In fact, in younger subjects, the GH concentration curves closely followed the mianserin plasma levels while this did not happen in the elderly where, despite higher drug plasma concentrations, the secretion of GH was lower and poorly related to mianserin plasma levels (Fig. 3).

In advanced age, impairment in physiological functions of important organs leads to alterations in pharmacokinetic parameters such as bioavailability, distribution, and clearance (Fig. 4). Consequently, steady-state plasma concentrations achieved are significantly higher, and lower standard daily doses should be used to avoid overdosing phenomena (Altamura et al. 1982, 1983, 1986; Bareggi et al. 1990; Cazzullo and Altamura 1985; Gram et al. 1978).

The higher incidence of side effects, such as anticholinergic reactions, can aggravate the somatic problems of the elderly, further decreasing the quality of life of the patients. Often side effects such as blurred vision, constipation, and tremors can counteract the antidepressant effects of drugs also leading to a loss of compliance in elderly patients (Montgomery 1982; Robinson 1983).

The new generation of antidepressants, because of fewer anticholinergic and cardiotoxic side effects, in principle cause less exacerbation of the baseline

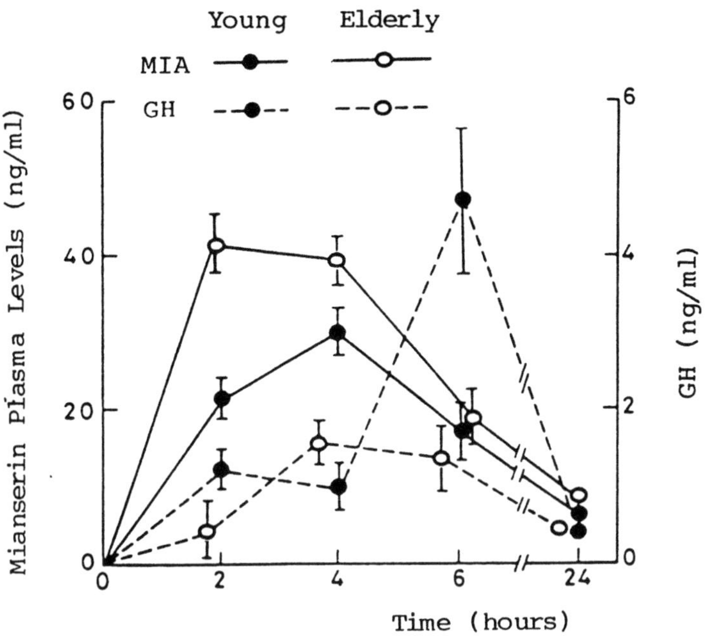

Fig. 3. Mianserin and GH plasma concentrations (ng/ml) after acute administration of mianserin (30 mg po) in young and elderly subjects

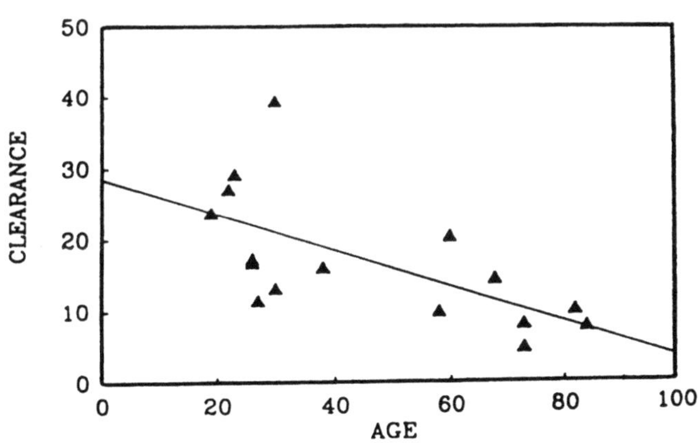

Fig. 4. Clearance of dothiepin (ml/min/kg) as a function of age (years), also shown in the regression line ($r = -0.67$; $P < 0.01$). (Bareggi et al. 1990)

problems of aging and are generally better tolerated than "classic" antidepressants (Altamura and Mauri 1991). The utilization of compounds with minimal side effects leads to an indistinguishable clinical response between adult and elderly depressed patients, although in the latter, the therapeutic setting seems to

Table 1. Strategies to counteract pharmacotherapy problems of elderly depressed patients

Problem	Strategy
Drug disposition age-related differences in pharmokinetic profile	a) Prediction of steady-state plasma levels (by using single loading dose studies) b) Drug plasma monitoring to avoid toxic levels during chronic treatments and to evaluate level-response and side effects relationhip
Drug efficacy by age group	Controlled clinical studies vs reference drugs in different age populations and settings (i.e. adult vs elderly, ambulatory vs hospitalized patients
Tolerance	a) More closer side-effects checking b) Use of alternative compounds: nontricyclic drugs (atypical antidepressants)
Compliance	Clearly written posological schemes and reduced daily drug administrations
Drug interactions	Reduced polypharmacotherapy

more consistently influence the clinical outcome. In fact, in our study, the inpatients' or outpatients' condition did not appear to affect the clinical response significantly in younger patients, while the elderly outpatients did significantly better than the inpatients. This was not due to a diagnostic imbalance or to significant differences in plasma levels and in L/D ratios between in- and outpatients. In other words, outpatient treatment seems to be even more appropriate than hospitalization in the management of elderly depression, probably since it avoids rooting out subjects, with a reduced rate of adaptation, from their own environment (Altamura et al. 1986; Comfort 1982). In fact, hospitalization is particularly stressful in old age, since it frequently creates emotional problems or exacerbates existing psychiatric disorders (Ruskin 1985). According to Millard (1983), better results could be obtained in elderly depressives "if the hospital went to the home."

The strategies to counteract the problems with pharmacological management of elderly depression are summarized in Table 1.

Conclusions

From the above-mentioned data, it clearly emerges that detection, assessment, and treatment of elderly depression is one of the most complex topics to deal with in clinical practice although less frustrating than other elderly pathological states such as dementia or late paraphrenia, which respond poorly to drug treatments. Moreover, keeping in mind the multidetermined pathogenesis of elderly depressive states, treatment of depression in the aged should not be based exclusively on drugs, but involve, particularly in non-organogenetic/reactive forms, early environmental and/or socio-psychotherapeutic interventions.

References

Altamura AC (1987) Anxious-depressive syndromes in the elderly: assessment, clinical course and treatment. In: Racagni G, Smeraldi E (eds) Anxious depression: assessment and treatment. Raven, New York, pp 209–216

Altamura AC, Mauri MC (1991) Aspects of treatment of elderly depression. The fluoxetine experience. In: Freeman HL (ed) The uses of fluoxetine in clinical practice. Royal Society of Medicine Services, London, pp 53–59

Altamura AC, Melorio T, Invernizzi G, Colacurcio F, Gomeni R (1983) Age-related differences in kinetics and side effects of viloxazine in man and their clinical implications. Psychopharmacology 81: 281–85

Altamura AC, Mauri MC, Guercetti G (1986) Age, therapeutic "milieu" and clinical outcome in depressive patients treated with viloxazine: a study with plasma levels. Prog Neuropsychopharmacol Biol Psychiatry 10: 67–75

Altamura AC, Mauri MC, Rudas R et al. (1989) Clinical activity and tolerability of trazodone, mianserin, and amitriptyline in elderly subjects with major depression: a controlled multicenter trial. Clin Neuropharmacol 12(S1): 25–33

Altamura AC, Gianetti S, Masserini C, Percudani M, Pugnetti L (1990) Neuromorphological and biochemical patterns of Alzheimer's disease. In: Stefanis CN, Soldatos CR, Rabavilas AD (eds) Psychiatry: a world perspective, vol. 2. Excerpta Medica, Amsterdam, pp 455–459

Bareggi SR, Cavallaro R, Pirola R, Altamura AC (1990) Pharmacokinetics and adverse effects of single doses of dothiepin in young and elderly subjects. Prog Neuropsychopharmacol Biol Psychiatry 14: 163–170

Blazer D, Huges DC, George LK (1987) The epidemiology of depression in an elderly community population. Gerontologist 27: 281–287

Blazer DG, Williams CD (1980) The epidemiology of dysphoria and depression in an elderly population. Am J Psychiatry 137: 439–444

Borson S, Barnes RA, Kukull WA, Okimoto JT, Veith RC, Inui TS, Carter W, Raskind MA (1986) Symptomatic depression in elderly medical outpatients: 1. Prevalence, demography and health services utilization. J Am Geriatr Soc 34: 341–347

Brown RP, Sweeney J, Frances A et al. (1983) Age as a predictor of treatment response in endogenous depression. J Clin Psychopharmacol 3: 176–178

Carlsson A (1986) Brain neurotransmitters in normal and pathological aging. In: Scheibel AB, Wechsler B, Brazier C (eds) The biological substrates of Alzheimer's disease. Academic, New York, pp 193–204

Cazzullo CL, Altamura AC (1985) Bioavailability of some atypical antidepressants and therapeutic management of late life depressive states. Integr Psychiatry 3S: 50–57

Cheah KC, Beard OW (1980) Psychiatric findings in the population of a geriatric evaluation unit: implications. J Am Geriatr Soc 28: 153–156

Clark DC, Cavanaugh SV, Gibbons RD (1983) The core symptoms of depression in medical and psychiatric patients. J Nerv Ment Dis 171: 705–713

Comfort A (1982) Anxiety in old age. In: Wheatley D (ed) Psychopharmacology of old age. University Press, Oxford, pp 159–164

Dovenmuehle RH, Reckless JB, Newman G (1970) Depressive reactions in the elderly. In: Palmore E (ed) Normal aging: reports from the Duke longitudinal study, 1955–1969. Duke University Press, Durham, pp 90–97

Fassler RB, Gaviria M (1978) Depression in old age. J Am Geriatr Soc 26: 471–475

Gibson GE, Peterson C, Jender DJ (1981) Brain acetylcholine synthesis declines with senescence. Science 213: 674–676

Gram LF, Reisby N, Bech P, Nagy A, Christiansen J (1978) Factors influencing pharmacokinetics and clinical effects of tricyclic antidepressants. In: Garattini S (ed) Depressive disorders. Schattauer, Stuttgart, pp 337–346
Grimmson A, Idanpaan-Heikkila J, Lunde PK, Olafsson O, Westerholmm M (1977) Ferbrukninger aw psykofarmaka i Finldan, Island, Norge, och Sverige. Nord Med 92: 49–54
Gurland BJ, Dean L, Cross P, Golden R (1980) The epidemiology of depression and dementia in the elderly: the use of multiple indicators of these conditions. In: Cole JO, Barrett JE (eds) Psychopathology of the aged. Raven, New York, pp 37–60
Klerman GL, Lavori PW, Rice J, Reich T, Endicott J, Andreasen NC, Keller MB, Hirschfield RMA (1985) Birth-cohort trends in rates of major depressive disorder among relatives of patients with affective disorder. Arch Gen Psychiatry 42: 689–693
Kraepelin E (1907) Lehrbuch der Psychiatrie, 7th edn. McMillan, New York
McGarvey B, Gallagher D, Thompson LW, Zelinski E (1982) Reliability and factor structure of the Zung self-rating depression scale in three age groups. Essence 5: 141–151
Millard PH (1983) Depression in old age. Br Med J 287: 375–376
Moffic HS, Paykel ES (1975) Depression in medical inpatients. Br J Psychiatry 126: 346–353
Montgomery SA (1982) Treatment of depression in old age. In: Wheatley D (ed) Psychopharmacology of old age. Oxford University Press, Oxford, pp 165–172
Musetti L, Perugi G, Soriani A, Rossi VM, Cassano GB, Akiskal HS (1989) Depression before and after age 65. Br J Psychiatry 155(3) : 330–336
Myers JK, Weissman MM, Tischler GL, Holzer CE, Leas PJ, Orvaschel H, Anthony JC, Boyd JH, Burke JB, Kramer M, Stoltzman R (1984) Six-month prevalence of psychiatric disorders in three communities, 1980–1982. Arch Gen Psychiatry 41: 959–967
Nielsen AC, Williams TA (1980) Depression in ambulatory medical patients: prevalence by self-report questionnaire and recognition by nonpsychiatric physicians. Arch Gen Psychiatry 37: 999–1004
Norris J, Gallagher D, Wilson A, Winograd CH (1987) Assessment of depression in geriatric medical outpatients: the validity of two screening measures. J Am Geriatr Soc 35: 989–995
Post F (1976) Diagnosis of depression in geriatric patients and treatment modalities appropriate for the population. In: Gallant DM, Simpson GM (eds) Depression: behavioral, biochemical, diagnostic and treatment concepts. Spectrum, New York, pp 205–231
Rich CL, Young D, Fowler RC (1986) San Diego suicide study. Arch Gen Psychiatry 43: 577–582
Riege WH, Metter J (1988) Cognitive and brain imaging measures of Alzheimer's disease. Neurobiol Aging 9: 69–86
Robinson DS (1983) Aging and neuropsycopharmacology. In: Yetiv JZ, Bianchine JR (eds) Recent advances in clinical therapeutics. Grune and Stratton, New York, pp 127–157
Ruskin PE (1985) Geropsychiatric consultation in a university hospital: a report on 67 referrals. Am J Psychiatry 142(3S) : 333–336
Sunderland T, Lawlor BA, Molchan SE, Martinez RA (1988) Depressive syndromes in the elderly: special concerns. Psychopharmacol Bull 24(4): 567–576
Thompson LW, Futterman A, Gallagher D (1988) Assessment of late-life depression. Psychopharmacol Bull 24: 577–586
Yesavage J (1986) The use of self-rating depression scales in the elderly. In: Poon LW, Crook T, Davis KL, Eisdofer C, Gurland BJ, Kasziniak AW, Thompson LW (eds) Handbook for clinical memory assessment of older adults. American Psychological Association, Washington DC, pp 213–217
Yesavage J, Brink T, Rose T, Lum O, Huang O, Adey V, Leirer V (1983) Development and validation of a geriatric screening scale: a preliminary report. J Psychiatr Res 17: 37–49

Recurrent Major Depression: Catamnestic Evaluation of Inpatients

L. Ravizza, F. Bogetto, C. Cappa, M. Dalmotto, M. Spagnolini, and R. Torta

Introduction

Depression is one of the most important psychiatric disorders of late life, but the true prevalence of depressive symptoms in the community is unknown, even though estimates range from less than 5% to 44%. There has been less variability in the reported prevalence of major affective disorders: estimates range from 1% to 3%.

Significant progress in understanding late-life depression has been made during the past decade. Considerably more is known about the biological correlates, diagnosis, and treatment of depression. The term "depression" has been used to describe a variety of mood disorders, ranging from commonly occurring transient negative feelings of no clinical consequence to a seriously debilitating life-threatening psychiatric illness. Until recently it was thought that major depression not only occurred more frequently in older than in younger people, but that it was more severe. It has been believed that "depression" was a natural response to the problems associated with aging. Advances in nosology, however, have made the identification and diagnosis of symptoms more reliable. Thus recent investigations, employing newer criteria, have demonstrated that major depression is less prevalent in aged than in younger individuals or that, in terms of recovery and remission, older adults do not differ from their middle-aged counterparts (Blazer and Williams 1984; Bland et al. 1988). Furthermore, in its melancholic form, geriatric depression presents a symptom profile similar to that of younger depressed patients and responds to treatment (Blazer et al. 1987). Other epidemiologic studies have demonstrated that a variety of less severe depressive symptoms are quite prevalent in a geriatric population residing in the community or in an institution. There is no general consensus on a definitive classification of these depressive subtypes, on their clinical import, or on their responsiveness to treatment. This may be true even for major depression. An explanation of this phenomenon may derive from several factors. The presence of concomitant medical diseases may complicate the diagnosis of depression.

Investigations on elderly depression should include such subtypes as age-related dysthymia or dysphoria, depression presenting as dementia or associated with it, depression occurring with medical illness, and depression associated with previous alcohol abuse.

The syndrome of depression may be more difficult to distinguish in its various clinical presentations in elderly individuals. Meyers and Greenberg (1986) suggest that late-onset depression may be a specific subtype, that age onset may influence the presentation of depression, and that depression occurring in later life may be associated with degenerative changes in the brain, resulting in cognitive disturbances.

Bipolar I and Bipolar II disorders and recurrent unipolar major depression typically arise before the age of 65 and show high familiar prevalence of mood disorders. Single episode depression, by contrast is significantly more common after the age of 65; environmental factors are more common in this subtypes.

According to Gross et al. (1989), elderly individuals with a depressive disorder for the first time in their life may be incorrectly diagnosed as having a generalized anxiety disorder and treated with anxiolytics, which may temporarily decrease the symptoms but do little to lessen the underlying cause of agitation. Major depression as a diagnosis takes precedence over anxiety disorder.

Masked depression is thought to be more common in the elderly (Nott and Fleminger 1975). The term "masked depression" has been used to refer to patients who deny apparent dysphoria while voicing excessive somatic complaints or displaying primarily signs of cognitive decline (LaRue et al. 1983). Depression with cognitive impairment is in fact the disorder most often misdiagnosed as primary degenerative dementia (Ron et al. 1979; Kay et al. 1955).

Although it has been generally believed that the incidence of mood disorders rises with age, recent studies have questioned this assumption (Blazer 1983). Patients suffering from late-life depression with melancholia often have a history of multiple depressive episodes, followed by complete or nearly complete recovery. Angst (1990) found that the course of endogenous affective psychoses is characterized by a decrease in the average length of the cycles with an increase in the number of episodes, instead of what was generally believed that the episodes of depression in late life last longer than the episodes at earlier times during the life cycle.

Melancholic depression in late life has been thought to be different from midlife depression in a number of ways: in late life depressed mood and guilt are less common (Busse 1965: Winokur et al. 1980), while hypochondrial symptoms (de Alarcon 1964), decreased self-esteem (Post 1965), and lethargy (Gaitz and Scott 1972) are more common. Musetti et al. (1989) have not found the generally believed characteristics in the old depressed patients, such as greater agitation, hypochondria, somatic symptoms, tendency to psychotic symptoms, and cronicity.

Four clinical entities are listed under the affective disorders in DSM III-R relevant to the clinical manifestation of depression in the elderly. They are: (1) bipolar disorder (manic, depressed, and mixed); (2) major depression (single episode, recurrent, with or without melancholia, with or without psychotic features, (3) dysthymic disorder (depressive neurosis), and (4) atypical depression.

The purpose of this presentation is to evaluate the prevalence, the course, and some clinical characteristics of the recurrent unipolar major depression in patients with illness onset before the age of 60 years in comparison to those who had their first depressive episode after the age of 60.

Method

The present investigation examined the clinical documentation of 3074 inpatients of the Institute of Clinical Psychiatry of the University of Turin from 1969 to 1989. According to the DSM III-R criteria, 609 patients were framed in a major depressive disorder; of those 609, 255 (89 males, 166 females) were found to meet the criteria for a diagnosis of recurrent major depressive disorder.

On the basis of the data obtained it was possible to subdivide our 255 patients into two main groups: those who had their first depressive episode onset before 60 years old and those whose onset occurred after 60. Patients with concomitant somatic pathology and those with extensive premorbid psychopathology were excluded. Family history for major depressive disorder and life events (familiar, occupational, financial, health, and mourning) were taken into account.

Following a semistructured interview and the Hamilton Rating Scale for Depression, patients have been examined for these symptoms: hypochondria, psychomotor retardation, anxiety, somatoform symptoms, and memory impairment. The mean frequency of the depressive episodes (number of episodes/years from illness onset), its variation, the mean length and its variation have been studied. The severity of depression has been classified, using the criteria established by the DSM III-R, into mild, moderate, severe, severe with mood congruent psychotic features (guilt, poverty, disease), and severe with mood incongruent psychotic features (control, persecutory). Finally we reported the variation in the mean frequency and mean length of a group of 27 patients with the first depressive episode onset before 60 years old.

A statistical analysis of the data obtained was carried out with Student's *t* test and chi-square test.

Results

The data displayed in the accompanying tables compare the population of recurrent depressed patients who had their first depressive episode onset before 60 years old and the population of patients who had their first depressive episode onset after 60.

According to the literature we found a higher incidence of women who suffer from recurrent depressive disorder. The illness onset appears to be higher before 60 years old (Table 1). The comparison of different parameters in the two

Table 1. Onset of first depressive episode

	age < 60 years		age > 60 years	
	n	%	*n*	%
Total: 255	217	85	38	15
Male: 89	74	83	15	17
Female: 166	143	86	23	14

population has given the following results:

– No difference in family history for major depressive disorder has been reported between the two populations. First degree relatives show a lower incidence of depressive disorders when compared to the other relatives (Table 2).

– Life events play important roles in patients with an early onset of recurrent depression mostly concerning familiar problems. In the older patients recurrent depression is often related to mourning. Life events such as occupational problems and health are substantially the same in both groups (Table 3).

– Considering the main symptoms a significant statistical difference has been found between the two populations when psychomotor retardation, which is prevalent in patients with the illness onset after 60 years old, is examined. Senile patients also show a higher incidence of hypochondria and memory impairment but we failed to find any statistical significance relating to these

Table 2. Family history of major depressive disorders

Relatives	age < 60 years		age > 60 years		X^2	*p*
	n	%	*n*	%		
First degree	14	35	1	33.3	0.023	ns
Others	26	65	2	66.6	0.010	ns

Table 3. Life events and recurrent major depressive episodes

Life events	age < 60 years		age > 60 years	
	n = 136	(100%)	*n* = 36	(100%)
Familiar	42	(30%)	0*	
Occupational	19	(13.9%)	3	(8.3%)
Financial	12	(8.8%)	3	(8.3%)
Health	40	(29.4%)	9	(25%)
Mourning	23	(16.9%)	21	(58.3%)
Life events-related episodes/total episodes		136/539 (25%)		36/67 (54%)

* $p < 0.01$

symptoms. Anxiety and somatoform symptoms show approximately the same incidence in both populations (Table 4).

– The mean frequency of the episodes is slightly higher in patients with their first depressive episode onset after the age of 60 (Table 5).

– The mean length of the depressive episodes is higher in the younger population but it is not of statistical significance (Table 6).

– Looking at the severity of the depressive episodes it has been found that patients with illness onset before the age of 60 show a higher incidence of depressive episodes without psychotic features, compared to the patients whose depressive disorder onset has been after the age of 60. There is a prevalence in the younger patients of mild, moderate, and severe types of depression; this prevalence is statistically significant for moderate and severe types. In the older patients there is a higher frequency, statistically significant, of severe depression with mood congruent psychotic features, with delusions of poverty and disease (Table 7).

– The variation in mean frequency and length of the depressive episodes during the life span of a group of 27 patients with their first depressive onset before the age of 60 is reported in Tables 8 and 9. The frequency rises significantly and the length of the episodes is slightly longer in older age.

Table 4. Main symptoms of major dpressive disorder

	age < 60 years		age > 60 years		X^2	p
	n	%	n	%		
Hypochondria	14	9.7	3	15.7	0.64	ns
Psychomotor retardation	86	60.0	18	94.7	7.29	< 0.001
Anxiety	78	54.5	9	47.3	0.12	ns
Somatoform symptoms	56	39.0	8	42.1	0.0	ns
Memory impairment	8	5.5	2	10.5	0.70	ns

Table 5. Recurrent major depressive episodes mean frequency

Age < 60 years ($n = 99$)	Age > 60 years ($n = 20$)	t	p
$f = 0.93 \pm 1.08$	$f = 1.34 \pm 0.91$	1.34	ns

Table 6. Recurrent major depressive episodes: mean length (L, months)

Age < 60 years ($n = 217$)	age > 60 years ($n = 38$)	t	p
L = 5.896 ± 5.498	L = 4.66 ± 2.78	1.008	ns

Table 7. Recurrent major depression episodes (DSM III-R)

	age < 60 years		age > 60 years	
	n	%	*n*	%
Mild	17	3.2	1	1.5
Moderate	164	30.4	7*	10.5
Severe	277	51.4	23**	34.3
Severe with mood-congruent psychotic features:				
– guilt	21	3.9	6	9.0
– poverty	26	4.8	15*	22.4
– disease	9	1.7	6*	9.0
Severe with mood-incongruent psychotic features:				
– control	8	1.5	4	6.0
– persecution	17	3.2	5	7.5
Total	539	100	67	100

* $p < 0.001$; ** $p < 0.01$

Table 8. Major depressive episodes: frequency variations during life-course (sample of 27 patients with first episode onset before 60 years)

Frequency before 60 years	Frequency after 60 years	*t*	*p*
$f = 0.35 \pm 0.63$	$f = 1.1 \pm 0.96$	3.30	< 0.001

f, no. of episodes/years from onset of illness.

Table 9. Major depressive epidsode mean length (L, months): variations during life-course (sample of 27 patients with first before 60 years)

Length before 60 years	Length after 60 years	*p*
$L = 6.83 \pm 10.52$	$L = 9.63 \pm 13.91$	ns

Conclusions

The data obtained from the comparison of the population with their first depressive episode onset before the age of 60 and the population with the onset after the age of 60 lead to some considerations. No significant differences between the two populations have been found concerning the incidence of family history of major depressive disorders.

Life events become an important factor in the population with illness onset after the age of 60, especially relating to mourning. In the patients with an earlier onset family problems play an important role as a life event. In both groups we have noted a high incidence of health problems. In the two populations we noticed a high rate of anxiety. In patients with later onset a higher prevalence of psychomotor retardation has been found. Such symptoms as hypochondria, somatic symptoms, and memory impairment did not differ from the population with the earlier onset. These findings disagree with some assumptions in traditional literature that assign such characteristics as greater agitation, atypical masked features, somatic symptoms, hypochondrial worries, suspicious attitude and chronic evolution to the geriatric depressed patient. Nevertheless if we take into consideration depression as a whole in the population with a later illness onset we find a high statistically significant percentage of severe depression with congruent psychotic features. Therefore, even if there is a low incidence of somatoform symptoms and hypochondria, the high frequency of hypochondrial delusions in the population with illness onset after 60 should be taken into consideration.

The higher frequency of hospitalization of patients with the illness onset before the age of 60 for a mild, moderate, or severe depression without psychotic features than the older population, leads us to look at two different ways in which to consider the recurrent depressive disorder in relation to the age at onset. As a matter of fact the patients with illness onset before the age of 60 are hospitalized before the disorder becomes severe; in contrast, in geriatric patients depression is often under evaluated and underestimated. This leads to late hospitalization, when the disorder has already become severe, particularly when it has been complicated with psychotic features.

No relevant differences have been found between the two populations regarding the frequency and length of the depressive episodes, even if the frequency rises slightly in the population with the first depressive onset after the age of 60.

Finally, when considering the variation in frequency and length of the depressive episodes in a sample of 27 patients with their first episode before the age of 60 it has been found that the frequency rises significantly after the age of 60, and the length of the episodes seems to be slightly longer. This leads to the supposition that there is a tendency towards chronicity of recurrent depressive episodes in late life. These data agree with the current literature.

In conclusion, in this study no relevant differences have been found between the two populations with recurrent major depressive disorder relating to the symptomatology, even if some data, such as the severity of depression, should be further investigated.

References

Angst J (1990) Course as classifier for depression. In: Proceedings of the international symposium on recurrent mood disorders, March 23–25 1990, Monte Carlo

Bland RC, Newman SC, Orn H (1988) Age of onset of psychiatric disorders. Acta Psychiatr Scand Suppl 338: 43–49

Blazer D (1983) Impact of late life depression in the social network. Am J Psychiatry 140: 162–166

Blazer D, Williams CD (1984) The epidemiology of dysphoria and depression in an elderly population. Am J Psychiatry 137: 439

Blazer D, Bachar JR, Hughes D (1987) Depression with melancholia: a comparison of middle aged and elderly adults. J Am Geriatr Soc 35: 927–932

Busse EW (1965) Research on aging: some methods and findings. In: Berezin MA, Cath SH (eds) Geriatric psychiatry: grief loss and emotional disorders in the aging processes. International University Press, pp 73–95

De Alarcon RD (1964) Hypochondriasis and depression in the aged. Gerontol Clin 6: 266–277

Gaitz C, Scott J (1972) Age and measurement of mental health. J Health Soc Behav 13: 55–67

Gross PL, Fitten LJ, Morley JE, Petry SD, Cole KD (1989) Depression. UCLA geriatirc grand rounds. J Am Geriatr Soc 37: 459–472

Kay DWK, Roth M, Hopkins B (1955) Affective disorders arising in the senium. J Ment Sci 101: 302–318

LaRue A, Dessonville C, Jarvik LF (1983) Aging and mental disorders. In: Birren JE, Schaide KW (eds) Handbook of psychology of aging. Van Nostrand Reinhold, New York, pp 66, 702

Meyers BS, Greenberg R (1986) Late-life delusional depression. J Affective Disord 11: 133–137

Musetti L, Perugi G, Soriani A, Rossi VM, Cassano GB, Akiskal HS (1989) Depression before and after age 65. A re-examination. Br J Psychiatry 55: 330–336

Nott PN, Fleminger JS (1975) Presenile dementia: the difficulty of early diagnosis. Acta Med Scand 51: 210–217

Post F (1965) The clinical psychiatry of late life. Pergamon, New York

Ron MA, Toone BK, Garralda ME et al (1979) Diagnosic accuracy in presenile dementia. Br J Psychiatry 134: 161

Winokur G, Behan D, Schlesser M (1980) Clinical and biological concepts of depression in the elderly. In: Cole JO, Barret JE (eds) Psychopathology in the aged. Plenum, New York, p 145

Psychotic Mixed State: Clinical-Anamnestic and Familial Comparisons with Nonpsychotic Mixed, Psychotic Manic, and Schizoaffective Disorders

L. Dell'Osso, G.F. Placidi, P. Freer, R. Nassi, and G.B. Cassano

An extreme variability and polymorphism in the clinical picture, a frequency of psychotic features, prolonged duration, and resistance to lithium treatment often conceal the affective nature of bipolar mixed episodes, leading to a misdiagnosis of schizophrenia. The extent of the unsolved diagnostic dilemmas is reflected in the latest edition of the formal classificatory systems, DSM-III-R (American Psychiatric Association 1987) and ICD-10 Draft (1989), where the mixed state appears as the vaguest category of mood disorders, with inadequate diagnostic criteria. These criteria do not allow distinction from rapid cycling, nor the recognition of a mixed episode at the onset of bipolar illness; they ignore the low-grade forms and do not encompass the variable and shifting symptomatology, leaving the boundary with most mental disorders, from the neurotic to the schizophrenic, quite fluid. The longitudinal criterion may be useful in many of these conditions: family history, the previous course, characterized by typical mood episodes, usually depressive, alternated with intervals free from psychopathologic symptoms, generally allow the identification of the affective nature and guide us towards a correct interpretation of these forms.

Sometimes a mixed episode appears in concomitance with alcohol, sedative, or other substance abuses, considered as kindling factors which often complicate the course of bipolar illness. Moreover a preexisting depressive temperament, adding a dysphoric component to the excited state, may favor mixed recurrences (Dell'Osso et al. 1991); thereby the mixed state often substitutes the manic episode in the course of the manic-depressive cycle (Kraepelin 1991).

In a previous study it was observed that the mixed state represents a specific longitudinal pattern of manic-depressive illness which, compared to "pure" bipolar (i.e., a course with depressive or manic episodes alone), is characterized by a heavier family affective loading – often depressive –, a lower frequency of hyperthymic temperament, and a tendency to recur true to type, often with psychotic mood-incongruent features. The strong affective coloring, the frequent total remission of the episode, and the good interepisodic adjustment give evidence of the bipolar nature of this form, despite the frequent psychotic presentation (Dell'Osso et al. 1991).

The present chapter contributes to the clinical anamnestic characterization of mixed state by comparing two subtypes of this form, i.e., the psychotic versus the nonpsychotic mixed state, the aim being to evaluate the impact of psychoticism in the course of this kind of presentation of the bipolar illness, the well-known polymorphism of which is often a source of misdiagnosis. Moreover, in order to shed light on differential diagnostic features between psychotic mixed states and two categories within the psychotic bipolar spectrum, i.e., psychotic mania and schizoaffective disorder, bipolar type, further comparisons were performed.

Patients and Method

Patient Population. This study is part of the collaborative research on recurrent mood disorders conducted by the Universities of Pisa, Italy and Memphis, Tennessee, United States. The project has an ambulatory component (Cassano et al. 1989) as well as the inpatient one (Dell'Osso et al. 1990) from which the present paper derives.

To date we have investigated 229 patients suffering from a primary mood disorder or a schizoaffective disorder consecutively admitted to the female ward of the Psychiatric Clinic of the University of Pisa for a mood episode (manic, depressive, or mixed).

In this contribution, data are reported on 41 patients suffering from a mixed episode (21 with psychotic features and 20 without), 17 from a manic episode with psychotic features, and 16 from a schizoaffective disorder.

Assessment and Measures. Data were collected on familial, temperamental, anamnestic, and clinical parameters based on an Italian adaptation (Dell'Osso et al. 1989) of the Mood Clinic Data Questionnaire (MCDQ) by Akiskal et al. (1978). We used a semistructured face-to-face interview lasting 60–120 min. Data concerning psychiatric history were also collected from family members and all other relevant sources, (i.e. social workers and physicians) and systematically recorded. Previous hospital records and physicians' clinical notes completed the collection of retrospective data. The family history concerning psychiatric disturbances was investigated using the Research Diagnostic Criteria–Family History Version by Andreasen et al. (1977).

The affective temperaments were assessed using Akiskal and Mallya's criteria (1987) derived from Schneider's (1958) description of depressive and hyperthymic types.

Onset of illness was defined in three ways, according to Roy-Byrne et al. (1985): first subjective symptoms, first treatment, and first hospitalization. With regard to the course of illness, we included only the episodes that required psychiatric observation and treatment.

As for cross-sectional features, we assessed many variables, such as age, latency of hospitalization, (i.e., interval between onset of episode and admission to hospital), duration of episode, psychosocial stressors and psychopathological and social functioning just before the index episode (using the GAF scale of DSM III-R, 1987). The psychopathologic cross-sectional profile was assessed by the Clinical Global Improvement Scale (CGI), the Brief Psychiatric Rating Scale (BPRS) and the Hamilton Rating Scale for Depression (HRSD).

Diagnostic Criteria. The psychotic manic episode was diagnosed according to DSM-III-R (American Psychiatric Association 1987) criteria which include psychotic features, congruent and incongruent, because current evidence has confirmed the acute presence of first-rank symptoms in patients defined as manics. In this study manic patients who had no mixed episodes in their history of illness were isolated because for our study a sample of "pure" bipolar patients was necessary.

As for mixed states, the diagnosis was made in those cases characterized by a major depressive syndrome in the context of a classic manic picture (according to DSM-III-R criteria); the depressive component was assessed on the basis of the HRSD score (Hamilton 1967) – more than 15 in the first 17 items. Opposite affective symptoms had to coexist for at least 2 weeks; following Prien et al. (1988), the DSM-III-R criterion A of alternating manic and depressive features was not used, because of the possible overlap with rapid cycling bipolar illness. According to the ICD-10 Draft (1989), at least one prior manic episode was required to differentiate this condition from non-affective psychoses. The diagnosis of schizoaffective disorder was made in the presence of a full depressive or manic syndrome associated with at least one schneiderian first-rank symptom (Research Diagnostic Criteria, Spitzer et al. 1975), and, on the basis of DSM-III-R, a prior episode characterized by psychotic symptomatology with no relevant affective symptoms for more than 2 weeks was also required.

Statistical Analyses. The data were processed at the Center for Clinical Psychopharmacological Data Documentation (CCPDD) of the Institute of Psychiatry of Pisa University, Italy (Cassano et al. 1985), by Statistical Analysis System (SAS), with Student's t test, chi-square test, Fisher's exact test (second tail), and analysis of variance. We conservatively used two-tailed statistics. Two types of analyses were carried out:

1. Psychotic mixed versus nonpsychotic mixed patients: data on the 21 patients suffering from a mixed episode with psychotic features (PM) were compared to those of 20 mixed patients without psychotic features (NPM).

2. Psychotic mixed versus psychotic manic versus schizoaffective patients: 54 patients who presented a severe compromise of reality testing at hospitalization, as demonstrated by delusion, hallucinations, incoherence, marked loosening of associations, catatonic stupor or excitement, and bizarre behavior (psychotic bipolar spectrum). In this group 21 patients (38.9%) met criteria for a PM, 17 (31.5%) for a psychotic manic (PMan) episode, and 16 (29.6%) for a schizoaffective disorder, bipolar type (SA). Clinical anamnestic features were compared in the three groups.

Results

Psychotic-Mixed Versus Nonpsychotic-Mixed Patients

From the comparison of PM ($n = 21$) and NPM ($n = 20$), no significant differences emerged regarding depressive and hyperthymic temperaments; however, a double diagnosis of cyclothymia was made in 40% of NPM vs 4.8% of PM (Fisher's exact test, two-tail, $p = 0.0009$).

Table 1. Index episodes

	PM[a] ($n = 21$)	NPM[a] ($n = 20$)	T	p
Age (years)	41.0 ± 16.0	40.3 ± 16.0	0.13	NS
Length of hospitalization (weeks)	2.8 ± 2.2	5.1 ± 6.5	−1.54	NS
Length of episode (months)	2.8 ± 1.7	6.1 ± 7.2	−2.02	0.05
Severity (CGI)	5.6 ± 0.7	5.4 ± 0.7	0.80	NS
Length of interepisodic phase (months)	21.1 ± 27.8	24.7 ± 33.3	−0.38	NS
Axis V (GAF scale)	47.3 ± 27.0	51.1 ± 23.5	−0.48	NS

[a] Results are mean ± standard deviation.

Family history clearly distinguished PM and NPM with a significant prevalence in PM first-degree relatives of bipolar (23.8%) and depressive disorders (42.9%) vs NPM ones (bipolar 10% and depressive 25%; $p = 0.009$ and 0.007 respectively), as well as of a higher rate of suicidal behaviors (PM = 33.3% vs NPM = 5%, $p < 0.0001$).

The course of illness did not significantly differ in the two groups, except for the repetition of episodes similar to the index one ($p = 0.0001$): in PM 97.4% of the mixed anamnestic episodes showed psychotic features, mood congruent or incongruent, vs 19% of prior psychotic mixed episodes in NPM.

As for cross-sectional features, as shown in Table 1, psychotic-mixed states differed significantly from the nonpsychotic ones by shorter duration of the index episode; because of the homogeneity of the sample formed by inpatients, the severity of symptomatology, assessed by CGI was not significantly different, although PM showed slightly higher scores; the same is true for BPRS total scores (47.3 ± 9 in PM vs 44.5 ± 6.5 in NPM) and HRSD total score (24.1 ± 6.5 in PM vs 23.4 ± 5.7 in NPM).

Significant differences were also observed as regards the latency of hospitalization, shorter in PM (4.7 weeks vs 17.7; T = − 2.20, $p = 0.03$), and the rate of psychosocial stressors preceding the index episode (negative events according to Paykel et al.'s classification, 1971), higher in NPM (21.9%) vs PM (7.3%; $df = 1$, X^2 4.668, $p = 0.031$); finally no significant differences were found in the score on axis V.

Psychotic-Mixed Versus Psychotic Manic Versus Schizoaffective Patients

Mean age was 41 years (±16) in PM, 39.5 years (±14.5) in PMan and 34.6 years (±8.4) in SA. A premorbid depressive temperament was recorded in 19% of PM, in 18.7% of SA, and in 0% of the PMan ($p = 0.158$); hyperthymia was found in 9.5% of PM, in 6.2% of SA, and in 52.9% of PMan ($p = 0.001$). As for family history, a statistically significant difference among the three groups was

Table 2. Rates of family history

	PM ($n = 21$) %	PMan ($n = 17$) %	SA ($n = 16$) %	*df*	X^2	*p*
Bipolar disorders	23.8	29.4	18.7	2	0.51	NS
Depressive disorders	42.9	5.9	12.5	2	8.7	0.01
Schizophrenia	0.0	0.0	12.5	2		
Unspecified hospitalized psychotic disorders	14.3	5.9	6.2	2	1.035	NS
Suicide/suicide attempts	28.6	17.6	6.2	2	3.011	NS

Table 3. Index episodes

	PM[a] ($n = 21$)	PMan[a] ($n = 17$)	SA[a] ($n = 16$)	*F*	*p*
Age (years)	41.0 ± 16.0	39.5 ± 14.5	34.6 ± 8.4	1.02	NS
Length of hospitalization (weeks)	2.8 ± 2.2	3.4 ± 2.4	3.6 ± 2.9	0.38	NS
Length of episodes (months)	2.8 ± 1.7	2.9 ± 2.2	3.4 ± 2.3	0.48	NS
Severity (CGI)	5.6 ± 0.6	5.6 ± 1.3	5.8 ± 0.8	0.58	NS
Length of interepisodic phase (months)	21.1 ± 27.8	15.1 ± 22.9	28.8 ± 31.6	1.02	NS
Adjustment (GAF scale)	47.3 ± 27.0	37.5 ± 25.3	49.1 ± 21.5	1.08	NS

[a] Results are mean ± standard deviation.

observed regarding the rate of depressive disorders in first-degree relatives (Table 2). Psychopathological and clinical features at index episode did not significantly differ in the three groups (Table 3).

As regards the onset of illness, a much lower age of first hospitalization was observed in SA (23.4 ± 6.3) vs PM (33.8 ± 11.7) and PMan (32.8 ± 12.6). With respect to the course of illness there were no significant differences among the three groups as regards the length of illness (12.9 ± 11.3 in PM vs 11.0 ± 8.9 in PMan vs 12.9 ± 9.4 in SA), the number of mood episodes (7.1 ± 6.9 in PM vs 5.1 ± 4.2 in PMan vs 5.9 ± 3.8 in SA), the number of hospitalizations (3.4 ± 4.2 in PM vs 3.6 ± 2.8 in PMan vs 4.6 ± 3.4 in SA), the number of suicidal attempts (0.5 ± 1 in PM vs 0.5 ± 0.8 in SMan vs 0.1 ± 0.3 in SA). As regards prior episodes, 38.4% of all episodes in PM, 33.9% in PMan, and 35.8% in SA were depressive. The analysis of prior manic episodes shows a rate (34.9%) of pure manic episodes in PM, intermediate between PMan (63.1%) and SA (10.8%). Mixed episodes represented 26.7% of all previous episodes in PM and 15.6% in

SA. Psychotic features were prevalently mood incongruent in PM and SA and prevalently mood congruent in PMan.

Significant differences ($p = 0.001$) on circannual cyclicity of the episodes were noticed, with a summer-autumn prevalence in the PMan (70.6% vs 42.9% in PM and 37.4% in SA) and a winter prevalence in SA (43.7%) and in PM (42.9% vs 11.8% in PMan).

Discussion

Compared to the nonpsychotic mixed, the psychotic subgroup tends to recur true to type, i.e., with psychotic features, mainly incongruent; furthermore it is characterized by a heavier familial loading for mood disorders, particularly depressive, and for suicidal behavior. Despite severe psychopathological impairment during acute episodes, and a higher frequency of recurrences, the duration of the psychotic mixed episode is shorter than that of the nonpsychotic one and hospitalization is less frequently required. Finally, the psychotic mixed episode appears to be seldom triggered by psychosocial stressors.

The psychotic mixed state is more clearly demarcated by findings derived from a comparison with psychotic mania and schizoaffective disorder – family history emerges as the most differentiating. In fact a specific pattern typical for each subtype was found; compared to the other two groups, relatives of psychotic-mixed patients show the highest percentage of mood disorders, particularly depressive, sometimes even with double heredity (depressive and bipolar disorders on different sides of the family), and the highest familial risk for suicide; only schizoaffective patients show familial predisposition to schizophrenia, though often in association with affective family history; finally in psychotic manics, family history shows the highest rate of typical bipolar disorders and the lowest rate of depression, whereas suicide risk is intermediate between the other two groups.

As for annual cyclicity, MP just like SA shows prevalently winter recurrences while PMan shows a clear prevalence of summer-autumn episodes.

Interesting differences have also been observed concerning premorbid temperament: a depressive one was found in one of five PM and SA and in none of PMan; instead the latter show a very high rate of hyperthymia.

As can be deduced from these data, longitudinal data clearly differ in the three groups, particularly those on family history, premorbid temperament, and seasonality of recurrences. The findings that emerge from the comparison between the subgroups included in the bipolar psychotic spectrum suggest that psychoticism does not interfere significantly with the course of bipolar illness. On the contrary, regarding the cross-sectional aspects, index episode features like rapidity of onset (latency of hospitalization), duration of episode, and the occurrence of psychosocial stressors in the year preceding the index episode do not show significant differences. These observations derive from retrospective methodology; psychotic features may ultimately exercise powerful impact on the longterm prospective course of these patients.

The data and considerations presented in this paper are part of ongoing studies and larger case material might alter them in significant ways. Finally, a limitation of this study is that it is based on female gender. Although women are more at risk for mixed states, it would be nonetheless important to repeat these observations on male bipolar patients.

References

Akiskal HS, Mallya G (1987) Criteria for the soft bipolar spectrum: treatment implications. Psychopharmacol Bull 23: 68–73
Akiskal HS, Bitar AH, Puzantian VR, Rosenthal TL, Walker PW (1978) The nosologic status of neurotic depression: a prospective three-to-four year examination in light of the primary-secondary and unipolar-bipolar dichotomies. Arch Gen Psychiatry 35: 756–766
American Psychiatric Association (1987) Diagnostic and statistical manual of mental disorders, 3rd edn, revised. American Psychiatric Association, Washington
Andreasen NC, Endicott J, Spitzer RL (1977) The family history method using diagnostic criteria. Arch Gen Psychiatry 34: 1229–1235
Cassano GB, Conti L, Musetti L, Mauri M, Dell'Osso L (1985) CCPDD – un centro per la documentazione dei dati in psicofarmacologia clinica. Riv Psichiatr 20: 1–17
Cassano GB, Akiskal HS, Musetti L, Perugi G, Soriani A, Mignani V (1989) Psychopathology, temperament, and past course in primary major depressions: II. Toward a redefinition of bipolarity with a new semi-structured interview for depression (SID). Psychopathology 22: 278–288
Dell'Osso L, Conti L, Meschi M, Sebastiani P, Toschi D, Placidi GF (1989) Predittori di decorso nei disturbi ricorrenti dell'umore: dati preliminari. In: Placidi GF, Dell'Osso L, Faravelli C (eds) La malattia depressiva. Idelson, Napoli, pp 53–68
Dell'Osso L, Placidi GF, Nassi R, Freer P, Cassano GB, Akiskal HS (1991) The manic-depressive mixed state: familial, temperamental and psychopathologic characteristics in 108 female inpatients. Eur Arch Psychiatry Clin Neurosci 240: 234–239
Hamilton M (1967) Development of a rating scale for primary depressive illness. Br J Clin Psychol 6: 278–296
ICD-10 Draft (1989) Mental and behavioural disorders. World Health Organization, Geneva
Kraepelin E (1921) Manic-depressive Insanity and Paranoia. Livingstone, Edinburg
Prien R, Himmelhoch JM, Kupfer DJ (1988) Treatment of mixed mania. J Affective Disord 15: 9–15
Roy-Byrne P, Post RM, Udhe TW, Poren T, Davis D (1985) Longitudinal course of recurrent affective illness: life chart at the NIMH. Acta Psychiatr Scand 71 [Suppl 317]: 1–34
Schneider K (1958) Psychopathic personalities. Cassell, London
Spitzer RL, Endicott J, Robins E (1975) Research Diagnostic Criteria (RCD) for a selected group of functional disorders. Biometrics Research, New York

Heterogeneity of Course and Outcome in Subjects with a Cross-Sectional Diagnosis of Schizoaffective Disorder

M. Maj

Introduction

The long-term course of the disorders defined cross-sectionally as schizoaffective has been paid little attention during the past years. In fact, longitudinal studies have usually focused on the onset and the outcome of these conditions, disregarding what happens in between, that is, "the whole gestalt of the course over lifetime" (Angst 1986).

This state of things is particularly disappointing, since a careful assessment of course is likely to provide a clue to a better understanding of schizoaffective disorders, and of their relationship to schizophrenia and to major affective disorders, and some useful information on the more general issue of stability of diagnosis over time in major psychiatric disorders.

Indeed, the few studies providing such an assessment (Angst et al. 1980; Brockington et al. 1980a, b; Maj 1985; Marneros et al. 1988) have shown that patients defined cross-sectionally as schizoaffective turn out to represent a very heterogeneous group when they are followed up longitudinally. Bipolarity of course and/or occurrence of pure affective episodes in addition to the schizoaffective ones seem to characterize schizoaffective forms with a long-term outcome similar to major affective disorders (Brockington et al. 1980b; Maj et al. 1987; Marneros et al. 1988), whereas the onset of schizoaffective episodes against the background of previous schizophrenic symptoms appears to be associated with a poor outcome (Brockington et al. 1980a; Maj et al. 1987).

These two extreme patterns of course correspond to the affective and the schizophrenic subtypes identified by Maj and Perris (1985) on the axis 2 (course) of their multiaxial classification of schizoaffective disorders. Moreover, the latter pattern has much in common with schizoaffective disorder as characterized in DSM-III-R (American Psychiatric Association 1987).

Whether further subtypes of the above disorders can be singled out on the basis of long-term course remains an open research issue, which was approached by the present study.

Methods

The study was conducted on two samples of patients. The former (schizoaffective group) included 77 subjects who: (a) were referred to the Centre for Prevention and Treatment of Affective Disorders at the First Psychiatric

Department of Naples University during the period from 1 January 1979 to 30 June 1986; (b) fulfilled, on the occasion of the first visit, Research Diagnostic Criteria (RDC, Spitzer et al. 1975) for schizoaffective disorder; and (c) could be examined prospectively for at least 3 years and on the whole (i.e., considering retrospective and prospective assessment) for at least 10 years. This sample included 35 males and 42 females, with an age ranging, at the time of the first visit, from 20 to 51 years. Cross-sectional RDC diagnosis was schizoaffective disorder, manic type in 30 of them, and schizoaffective disorder, depressed type in 47.

The latter sample (affective group) consisted of the first 30 patients with a cross-sectional RDC diagnosis of manic disorder and the first 47 patients with a RDC diagnosis of major depressive disorder referred to the above Centre since 1 January 1979 who could be examined prospectively for at least 3 years and on the whole for at least 10 years. They were 33 males and 44 females, with an age ranging from 26 to 56 years. The duration of the observation period ranged from 10 to 28 years (mean $\pm$ SD 14.9 $\pm$ 11.6) in the schizoaffective group and from 10 to 30 years (mean $\pm$ SD 16.5 $\pm$ 13.0) in the affective one.

In each patient, retrospective assessment was made on the occasion of the first visit by means of the Schedule for Affective Disorders and Schizophrenia (SADS, Endicott and Spitzer 1978). The interview was supplemented by the collection of all available information from relatives, health care providers, and medical records. Previous episodes were classified, when possible, according to RDC. Prospective evaluation was made by interviewing the patient monthly or bimonthly by the SADS, and assessing his/her psychopathological state by the Comprehensive Psychopathological Rating Scale (CPRS, Asberg et al. 1978). New morbid episodes were recorded and classified according to RDC. Interepisodic symptoms were also recorded: they were defined as the symptoms occurring during the periods in which the patient did not fulfill RDC for any psychiatric disorder (excluding the last visit before and the first visit after an episode).

At the end of the follow-up period, the psychopathological and the psychosocial outcome were evaluated in each patient by means of the Strauss-Carpenter Outcome Scale (Strauss and Carpenter 1972) and the Disability Assessment Schedule (DAS, Jablensky et al. 1980). On the basis of the score on the section 5 ("global evaluation of social adjustment") of the DAS, the psychosocial outcome was rated as good (score of 1 or 2), intermediate (score of 3), or poor (score of 4, 5, or 6).

Statistical analysis was made by Student's paired t test and the χ^2 method with Yates' correction, as indicated.

Results

The morbid episodes recorded during the observation period in patients defined cross-sectionally as either schizoaffective or affective are summarized in Table 1. In patients diagnosed as schizoaffective, 49.7% of the episodes were schizoaffective, 30.1% affective, and 12.6% schizophrenic; 2.9% of the episodes could

Table 1. Episodes recorded during the observation period in patients defined cross-sectionally as either schizoaffective or affective

Type of episode (according to RDC)	Schizoaffectives		Affectives	
	Episodes (*n*)	(%)	Episodes (*n*)	(%)
Manic	36	10.3	135	34.0
Major depressive	69	19.8	219	55.2
Schizomanic	61	17.5	10	2.5
Schizodepressive	112	32.2	15	3.8
Schizophrenic	44	12.6	4	1.0
Other	10	2.9	8	2.0
Not classifiable	16	4.6	6	1.5

not be classified according to RDC (mostly because the number of affective symptoms was not sufficient to fulfill the criterion B for a schizoaffective disorder), whereas for 4.6% of the episodes information was not sufficient to allow classification. In patients defined as affective, 55.2% of the episodes were depressive, 34.0% were manic, 6.3% were schizoaffective, 1.0% were schizophrenic, 2.0% did not fulfill criteria for any RDC category, and 1.5% could not be classified due to the lack of sufficient information.

A course definable as "polymorphous" (i.e., characterized by the occurrence of at least two types of episodes among the following: schizoaffective, affective, schizophrenic, and other) was observed in 59.7% of patients defined cross-sectionally as schizoaffective and in 16.9% of those defined cross-sectionally as affective. This difference is statistically significant ($\chi^2 = 28.135$; $df = 1$; $p < 0.001$). On the other hand, a bipolar course (i.e., a course marked by the appearance of both manic or schizomanic and depressive or schizodepressive episodes) was significantly more frequent in affective than in schizoaffective patients (57.1% vs 29.9% of cases; $\chi^2 = 10.568$; $df = 1$; $p < 0.01$).

The patterns of course which could be identified in patients defined cross-sectionally as schizoaffective are summarized in Table 2. The most frequent pattern was the bipolar one marked by the appearance of schizomanic and depressive or of schizomanic, manic, and depressive episodes (27.3% of cases), followed by that characterized by the occurrence of schizodepressive episodes only (22.1%), and by that marked by the appearance of schizodepressive and schizophrenic episodes (15.6%).

Table 3 shows the depressive, manic, and "schizophrenic" CPRS items (from the list proposed by Maj and Perris 1985) which were the most frequently rated during the interepisodic periods in patients defined cross-sectionally as schizoaffective. Four items were rated in at least six visits in more than one-quarter of patients: reduced sleep, reduced appetite, lassitude, and concentration difficulties. Only two schizophrenic items were rated in at least six visits in more than ten patients: withdrawal and lack of appropriate emotion; 7 of the 13 patients with the former symptom and 6 of the 12 patients with the latter showed the pattern of course indicated as C in Table 2 (occurrence of schizodepressive and schizophrenic episodes).

Table 2. Patterns of course in patients defined cross-sectionally as schizoaffective

Pattern of course	Patients	
	(*n*)	(%)
A = Occurrence of schizomanic and depressive or of schizomanic, manic, and depressive episodes	21	27.3
B = Occurrence of schizodepressive episodes only	17	22.1
C = Occurrence of schizodepressive and schizophrenic episodes	12	15.6
D = Occurrence of schizomanic episodes only	6	7.8
E = Single schizoaffective episode	6	7.8
F = Occurrence of schizodepressive and depressive episodes	5	6.5
G = Occurrence of schizoaffective episodes and of "mixed" psychotic episodes not fulfilling RDC for schizoaffective disorder	4	5.2
H = Occurrence of schizomanic and schizophrenic episodes	2	2.6
I = Occurrence of schizomanic and schizodepressive episodes	2	2.6
J = Occurrence of affective, schizoaffective, and schizophrenic episodes	2	2.6

Table 3. Most frequent interepisodic symptoms in patients defined cross-sectionally as schizoaffective

CPRS item	Patients in whom the item was rated in at least six visits	
	(*n*)	(%)
Reduced sleep	32	41.5
Reduced appetite	28	36.4
Lassitude	26	33.8
Concentration difficulties	22	28.6
Inability to feel	17	22.1
Failing memory	15	19.5
Withdrawal	13	16.9
Pessimistic thoughts	12	15.6
Lack of appropriate emotion	12	15.6
Agitation	10	13.0

At the end of the follow-up period, the mean global score on the Strauss-Carpenter Outcome Scale was significantly lower in patients defined cross-sectionally as schizoaffective than in those defined as affective (12.5 ± 2.8 vs 13.7 ± 2.8; $t = 2.66$; $p < 0.01$). As shown in Table 4, within patients defined cross-sectionally as schizoaffective, those with a unipolar monomorphous course (patterns B and D of Table 2) and those with a course characterized by schizoaffective and schizophrenic episodes (patterns C and H) also had a poorer outcome than patients defined cross-sectionally as affective, whereas subjects

Table 4. Mean global scores on Strauss-Carpenter Outcome Scale in patients defined cross-sectionally as either schizoaffective (subdivided on the basis of pattern of course, see Table 2) or affective

Patient group	*n*	Global score on Strauss-Carpenter Outcome Scale (mean ± SD)
Schizoaffective disorder	77	12.5 ± 2.8[a]
Pattern of course A	21	13.2 ± 3.0
Pattern of course B + D	23	12.4 ± 2.8[b]
Pattern of course C + H	14	11.6 ± 3.6[c]
Major affective disorder	77	13.7 ± 2.8

[a] Significantly lower than affective patients ($t = 2.66$; $df = 142$; $p < 0.01$)
[b] Significantly lower than affective patients ($t = 1.95$; $df = 98$, $p < 0.05$)
[c] Significantly lower than affective patients ($t = 2.26$; $df = 89$; $p < 0.05$)

Table 5. Psychosocial outcome in subgroups of patients defined cross-sectionally as schizoaffective, identified on the basis of pattern of course (see Table 2)

Pattern of course	Patients (*n*)	Psychosocial outcome		
		Good	Intermediate	Poor
A	21	16	4	1
B	17	7	8	2
C	12	3	4	5
D	6	3	3	0
E	6	4	2	0
F	5	2	3	0
G	4	3	1	0
H	2	1	0	1
I	2	0	2	0
J	2	0	1	1

with a bipolar course marked by the presence of pure affective episodes (pattern A) had an outcome not significantly different from affective patients.

The psychosocial outcome of patients defined cross-sectionally as schizoaffective was good in 39 cases (50.6%), intermediate in 28 (36.4%), and poor in 10 (13.0%). The corresponding figures in patients defined cross-sectionally as affective were 60 (77.9%), 13 (16.9%), and 4 (5.2%), the difference being statistically significant ($\chi^2 = 12.510$; $df = 2$; $p < 0.01$). The psychosocial outcome in the different schizoaffective groups identified on the basis of the pattern of course is shown in Table 5. In patients whose course was bipolar with pure affective episodes (pattern A) the outcome was not significantly different from affective patients, whereas in those with a unipolar monomorphous course (patterns B and D) or with schizoaffective and schizophrenic episodes (patterns C and H) it was significantly poorer than in affective patients ($\chi^2 = 10.427$; $df = 2$; $p < 0.01$; and $\chi^2 = 20.258$; $df = 2$, $p < 0.001$, respectively).

Discussion

The present study confirms that the conditions defined as schizoaffective according to cross-sectional criteria turn out to be very heterogeneous when studied longitudinally and that a polymorphous course (i.e., a course marked by the occurrence of at least two different types of episodes among the following: schizoaffective, affective, schizophrenic, and other) is significantly more frequent in these conditions than in major affective disorders.

Bipolarity was found to be common in schizoaffectives, although the observed percentage of bipolar cases was lower than that reported in some previous investigations (Angst et al. 1980; Marneros et al. 1988) : this is probably in part due to a definition of bipolarity requiring the occurrence of both manic or schizomanic and depressive or schizodepressive episodes, whereas (contrary to some previous studies) a course characterized by schizomanic episodes only was not defined as bipolar.

It was confirmed that in patients defined cross-sectionally as schizomanic a frequent pattern of course is the bipolar one with occurrence of schizomanic and depressive, or schizomanic, manic and depressive episodes. In these forms, intervals between the episodes are usually free from schizophrenic symptoms (although residual affective symptoms may be present), and the outcome is not different from that of pure major affective disorders. In some patients of this group, schizomanic episodes are only a sporadic occurrence within a course dominated by pure affective episodes: in these cases, schizoaffective attacks tend to be more frequent in the earlier years of the illness.

Analogous to this first pattern of course may be that characterized by the appearance of schizodepressive and pure depressive episodes: in the present study, this type of course was observed only in five patients, who did not show any schizophrenic symptomatology between the episodes and had a good or intermediate outcome.

The other extreme pattern of course whose existence was confirmed by the present study is that marked by the appearance of schizodepressive and schizophrenic episodes. In this subtype of schizoaffective disorder, the frequency of interepisodic schizophrenic symptoms is high (58.3% of patients had withdrawal and 50.0% of them had lack of appropriate emotion in at least six visits), and the outcome is significantly poorer than that of pure major affective disorders, from both the psychopathological and the psychosocial viewpoint. The literature on "depression in schizophrenia" and its multiple determinants (Galdi 1983) may be relevant in this context. On the other hand, it should be stressed that the distinction between depressive symptoms and the "negative" symptoms of schizophrenia may be sometimes difficult (Kulhara et al. 1989), so that a proportion of patients of this group may be schizophrenics with prominent negative symptoms, either primary or secondary to psychotic experiences or neuroleptic treatment (Carpenter et al. 1985).

Our data confirmed that schizoaffective disorders with a "monomorphous" course (i.e., characterized by schizoaffective episodes only) are not uncommon. The most frequent pattern is that marked by the occurrence of multiple schizodepressive episodes, whereas the occurrence of multiple schizomanic episodes or a bipolar course with schizodepressive and schizomanic episodes are much rarer. The interpretation of these patterns remains problematic. Nevertheless, the outcome of these forms is clearly poorer in comparison not only with pure major affective disorders but also with the conditions in which schizoaffective episodes alternate with pure affective ones. Recurrent schizodepressive disorders may partially overlap with "delusional depressions" repeatedly described in the literature (Kantor and Glassman 1977), although it should be specified that delusions may not be the only psychotic symptoms in these schizodepressive forms. Some cases of this group may also be the result of the superimposition of a manic or depressive syndrome on the substrate of a schizotypal personality, characterized by peculiarities and oddities of ideation, perception, and behavior, whose presence during the acute episode may prompt a diagnosis of schizoaffective disorder, and whose persistence after recovery may be interpreted as a residual schizophrenic symptom (Akiskal and Puzantian 1979).

A relatively infrequent pattern of course identified in the present study was that characterized by the occurrence of schizoaffective episodes and of "mixed" episodes not fulfilling RDC for schizoaffective disorder (mostly because the number of affective symptoms was not sufficient to meet the criterion B). This pattern may pertain to the borderline between schizoaffective and cycloid disorders. According to the diagnostic criteria provided by Perris and Brockington (1981), cycloid episodes are marked by "mood swings not so pronounced as to justify a diagnosis of affective disorder," in addition to mood incongruent delusions and/or hallucinations and perplexity or puzzlement. Although these episodes tend to recur with the same characteristics in a given patient, it has been documented (Maj 1988) that cycloid episodes may occur in patients defined cross-sectionally as schizoaffective, and that schizoaffective episodes may be recorded in patients diagnosed cross-sectionally as cycloid.

Finally, a very rare pattern of course is that marked by the appearance of pure affective, schizoaffective, and pure schizophrenic episodes. In these cases, one or two schizoaffective episodes may represent an intermediate stage in the transition from an affective to a schizophrenic syndrome (or vice versa) or, in other terms, a "concurrent" schizoaffective disorder may be part of the development of a "sequential" (Maj and Perris 1985) one.

It cannot be excluded that the results of the present study have been conditioned by the short duration of the observation period and by the relatively small size of the patient sample. In particular, the former factor may have biased the patterns of course identified in the study, while the latter may have produced an over- or underestimation of the frequency of the various patterns. Moreover, as always in research concerning schizoaffective disorders, hidden selection factors may have been at work in patients' recruitment (for instance, the fact that the unit in which patients were enrolled is designed for prevention and treatment of affective disorders may have produced a bias in favor of the subtypes of schizoaffective syndromes with a predominant affective component)

Anyway, the results of the study confirmed that a careful assessment of long-term course in patients defined cross-sectionally as schizoaffective can provide a clue to the identification of more homogeneous subtypes of schizoaffective disorders. They suggested that the currently predominant cross-sectional approach to the diagnosis and classification of these conditions may be inadequate, and that future diagnostic criteria should pay more attention to the variable represented by the course of the illness.

References

Akiskal HS, Puzantian VR (1979) Psychotic forms of depression and mania. Psychiatr Clin North Am 2: 419–439

American Psychiatric Association (1987) Diagnostic and statistical manual of mental disorders, 3rd edn, revised. American Psychiatric Association, Washington DC

Angst J (1986) The course of schizoaffective disorders. In: Marneros A, Tsuang MT (eds) Schizoaffective psychoses. Springer, Berlin Heidelberg New York

Angst J, Felder W, Lohmeyer B (1980) Course of schizo-affective psychoses: results of a follow-up study. Schizophr Bull 6: 579–585

Asberg M, Perris C, Schalling D, Sedvall G (1978) Comprehensive Psychopathological Rating Scale: CPRS. Acta Psychiatr Scand [Suppl] 271: 5–27

Brockington IF, Kendell RE, Wainwright S (1980a) Depressed patients with schizophrenic or paranoid symptoms. Psychol Med 10: 665–675

Brockington IF, Wainwright S, Kendell RE (1980b) Manic patients with schizophrenic or paranoid symptoms. Psychol Med 10: 73–83

Carpenter WT, Heinrichs DW, Alphs LD (1985) Treatment of negative symptoms. Schizophr Bull 11: 440–452

Endicott J, Spitzer RL (1978) A diagnostic interview: the schedule for affective disorders and schizophrenia. Arch Gen Psychiatry 35: 837–862

Galdi J (1983) The causality of depression in schizophrenia. Br J Psychiatry 142: 621–625

Jablensky A, Schwarz R, Tomov T (1980) WHO collaborative study on impairments and disabilities associated with schizophrenic disorders. Acta Psychiatr Scand [Suppl] 268: 152–163

Kantor SJ, Glassman AH (1977) Delusional depression: natural history and response to treatment. Br J Psychiatry 131: 351–360

Kulhara P, Avasthi A, Chadda R, Chandiramani K, Mattoo SK, Kota SK, Joseph S (1989) Negative and depressive symptoms in schizophrenia. Br J Psychiatry 154: 207–211

Maj M (1985) Clinical course and outcome of schizoaffective disorders. A three-year follow-up study. Acta Psychiatr Scand 72: 542–550

Maj M (1988) Clinical course and outcome of cycloid psychotic disorder: a prospective study. Acta Psychiatr Scand 78: 182–187

Maj M, Perris C (1985) An approach to the diagnosis and classification of schizoaffective disorders for research purposes. Acta Psychiatr Scand 72: 405–417

Maj M, Starace F, Kemali D (1987) Prediction of outcome by historical, clinical and biological variables in schizoaffective disorder, depressed type. J Psychiatr Res 21: 289–295

Marneros A, Deister A, Rhode A, Jünemann H, Fimmers R (1988) Long-term course of schizoaffective disorders. Part I: definitions, methods, frequency of episodes and cycles. Eur Arch Psychiatry Neurol Sci 237: 244–257

Perris C, Brockington IF (1981) Cycloid psychoses and their relation to the major psychoses. In: Perris C, Struwe G, Jansson B (eds) Biological psychiatry 1981. Elsevier, Amsterdam
Spitzer RL, Endicott J, Robins E (1975) Research Diagnostic Criteria (RDC) for a selected group of functional disorders, 2nd edn. Biometrics Research, New York
Strauss JS, Carpenter WT (1972) The prediction of outcome in schizophrenia: I. Characteristics of outcome. Arch Gen Psychiatry 27: 739–746

Old and New Treatments and Prophylaxis

Testing Efficacy and Safety of Long-Term Treatment in Manic-Depressive Illness: Past and Present Problems

M. Schou

The testing of treatment efficacy is a far-reaching topic to discuss; the testing of treatment safety no less so. Add to these the time dimension of long-term or maintenance or prophylactic treatment, and you will understand that this brief presentation must limit itself to main issues and selected examples.

Efficacy

When the prophylactic or relapse-preventive properties of lithium in recurrent manic-depressive illness were first discovered, strategies for testing such drug actions were not available and had to be elaborated. Observations in individual patients (Schou 1956) were followed by studies on small groups of patients (Baastrup 1964; Hartigan 1963). Then came systematic observation of large groups of patients followed over many years, first without and then with lithium maintenance treatment, so that the patients served as their own controls (Baastrup and Schou 1967). These so-called *one-group mirror-design studies* were later supplemented with placebo-controlled double-blind trials, which were of two kinds, namely those where patients having been on lithium for some time were switched double-blind and randomly to either placebo or continued lithium (Baastrup et al. 1970), the *two-group trials of discontinuation design*, and those where patients were started simultaneously on either lithium or placebo, randomly allocated (e.g. Coppen et al. 1971; Hullin et al. 1972), the *two-group trials of start design.*

These early studies dealt with problems that were new. Whereas in therapeutic trials the aim was to demonstrate that something happened, namely that the disease attack came to an end, the prophylactic trials aimed at demonstrating that something did not happen, namely that recurrences did not occur or occurred less frequently when treatment was given than when no treatment or dummy treatment was given. This necessarily involved large patient groups and long observation periods. The studies Baastrup and I carried out dealt with patient groups of close to 100 and observation periods of up to 6 years.

There were many difficulties to overcome in the early prophylactic era. Research was to some extent groping its way, and some of the trials were distinguished more by being executed at all – in the face of skepticism – than by infallibility of design. Nonetheless, lithium prophylaxis became established as a viable and valuable new treatment modality.

Today we are faced with different problems when testing efficacy of long-term treatments, and new strategies are required when we compare lithium treatments administered according to different regimens or in different combinations, and when we test the efficacy of prophylactic alternatives, be they antidepressants or carbamazepine or valproate or clonazepam or rubidium. Problems are now quantitative rather than qualitative, and since we are looking for relatively small differences, there is a substantial risk of type II errors unless patient groups are large.

Ethical problems must also be faced: Can we under present-day circumstances use placebo? To what extent are we justified in exposing our patients to a 50% risk of being given an experimental drug rather than a drug of proven prophylactic value? The very efficacy of lithium has turned out to be an impediment to the search for alternatives. Most studies on the latter have therefore been carried out on lithium nonresponders, and this is hardly satisfactory, because generalization is doubtful. When patients fail to respond to or do not tolerate therapy A and are thereafter given therapy B, this latter treatment almost unavoidably appears in the better light, for it cannot appear in a worse. Hence the claim that lithium is less effective in rapid cyclers than carbamazepine; they were never compared. Comparative conclusions can be based only on comparative trials with random allocation. Data analysis has revealed that blind trial designs are not of major importance in prophylactic studies (Schou et al. 1970), but random allocation of treatments undoubtedly is.

In future work on relapse prevention we must search for precise yet realistic operative definitions of not only response but gradations of response. We must use a variety of measures of prophylactic efficacy, including effects on life quality and social functioning during intervals. And we must investigate not only alternative treatments but also treatment combinations. Perhaps most important of all, we must combine prophylactic drug treatment with appropriate, individually tailored, psychological and social support. I believe it is in this latter field that the richest harvests can be reaped in terms of compliance, treatment efficacy, and the quality of treatment outcome as experienced by patients and family.

Safety

In the testing of drug safety, studies on animals are clearly indispensable, and it will be a major disaster for seriously ill patients if one day the more fanatical opponents to experimental animal work should get their way. On the other hand, animal studies can never replace close and careful clinical observation and laboratory monitoring of patients, especially when safety of long-term treatment is concerned.

The importance of single-case observations should not be overlooked, for they may alert attention and give clues to the design of systematic studies. But let me use this opportunity to warn against the lure of sensation-seeking alarm-crying. Nothing is easier than to use observation of a supposedly adverse reaction in a single or a few patients to gain glory by issuing warnings against the treatment. By cautioning, you prove yourself observant, responsible, and concerned with patient safety.

However, all too often warnings do not take into account the harm that may be inflicted on patients who because of the warnings are deprived of treatment that may be essential to their health and well-being, perhaps their survival. For some strange reason, persons who warn are never blamed for the unfortunate consequences of their action. On the contrary, it is well-nigh impossible to erase from memory, or from quoted references, one sensationally phrased warning, irrespective of the amount of reassuring evidence that may be collected and published afterwards.

As responsible physicians we should take a balanced view. A story of benefit is not complete without its counterpart tale of cost and risk, but cost and risk can only be assessed properly when seen in relation to the benefits conferred by giving the treatment and the risks involved in not giving it.

Lithium treatment has had its share of exigencies. As examples may be mentioned reports of development of blood dyscrasia, of the appearance of goiter or hypothyroidism, of adverse interaction with neuroleptics, and of the occurrence of morphological kidney changes. Each time such an observation was made, we had to ask ourselves: Is this caused by lithium, or is the finding coincidental? Do we perhaps buy the mental health of our patients at the expense of their blood-forming systems or thyroids or brains or kidneys?

The only way to answer such questions has been to collect more information, systematically and from many patients followed over a long time. Studies of this kind have taken up much of the lithium researchers' time, and in a way one can regret the consumption of effort and resources which perhaps could have been spent more profitably on studies of lithium's mode of action in the brain. On the other hand, work dealing with patient safety is not wasted, and it is gratifying to be able to conclude today that lithium treatment is a safe therapy provided a limited number of guidelines and precautions are followed.

Let me give two examples of adverse reactions to lithium, the first one real, the second imaginary. In the 1960s researchers in Denmark and Sweden (Schou et al. 1968; Sedvall et al. 1969) reported that lithium treatment may affect thyroid size and function. These findings have been confirmed in later studies, but the reported frequency of hypothyroidism ranges as widely as from 1% to 30%. This may have to do with geographical differences and with different definitions of what constitutes hypothyroidism. A major source of bewilderment is, however, that usually no distinction has been made between *incidence* and *prevalence*, that is, between the number of abnormalities that develop over a given period of time, in this instance time of exposure, and the number of abnormalities that are present in a population, in this case an exposed population, at a particular point of time.

Incidence studies have been carried out in Sweden and Denmark (Maarbjerg et al. 1987; Nilsson and Axelsson 1989; Smigan et al. 1984). They show that lithium-induced hypothyroidism requiring concurrent administration of thyroxine develops with a frequency of two cases per 100 years of lithium exposure. Other studies from other parts of the world may lead to different figures, but if they fail to distinguish between incidence and prevalence, nonsense and confusion are bound to ensue.

The second example deals with lithium and the kidneys. Observation in the 1970s of morphological changes in the kidneys of lithium-treated patients (Hestbech et al. 1977) generated grave concern among psychiatrists, who asked themselves whether patients given lithium for many years would eventually develop renal failure and die. Many centers decided to subject the matter to systematic scrutiny, and over the last decade the kidney function of more than 800 patients has been examined in longitudinal and of more than 2700 patients in cross-sectional studies.

I have reviewed the literature in detail (Schou 1988), and the outcome of the studies is remarkably clear and consistent. Study after study has shown that lithium treatment does not induce any change in the glomerular filtration rate. After more than 40 years of psychiatric lithium usage and after treatment of many thousands of patients, not a single case of renal failure has been observed which with any certainty can be ascribed to the therapy.

It has been known for many years that lithium may affect renal water handling. With the low lithium doses and serum levels in use today, this effect is moderate, but more importantly, rises in urine volume and falls in renal concentrating ability do not predict a fall of the glomerular filtration rate, for there is none. A large urine volume with complaints of frequent micturition may require that the lithium dose is reduced and the patient warned against dehydration, but a low renal concentrating ability does not constitute indication for discontinuing prophylactically effective and otherwise well-tolerated lithium treatment.

On the basis of the total evidence available today we may, indeed we must, conclude that lithium treatment, even when given for many years, does not lead to deterioration of the glomerular filtration rate, let alone renal failure. It is time that misleading and anxiety-inducing references to "the nephrotoxic effect of lithium" come to an end. Lithium treatment is not nephrotoxic, and psychiatrists can confidently use it for the benefit of their manic-depressive patients.

Concluding Comments

Efficacy and safety of long-term treatments are based on choice of drugs with the best possible benefit-risk ratio; they are no less dependent on best possible utilization of the drugs chosen. I have already referred to the value of combining drug treatment and supportive psychotherapy. When not in an episode, manic-depressive patients are not "sick," and to the extent of their ability they should be made coresponsible for the treatment that keeps them in health. This can be accomplished only when both physicians and patients are familiar with recommendations and caveats, with the "*do*'s" and "*don't*s" of the treatment. Nontechnical instruction books are available in several languages (Schou 1984a, b, 1986, 1987, 1990a, b, 1991a, b, 1993).

Recurrent mood disorders are devastating, dangerous, and disruptive for patient and family, and as responsible physicians we must do our utmost to combat them. Out patients are entitled to energetic, pragmatic, and sophisticated treatment.

References

Baastrup PC (1964) The use of lithium in manic-depressive psychosis. Compr Psychiatry 5: 396–408

Baastrup PC, Schou M (1967) Lithium as a prophylactic agent: its effect against recurrent depressions and manic-depressive psychosis. Arch Gen Psychiatry 16: 162–172

Baastrup PC, Poulsen JC, Schou M, Thomsen K, Amdisen A (1970) Prophylactic lithium: double-blind discontinuation in manic-depressive and recurrent-depressive disorder. Lancet 2: 326–330

Coppen A, Noguera R, Bailey J, Burns BH, Swani MS, Hare EH, Gardner R, Maggs R (1971) Prophylactic lithium in affective disorders: controlled trial. Lancet 2: 275–279

Hartigan GP (1963) The use of lithium salts in affective disorders. Br J Psychiatry 109: 810–814

Hestbech J, Hansen HE, Amdisen A, Olsen S (1977) Chronic renal lesions following long-term treatment with lithium salts. Kidney Int 12: 205–213

Hullin RP, McDonald R, Allsopp MNE (1972) Prophylactic lithium in recurrent affective disorders. Lancet 1: 1044–1046

Maarbjerg K, Vestergaard P, Schou M (1987) Changes in serum thyroxine and serum thyroid stimulating hormone during prolonged lithium treatment. Acta Psychiatr Scand 75: 217–221

Nilsson A, Axelsson R (1989) Effects of long-term lithium treatment on thyroid and renal function (serum creatinine and maximal urine osmolality) : a prospective study in psychiatric patients. Curr Ther Res 46: 85–102

Schou M (1956) Litiumterapi ved mani: Praktiske retningslinier. Nord Med 55: 790–794

Schou M (1984a) Le Lithium: Guide pratique pour les médecins et les patients. Presses Universitaires de France, Paris

Schou M (1984b) Lithium Treatment of Manic-Depressive Illness: A Practical Guide (Original title in Japanese). Igakushuppan-Sha, Tokyo

Schou M (1986) Il trattamento con litio della malattia maniaco-depressiva: una guida pratica. Athena Editrice, Roma

Schou M (1987) Lithium v léčbě maniodepresívního onemocnění. Avicenum, Praha

Schou M (1988) Effects of long-term lithium treatment on kidney function: An overview. J Psychiatr Res 22: 287–296

Schou M (1990a) Litiumbehandling av mano-depressiv sjukdom: En vägledning, 2nd edn. Astra, Södertälje

Schou M (1990b) Lithium Treatment of Manic-Depressive Illness: A Practical Guide (Original title in Greek). Zymel, Athens

Schou M (1991a) Lithiumbogen: Lithiumbehandling af manio-depressiv sygdom, 3rd edn. Welner & Rygaard, Copenhagen

Schou M (1991b) Lithium-Behandlung der manisch-depressiven Krankheit: Informationen für Arzt, Patient und Angehörige, 3rd edn. Thieme, Stuttgart

Schou M (1993) Lithium Treatment of Manic-Depressive Illness: A Practical Guide, 5th edn. Karger, Basel

Schou M, Amdisen A, Jensen SE, Olsen T (1968) Occurrence of goitre during lithium treatment. Br Med J 3: 710–713

Schou M, Thomsen K, Baastrup PC (1970) Studies on the course of recurrent endogenous affective disorders. Int Pharmacopsychiatry 5: 100–106

Sedvall G, Jönsson B, Pettersson U (1969) Evidence of an altered thyroid function in man during treatment with lithium carbonate. Acta Psychiatr Scand [Suppl] 207: 59–66

Smigan L, Wahlin A, Jacobsson L, von Knorring L (1984) Lithium therapy and thyroid function tests: a prospective study. Neuropsychobiology 11: 39–43

The Prophylaxis of Unipolar Depression

E.D. Peselow, D.L. Dunner, R.R. Fieve, and C. Di Figlia

Introduction

Over the last 15 years the focus of attention has shifted from the acute treatment of depression to long-term management of the depressive symptoms (Fieve and Peselow 1984). Since depression recurs, it is necessary to find treatments that lessen. the probability of relapses so that a patient will not have recurring depressive symptoms that interfere with his ability to function at his vocation or on an interpersonal basis. Since tricyclics are useful in acute depression, attempts were made to use these drugs to prevent relapse. In a comprehensive review of the literature Schou (1979) examined five double-blind studies of antidepressants vs placebo and noted a 35% relapse rate in 187 unipolar patients on tricyclics vs a 67% relapse rate in 187 unipolar patients on placebo over 1 year. In that same review, he examined nine double-blind studies of lithium carbonate, an agent with clear prophylactic action against recurrent bipolar and unipolar depression (Davis 1976) vs placebo in recurrent unipolar depression. Schou noted a depressive relapse rate of 22% in 76 unipolar patients on lithium, vs a 65% relapse rate in 77 unipolar patients on placebo. Though the numbers of patients are small and the definitions inexact (Task Force on Lithium Therapy 1975), the above evidence is strongly suggestive of the utility of these agents against recurrent unipolar depression.

Several questions remain to be answered. Is there any difference between lithium and antidepressants in the prophylaxis of unipolar depression? Does a lithium-antidepressant combination provide increased efficacy? Do these medications truly have a better chance than nothing of preventing a depressive episode? The purpose of this paper is two fold. First we will analyze through the longitudinal life-table method of Fleiss et al. (1976) and Mantel (1966) which of these treatments, lithium, antidepressants, a lithium-antidepressant combination, or placebo (or no treatment) given within the context of a naturalistic clinical setting, was most effective in the prophylaxis of unipolar illness. Second, and most important, using this longitudinal design, we will attempt to give the probability of remaining free of an affective episode over a 4-year course on these four treatments.

Method

The records of all patients who ever attended two outpatient facilities (The Foundation for Depression-Manic Depression and the New York State Lithium Clinic) through Jan 1, 1986 were examined (approximately 1400 patients in all). Patients selected for the study met Feighner et al.'s criteria (1972) for primary affective disorder, and Research Diagnostic Criteria, RDC (Spitzer et al. 1978) and DSM-III criteria (American Psychiatric Association 1980) for recurrent major depression. All patients had two discrete episodes of depression that had required previous treatment or hospitalization. All patients were seen at least once every month and rated by the Columbia-Milhauser Mood scale (a modified Biegel Mania scale; Biegel et al. 1971, Hamilton depression scale; Hamilton 1967), and a seven point global severity scale (one to three indicating severe, moderate, and mild depression, respectively, four indicating euthymia, and five to seven indicating mild, moderate, and severe mania, respectively).

To be included in the study, the patients had to have been observed and rated as having a euthymic mood and continued on the same regimen for 6 months. Once stable for 6 months on lithium, antidepressants, a lithium-antidepressant combination, or placebo (or no treatment), the patient was considered to have begun prophylaxis. While this time period is arbitrary (Quitkin et al. 1978), it is consistent with the work of Angst et al. (1979) who found the average length of time for a depressive episode to be 5.1 months. While some investigators required only 1 month of euthymia before assessing prophylaxis (Schou 1968; Fieve et al. 1975; Peselow et al. 1982), 6-months normothymia more definitively assures complete recovery and thus a subsequent depressive episode is a new attack rather than a continuation of an old one. The establishment of a 6-month normothymic period was important because it allowed for all patients to be brought to a common starting point, despite the fact that they entered the analysis at various points over a 10 year course.

Once stable on lithium (maintaining blood levels of 0.6–1.4 mEq/L), tricyclics (in this case amitriptyline or imipramine in doses of 75–300 mg/day – average dose 164 mg/day), lithium + tricyclics (amitriptyline or imipramine), or placebo (or no treatment) for 6 consecutive months the patients were then followed until one of three possible outcomes:

1. Termination well – if the patient remained continuously well until January 1, 1986 (the end of the study evaluation)
2. Failure – if the patient was rated depressed by the above global rating scales by both a nurse and a physician, and the symptoms were of such severity that the patient met RDC or DSM-III criteria for major depression and the patient now required either hospitalization or additional antidepressant treatment
3. Dropout

Since, as Fleiss et al. (1976) pointed out, it is impossible to know whether an individual dropped out well or dropped out because of depression, we made the same assumptions as Fleiss et al. (1976) and handled the dropouts in two ways. One assumption was that all dropouts failed (or had a depressive episode) in the month they dropped out. Fleiss considered this the pessimistic result as it gave the lowest probability of remaining free of a depressive episode. The other way to handle dropouts assumed that all dropouts left well, giving the optimistic result or highest probability of remaining free of a depressive episode. This method allows for the extreme ranges of probability with the true probability of remaining free of a depressive episode lying between the pessimistic (worst possible) and optimistic (best possible) results. For a complete description regarding calculations for the life-table and procedures for making statistical comparisons between life-tables from different samples, see Fleiss et al. (1976).

The decision as to which treatment a patient received varied. For about 10% of the cases the choice was made within the context of a double-blind placebo-controlled trial (lithium vs placebo). For the majority of patients, 90%, the treatment choice was open and based on clinical grounds. Clinical parameters used in determining treatment were past history of previous response to lithium, antidepressants, or lithium + antidepressants (in which case the treatment was used again), or sensitivity to side effects for these agents in which case another agent was used. Thus a severe tremor on lithium may have necessitated the use of antidepressants alone as prophylaxis. Individuals who received no treatment did so either because of severe side effects to the active agents or clinical stability on active treatment over several months time. As noted, all patients remained stable on the particular treatment that they received for 6 consecutive months prior to entry into the analysis. This indicated that they had responded to that particular treatment for an equivalent time period (6 months) with the presumption that they would continue to do equally well on the same treatment over longer time periods. Thus our clinical expectation, or bias, in this non-randomized evaluation as to choice of treatment was based on the hope of achieving the best possible result for the patient within a clinical setting.

In all, 61 patients on lithium alone, 75 patients on antidepressants alone, 56 patients on a lithium-antidepressants combination (lithium + amitriptyline, or lithium + imipramine), and 30 patients on either no treatment or placebo (20 patients on no treatment, 10 on placebo) were included in the analysis. The placebo-no treatment group will be analyzed separately and combined. All patients, following 6 months of euthymia, were evaluated over a 1 to 108-month-period (average time followed = 26.95 months, following 6 months of euthymia). All patients treated gave voluntary consent for treatment and for the accumulation of clinical data.

Results

Table 1 examines the demographic characteristics of the 222 total patients who were part of this analysis subdivided into four groups. As can be seen from this table, there was no difference among the four groups with respect to sex, age, and length of time depressed in the 2 years prior to treatment entry.

Table 1. Demographic characteristics of patients

	Lithium alone	Lithium and antidepressant combination	Antidepressants alone	Placebo or no treatment	Probability
No. of patients	61	56	75	30	
Males/females	19/42	23/33	38/37	13/17	$\chi^2 = 5.31$ 3 *df* $p = 0.15$
Age (years)	41.20 SD9.9	40.89 SD11.1	38.17 SD9.1	40.07 SD12.1	ANOVA (F(3,218) = 1.21 $p = 0.31$)
Average length of time depressed (months) prior 2 years	4.72 SD3.3	4.21 SD2.3	4.28 SD2.5	4.87 SD2.7	ANOVA (F(3,218) = 0.66 $p = 0.58$)
Average dose					
lithium (mmol/L)	0.87	0.83	154.4 (Imipramine)[b]		
antidepressant (mg)		160.7 (Imipramine)[a] 150.9 (Amitriptyline)[a]	174.3 (Amitriptyline)[b]		

[a] 28 Patients were on lithium + imipramine; 28 Patients were on lithium + amitriptyline.
[b] 40 Patients were on imipramine alone; 35 Patients were on amitriptyline alone.
SD, standard deviation; ANOVA, analysis of variance.

Table 2. Patients course during 6 month intervals

Interval (Months)	Starting interval well	Terminated well in interval	Dropped out in interval	Failed in interval	Probability of remaining well		
					Pessimistic result[a] %	Optimistic result[b] %	Average probability %
Lithium alone:							
Year 1	61	0	10	9	68.9	84.0	76.5
Year 2	42	2	5	9	45.4	64.8	55.1
Year 3	26	2	1	5	34.6	51.9	43.3
Year 4	18	0	1	1	30.7	48.9	39.8
Lithium + antidepressant combination:							
Year 1	56	1	10	8	67.8	83.7	75.8
Year 2	37	1	1	7	53.0	67.5	60.3
Year 3	28	2	2	5	39.0	53.8	46.4
Year 4	19	2	2	2	30.4	43.9	37.2
Antidepressants alone:							
Year 1	75	1	14	19	56.6	73.2	64.9
Year 2	41	1	4	8	41.1	59.8	50.5
Year 3	28	3	2	5	30.7	48.7	39.7
Year 4	18	2	2	2	23.2	42.7	33.0
Placebo or no treatment:							
Year 1	30	1	5	12	42.7	54.7	48.7
Year 2	12	1	1	4	24.7	35.0	29.9
Year 3	6	1	1	1	15.7	28.0	21.9
Year 4	3	0	0	1	10.5	18.7	14.6

[a] Pessimistic result: assuming dropouts failed in the interval they left treatment.
[b] Optimistic result: assuming dropouts left well.

Tables 2 evaluates the efficacy of the four groups with respect to prophylaxis against depression. Overall at each yearly interval, in this sample, it appears that lithium and the lithium-antidepressant combination are about 5%–10% more effective than the antidepressant alone (for either the pessimistic or optimistic outcome). However, at no point (1, 2, 3, or 4 years) did the trend in favor of lithium and the lithium-antidepressant combination over the antidepressant alone yield statistical significance, whether one assumed the optimistic or pessimistic result. Using the equation of Mantel (6), comparing the overall treatment using all points, one notes that there is no statistical difference in overall relapse rate among the three active treatments.

The pessimistic–optimistic probability for the no treatment group ($n = 20$) and placebo group ($n = 10$) were not significantly different (40.0%–55.6% for 1 year and 20.0%–39.7% for 2 years for the placebo group vs 45.0%–55.6% and 25.0%–34.7% for the no treatment group at 1 and 2 years respectively). Since these groups were not significantly different and since in essence both groups did not receive active prophylactic treatment, we combined the two groups and compared them against the active agents.

When one compares the three treatments (lithium, antidepressants, and the combination) versus the placebo-no treatment group at individual points over the 4 years (Table 2), one notes statistical significance for lithium and the lithium-antidepressant combination over the placebo-no treatment group at 1, 2, 3, and 4 years in both the optimistic and pessimistic cases. However, despite a trend, at all points, (1, 2, 3, or 4 years) the antidepressants alone were statistically superior to placebo-no treatment only at 2 years and 4 years if one

Table 3. Summary of clinical outcomes on the different treatment regimens

	Lithium alone	Lithium and antidepressant combination	Anti-depressants alone	Placebo or no treatment	Probability
No. of patients	61	56	75	30	
Course:					
Terminated well;					
<4 years	4	6	7	3	
>4 years	16	13	12	2	
					$\chi^2 = 5.20$ 6 *df* $p = 0.52$
Dropout <4 years	17	15	22	7	
Failed (had a depressive relapse)	24	22	34	18	
Average time (months) followed after 6 months' euthymia	31.03 SD29.0	30.52 SD27.3	25.25 SD26.4	15.73 SD21.1	ANOVA ($F(3.2181) = 2.67$ $p < 0.05$[a])

ANOVA, analysis of variance; SD, standard deviation.
[a] Statistically significant. Planned pairwise Fisher PLSD comparisons indicate that lithium and lithium-antidepressant groups remained euthymic statistically longer than the placebo-no treatment group ($p < 0.02$ for both lithium and lithium-antidepressant group vs placebo-no treatment).

assumed the optimistic result. At the other optimistic points (1 and 3 years) and at all pessimistic points the trend in favor of antidepressants alone vs placebo-no treatment did not reach statistical significance. In comparing the overall treatment using all points, lithium and the lithium-antidepressant combination were statistically superior to the placebo-no treatment group for both the pessimistic and optimistic cases. However, despite the trend, statistical significance was not achieved in the case of antidepressants alone over the placebo-no treatment group for either the pessimistic or optimistic cases.

The 4-year overall outcome (terminated well, dropout, or failure) indicated that the placebo-no treatment group had a greater percentage of dropouts and failures (total 83.3%) than the other three groups, but these differences over 4 years did not reach statistical significance (Table 3). The lithium and the lithium-antidepressant combination were able to remain euthymic for a longer period of time than the placebo-no treatment group.

Discussion

There have been very few controlled studies comparing lithium and antidepressants in the prophylaxis of unipolar illness (Table 4). Two studies (Prien et al. 1973; Glen et al. 1981) suggested that lithium was equal to antidepressants in prophylaxis with both agents being significantly better than placebo. Both studies, however, noted high relapse (33%–60%) rates despite active medication over 2–3 years of maintenance treatment.

Three other studies have yielded different conclusions. Coppen et al. (1976, 1978) compared lithium with two tetracyclic antidepressants – maprotiline and mianserin. In both cases lithium was statistically superior to the tetracyclic. Kane et al. 1982 looked at prophylactic efficacy over 2 years in 27 unipolar patients on lithium alone, lithium-imipramine combination, imipramine alone, and placebo. The conclusion, based on this small sample was that lithium did exert a statistically significant prophylactic effect versus placebo in unipolar illness whereas the antidepressant alone did not. The problem with the study was that the patients were followed for an average of 17 months and of the 13 patients in the four groups who remained free of a depressive episode, 11 were "terminated euthymic" before 2 years, as only two patients completed the designed 2-year trial free of a depressive episode.

The only study arguing against the prophylactic efficacy of lithium in unipolar illness was the NIMH study by Prien et al. (1984). In this study, of 148 patients who reached the maintenance phase (out of 343 patients who were treated for an index episode and for a minimum of 2 months after stability had been achieved), the relapse rate was 41% on imipramine alone, 32% on a lithium-imipramine combination, 57% on lithium alone, and 71% on placebo. Both imipramine and the lithium-imipramine combination were more effective than either lithium alone and placebo. However, the study did note that if the index episode that brought the patient into the study was not severe, lithium was

Table 4. Double-blind prophylactic studies in unipolar disorder

Study	Length (years)	No. of patients	Relapse rates			Comment
			Lithium	Anti-Depressant	Placebo	
Prien et al. (1973)	2	78	12/27 (44%)	12/25 (48%) (Imipramine)	24/26 (92%)	Li = Imi both > Pbo
Glen et al. (1981)	3	103 Severe depression	36/56 (64%)	31/47 (66%) (Amitripty-line)	–	Li = Ami only 19 pts completed 3-yr trial
		28 Mild depression	4/12 (33%)	4/7 (57%)	8/9 (89%)	Only 7/28 pts completed 3-yr trial
Kane et al. (1982)	2	27	2/7 (29%) Li alone 2/8 (25%) Li + imipramine combination	5/6 (83%) Imipramine	6/6 (100%)	Li > Pbo but Imi = Pbo only 2 pts completed 2-year trial. 11 pts terminated trial euthymic before 2 years
Coppen et al. (1976)	1	30	3/12 (25%) 3 dropouts	6/8 (75%) 7 dropouts (maprotiline)		Li > Maprotiline
Coppen et al. (1978)	1	41	0/15 (25%) 5 dropouts	7/13 (54%) 8 dropouts (mianserin)		Li > Mianserin
Prien et al. (1984)	2	148	21/37 (57%) Li alone 16/39 (41%) Li + imipramine combination	16/39 (41%) Imipramine	24/34 (71%)	Imi & Imi + Li combination > Li Li = Pbo only 54 pts stayed in trial and remained euthymic for greater than 1 yr

Li, lithium; Imi, imipramine; Pbo, placebo; pts, patients; Ami, amitriptyline.

not inferior to imipramine in preventing subsequent prophylactic efficacy. It must be noted that a significant percentage of patients who remained well terminated euthymic before the end of the study, as only 54 patients completed greater than 1 year of the designed 2-year trial free of a depressive episode.

The findings of our naturalistic life-table analysis suggest a slight trend in favor of lithium and the lithium-antidepressant combination versus antidepressants alone in the prophylaxis of unipolar illness. Obviously any conclusions regarding the relative efficacy among these treatments must be tentative based on the non-random and open design of the treatment. However a striking finding is evident from the analysis. It appears that despite active treatment acknowledged as efficacious (Consensus Development Panel 1985), relapses still occurred. Overall, 24 out of 61 patients (39.3%) on lithium alone, 34 out of 75 patients (45.3%) on antidepressants alone, 22 out of 56 patients (39.3%) on a lithium-antidepressants combination (lithium + amitriptyline or lithium + imipramine) were known to have a depressive episode that required either hospitalization or additional antidepressant treatment. Of particular note here are the findings at 2 years with a large percentage of the group still remaining. The 2-year average probability of remaining free of a depressive episode for all patients who took medication was 55% for patients on lithium alone, 50.5% for patients on antidepressants alone, and 60% for patients on a lithium-antidepressants combination. This was in agreement with the comprehensive review by Prien (1987), who, in examining six studies (Table 4) noted a combined 52% relapse rate on lithium and a 58% rate on antidepressants. Though our probability on active treatment was better than the 2-year average probability of 30% on placebo or no treatment it is hardly a panacea. Is a 20%–25% improvement in decreased frequency of depressive symptoms worth the risk of possible long-term effects such as lithium kidney toxicity (Jenner 1979) in addition to the troublesome anticholinergic and cardiovascular side effects of antidepressants (Boston Colloborative Drug Surveillance Program 1972).

Further systematic double-blind studies and naturalistic observations over longer time periods need to be carried out to determine the most efficient prophylactic treatment of unipolar illness. Since these agents are routinely prescribed for even longer periods of time than those studied, the above answers are sorely needed to allow clinicians to make adequate decisions concerning the risk/benefit ratio of prophylactic treatment for patients with recurrent unipolar depression.

References

American Psychiatric Association (1980) Diagnostic and statistical manual of mental disorders, 3rd edn American Psychiatric Association, Washington.

Angst J, Felder W, Frey R (1979) The course of unipolar and bipolar affective states. In: Schou M, Stromgren E (eds) Origin, prevention and treatment of affective disorders. Academic, London, pp 215–226

Biegel A, Murphy DL, Bunney WE (1971) The manic rating scale. Arch Gen Psychiatry 25: 256–262

Boston Collaborative Drug Surveillance Program (1972) Adverse reactions to tricyclic antidepressants. Lancet 1: 529–531

Consensus Development Panel (1985) Mood disorders: pharmacologic prevention of recurrences. Am J Psychiatry 142: 469–476

Coppen A, Montgomery SA, Gupta RK, Bailey JE (1976) A double-blind comparison of lithium and maprotiline in the prophylaxis of affective disorders. Br J Psychiatry 128: 479–485

Coppen A, Ghose K, Rao R, Bailey JE, Peet M (1978) Mianserin and lithium in the prophylaxis of depression. Br J Psychiatry 133: 206–210

Davis JM (1976) Overview: maintenance therapy in psychiatry: II. Affective disorders. Am J Psychiatry 133: 1–13

Feighner JP, Robins E, Guze S, Woodruff RA, Winokur G, Munoz R (1972) The use of research criteria in psychiatry. Arch Gen Psychiatry 26: 57–63

Fieve RR, Peselow ED (1984) Treatment of affective disorders. In: Endler NS, Hunt JM (eds) Personality and behavior disorders, vol 2. Wiley, New York, pp 975–1011

Fieve RR, Dunner DL, Kumbarachi T (1975) Lithium carbonate in affective disorders. A double-blind study of prophylaxis in recurrent unipolar depression. Arch Gen Psychiatry 32: 1541–1545
Fleiss JL, Dunner DL, Stallone F, Fieve RR (1976) The life-table: a method for analyzing longitudinal studies. Arch Gen Psychiatry 33: 107–112
Glen AMI, Johnson AL, Shepard M (1981) Continuation therapy with lithium and amitriptyline in unipolar depressive illness. A controlled clinical trial. Psychol Med 11: 409–416
Hamilton M (1967) Development of a rating scale for primary depressive illness. Br J Clin Psychol 6: 278–296
Jenner FA (1979) Lithium and the question of kidney damage. Arch Gen Psychiatry 36: 888–890
Kane JM, Quitkin F, Rifkin A, Ramos-Lorenzi JR, Nayak D, Howard A (1982) Lithium carbonate and imipramine in the prophylaxis of unipolar and bipolar illness. Arch Gen Psychiatry 39: 1065–1069
Mantel N (1966) Evaluation of survival data and two new rank order statistics arising from its consideration. Cancer Chem other Rep 50: 163–170
Peselow ED, Dunner DL, Fieve RR, Lautin A (1982) Lithium prophylaxis of depression in unipolar, bipolar II, and cyclothymic patients. Am J Psychiatry 139: 747–752
Prien RF (1987) Long-term treatment of affective disorders. In: Meltzer HY (ed) Psychopharmacology - the third generation of progress. Raven, New York, pp 1051–1059
Prien RF, Caffey EM, Klett CJ (1973) Lithium carbonate and imipramine in the prevention of affective episodes: a comparison in recurrent affective illness. Arch Gen Psychiatry 28: 337–341
Prien RF, Kupfer DJ, Mansky PA, Small JG, Tuason VB, Voss CB, Johnson WE (1984) Drug therapy in the prevention of recurrences in unipolar and bipolar affective disorders. Arch Gen Psychiatry 41: 1096–1104
Quitkin F, Rifkin A, Kane J, Ramos-Lorenzi JR, Klein DF (1978) Prophylactic effect of lithium and imipramine in unipolar and bipolar II patients. Am J Psychiatry 135: 570–572
Schou M (1968) Lithium in psychiatric therapy and prophylaxis. J Psychiatr Res 6: 67–95
Schou M (1979) Lithium as a prophylactic agent in unipolar depression. Arch Gen Psychiatry 36: 847–849
Spitzer R, Endicott J, Robins E (1978) Research diagnostic criteria: rationality and reliability. Arch Gen Psychiatry 35: 773–782
Task Force on Lithium Therapy (1975) The current status of lithium therapy. Report of the APA Task Force. Am J Psychiatry 132: 997–1001

Maintenance Therapies in Recurrent Depression: Psychotherapy and Combined Treatment*

E. Frank, D.J. Kupfer, and T. Hamer

Introduction

Unipolar illness follows a recurrent and episodic course for the majority of individuals afflicted (Angst 1973; Keller et al. 1982). A single episode of depression is disabling and often entails considerable economic cost and personal suffering; however, recurrent depression constitutes a major public health problem (Wells et al. 1989). Thus, the identification and prophylactic treatment of individuals who have a history of repeated episodes of depression should be high clinical priorities. The advent of well-defined diagnostic criteria has made the identification of the recurrent patient less difficult once the individual presents for treatment in a psychiatric setting. Unfortunately, however, many recurrent depressives accept their frequent episodes as natural, if debilitating, mood variation, never thinking to seek treatment for them. Still others are seen in general medical settings, treated for each acute episode and discharged, only to suffer another recurrence.

The last decade has seen increasing interest in the prophylaxis of future depressive episodes. In 1984, Prien et al. reported on 150 unipolar patients treated in a 2-year maintenance study. These patients were assigned to one of four maintenance treatment groups: (1) active imipramine and active lithium, (2) active imipramine, (3) active lithium, or (4) placebo. Also in 1984, Glen et al. published the results of a study of 131 unipolar patients followed in a 3-year maintenance trial in which they were assigned to one of three treatment groups: (1) active amitriptyline, (2) active lithium, or (3) placebo. A more recent study by Montgomery et al. (1988) analyzed 182 completers of a 1-year prophylactic study comparing an active fluoxetine treatment group to a placebo treatment group.

When considered in terms of the lifetime prognosis for the recurrent unipolar patient, the results of these studies have been quite discouraging. In the Prien et al. (1984) study, of the 88 unipolar patients whose index episode was considered severe, the most effective treatment group – active imipramine – had only a 48% success rate for the maintenance phase. The maintenance success rate for the severe recurrent depressives in the Glen et al. study was 32% for the active amitriptyline treatment group and only 30% for the active lithium

---

* Portions of this chapter have been excerpted from Frank (1991) and Frank et al. (1989, 1990)

treatment group. The Montgomery et al. (1988) study of fluoxetine vs placebo demonstrated 74% prophylaxis for the fluoxetine-treated group; however, 43% of the placebo-treated group also survived the year without a new episode of illness. This may be because only one previous episode within the last 5 years was required for study participation in the Montgomery et al. study and may have resulted in a less vulnerable population than those studied by Prien et al. and Glen et al.

The clear need for improved maintenance treatment strategies for patients with recurrent unipolar disorder led us to consider combined treatment approaches. The favorable findings of Klerman, Weissman and colleagues (Weissman et al. 1974; Klerman et al. 1974) and Simons (Simons et al. 1986) when psychotherapy was added to short-term or continuation treatment regimens suggested the possible value of combining one of the depression-specific psychotherapeutic approaches to maintenance pharmacotherapy. Because of the pronounced deficits in social adjustment we had observed even in those patients who remained well for 2 years (D.J. Kupfer and E. Buzzinoti, personal communication) in the Prien et al. (1984) protocol, we elected to modify interpersonal psychotherapy (Klerman et al. 1984) for use in a maintenance format in the hope of improving social adjustment and, thus, providing additional protection against future episodes.

Study Design

Our maintenance study of tricyclic antidepressants (imipramine hydrochloride) and the interpersonal psychotherapy (IPT) of Klerman et al. (1974, 1984) was designed to explore the relative efficacy of pharmacotherapy, a maintenance form of IPT, and their combination in the prevention of new episodes among patients at high risk of recurrence. The availability of data on those patients who experienced early recurrences in treatment cells involving no active medication offered an opportunity to ascertain whether specific pharmacological variables, clinical variables, or both might be responsible for the differential length of time to recurrence following withdrawal of medication. Since a majority of patients studied had onsets before the age of 30 years, all patients had had at least three previous episodes, and all had been well for 20 weeks at the time medication was discontinued, we anticipated that we would uncover other predictors of the length of the well interval once changes were made in the patients' medication regimen (Mindham et al. 1973). Several hypotheses were testable in this design. In particular, it was anticipated that patients with some residual symptoms, those taking particularly high dosages at the end of continuation treatment, and those who were also withdrawn from psychotherapy would show the earliest recurrence when withdrawn from active drug treatment.

To enter the maintenance therapies in recurrent depression protocol, subjects between the ages of 21 and 65 years were required to be seen initially in their third or greater episode of unipolar depression, with the immediately preceding episode being no more than 2 1/2 years before the onset of the present episode. A minimum Hamilton Rating Scale for Depression (HRSD) score of 15 and a minimum Raskin score of 7 were also required.

After a 2-week drug-free wash-out period, subjects were reevaluated with respect to severity of depression and then given a complete initial evaluation, which included biologic (all-night sleep electroencephalographic and neuroendocrine studies) and psychosocial (social adjustment and social support) measures. All subjects then received the same short-term treatment regimen consisting of imipramine hydrochloride (150–300 mg) and IPT (Klerman et al. 1984). Psychotherapy sessions were scheduled weekly for 12 weeks, then biweekly for 8 weeks, and then monthly. At whatever point in this short-term treatment regimen the patient had maintained a HRSD (Hamilton 1960) score of 7 or less and a Raskin (Raskin et al. 1969) score of 5 or less for 3 consecutive weeks, a second biologic and psychosocial evaluation was completed. Patients then continued receiving treatment for an additional 17 weeks, during which both HRSD and Raskin scores and imipramine dosages were required to remain stable. A third evaluation was then conducted, after which patients were randomly assigned to one of the five maintenance treatments described above for 3 years, or until they experienced a recurrence of illness.

A number of features of this research design were intended to maximize the probability that the question of treatment efficacy could be answered. First, since the period of the experimental study was to be 3 years, we increased the probability of observing recurrences during that period by including only those patients who were in at least their third episode of major depression, with the immediately previous episode being no more than 2 1/2 years earlier. Second, to obtain a relatively "pure" population, in which clear remissions and recurrences of illness could be observed, "double depressives" were excluded by our requirement that patients report a symptom-free interval of at least 10 weeks since their last episode. Third, in the hope that we could be certain that the index episode was fully treated and that any new episode of illness observed once our experimental manipulation began could be characterized as a recurrence rather than a relapse into the index episode, we required that patients remain relatively symptom-free (a HRSD score of ≤ 7 and a Raskin score of ≤ 5) for 20 weeks before entry into the experimental maintenance therapy phase of the study. Finally, so as not to bias patients regarding the probable efficacy of any of the five maintenance treatments to be studied, all patients were treated with the combination of drugs and psychotherapy throughout the short-term and continuation treatment phases.

Individual dosages of medication for continuation therapy were arrived at by using two guiding principles based on our clinical experience with more than 250 patients with recurrent depression – a target dose and a minimum plasma level. In general, the target dose was 200 mg. Dosages given to patients were typically raised in 50-mg increments over 3 weeks to a dosage of 200 mg. If the patient experienced substantial side effects, the dosage was lowered by 25- or 50-mg steps in an attempt to achieve comfort while still maintaining therapeutic effect; however, in no case was a patient permitted to enter the continuation phase with a combined imipramine-desimipramine hydrochloride plasma level of 125 ng/ml or less. If the patient failed to achieve remission at the 200-mg level, the dosage was adjusted upward in 50-mg steps to as high as 400 mg; however, in no instance was a patient permitted to remain on a dosage that resulted in a combined imipramine-desimipramine plasma level of 800 ng/ml or more.

Once the patients were assigned to maintenance therapy, the drug withdrawal schedules varied slightly depending on the actual number of pills the patient was taking at the time of random assignment. The general principle shaping the withdrawal schedule was a reduction of 33% per week for the first 3 weeks following random assignment. Thus, a patient receiving 300 mg would be reduced to receiving 200 mg by the end of the first week, to 100 mg by the end of the second week, and to all placebo or no pills by the end of the third week. The pharmacologic data for this report were drawn from determinations made at the last two clinic visits before maintenance treatment assignment.

Twenty six patients were assigned to maintenance interpersonal psychotherapy (IPT-M) alone cell, 26 were assigned to the IPT-M plus placebo cell, and 22 were assigned to the medication clinic with placebo cell.

Onset of a new episode during maintenance therapy was declared according to the following protocol. Any time a patient presented a state of substantial clinical worsening, the patient was observed and evaluated twice within a 7-day period. If the independent clinical evaluator and the treating clinician judged that the patient met the Research Diagnostic Criteria for major depressive disorder and the independent evaluator rated the patient as having the minimum HRSD (≥ 15) and Raskin (≥ 7) severity scores on both occasions, the patient was then seen by an independent senior psychiatrist, "blinded" to the patient's treatment assignment. A new episode was confirmed only when the scale evaluations completed by the independent evaluator and the clinical evaluation of the senior psychiatrist both indicated the presence of an episode of major depression. At the point of recurrence, the mean HRSD score for the patients described in this report was 21.9 (± 4.8) and the median score was 21.

The present report is intended to: (1) describe how IPT was adapted for use as a maintenance treatment (IPT-M), (2) describe IPT-M, (3) describe its application in a population of recurrent depressives, and (4) provide the results regarding the efficacy of IPT-M in the prevention of recurrence of depressive episodes from the Maintenance Therapies in Recurrent Depression protocol.

What Is Interpersonal Psychotherapy?

IPT (Klerman et al. 1984) is most commonly thought of as a well-defined, short-term intervention directed specifically at the amelioration of depressive symptoms; however, the first study of its efficacy occurred in what was described as a "maintenance" trial (Klerman et al. 1974; Weissman et al. 1974). This investigation, which today might be considered a continuation treatment trial, examined the effects of 8 months of psychotherapy in comparison to continued pharmacotherapy in depressed women who had remitted following 6–8 weeks of amitriptyline therapy. Until the present investigation, that study was the only controlled trial reported in the literature examining the *prophylactic* efficacy of psychotherapy.

IPT grows out of the work of the interpersonal and cultural schools; however, the therapeutic goals of IPT are somewhat different from those espoused by either school. The influence of early developmental experiences on adult patterns of interpersonal relationships is acknowledged, but reconstruction of the patient's early experiences is not considered essential for therapeutic response or protection against relapse or recurrence. IPT focuses on current interpersonal relationships, on the assumption that interpersonal experiences in the patient's family of origin are reflected in current interpersonal attitudes and behavior. IPT attempts to improve functioning within interpersonal relationships, not to restructure the patient's personality or character. This strategy is based on the premise that depression, regardless of biological vulnerability or personality traits, occurs in a psychosocial and interpersonal context. Exploration of the context associated with the onset of depression and examination of the possibility of renegotiating difficulties in current psychosocial/interpersonal domains are viewed as essential to recovery from a depressive episode. IPT helps the patient to develop more adaptive coping strategies for social and interpersonal problems associated with the onset of depressive symptoms. These major goals are achieved by (1) determining with the patient which of four common problems (grief, interpersonal disputes, role transitions, or interpersonal deficits) are related to the patient's index episode and (2) working with the patient to resolve the difficulties he or she is experiencing in the most prominent problem area.

In summary, the nature of IPT is interpersonal, as opposed to intrapsychic. The focus is on the present as opposed to early developmental experiences. The overall goals of treatment are to encourage mastery of current social roles and adaptation to problematic interpersonal interactions. A complete description of the development, goals, and strategies of IPT can be found in *Interpersonal Psychotherapy of Depression* (Klerman et al. 1984).

The Development of IPT-M

In adapting IPT to a maintenance format, it was critical that as much rigor be applied in the development of the maintenance treatment as the originators of IPT had employed in the development of the acute treatment strategies. We therefore began with the writing of a pilot treatment manual. This pilot manual was based largely on Klerman et al.'s *Interpersonal Psychotherapy Manual* since their book, *Interpersonal Psychotherapy of Depression*, (Klerman et al. 1984) had not yet been published.

Initial modifications in the manual focused on the following differences between IPT and the planned maintenance treatment: (1) according to the design of the study in which we planned to use IPT-M, all patients entering maintenance treatment would be fully remitted for a period of 20 weeks, (2) the goal of IPT-M was to maintain remission rather than to bring it about, and (3) the length of treatment would be 3 years, assuming the patient remained well. While retaining the four problem areas which distinguish IPT, as well as emphasizing a largely "here-and-now" orientation, we recognized that the number of problem areas likely to become the focus of one patient's treatment was greater than is the case in acute IPT and that the timing of the treatment sessions would have to be altered to suit the goals and the length of the planned maintenance treatment. We therefore settled on a more expansive treatment scope than had been possible in IPT and on a pattern of less frequent therapeutic contacts.

Only clinicians who had been trained by Dr. Bruce Rounsaville or Ms. Eve Chevron of the Yale University Depression Research Unit and who had been certified as competent acute IPT therapists by Drs. Klerman and Weissman were chosen for the pilot-testing of IPT-M. Each therapist was required to read the pilot manual and to attend several group meetings conducted by one of the authors (E.F.) at which both general issues of maintenance treatment and the specific application of IPT to maintenance treatment were discussed. Following this initial preparation, each therapist was required to treat a minimum of two pilot IPT-M cases for a period of 18 months, (i.e., 18 maintenance sessions of 45- to 50-min duration). Patients chosen as pilot IPT-M cases were fully remitted recurrent unipolar depressives who had previously been treated with a combination of imipramine (150-300 mg per day), and weekly IPT. All of these patients were continued on their acute treatment dose of imipramine throughout the maintenance treatment.

During the pilot-testing period, therapists met on a weekly basis in a group supervision format with Cleon Cornes, M.D., who had been certified as an acute IPT trainer by the Yale University training group. All pilot IPT-M sessions were videotaped in order to provide material for the group supervision sessions. Group supervision emphasized adherence to the basic techniques and strategies of IPT as well as exploration of dynamics peculiar to therapeutic intervention with patients in remission (see below).

Pilot sessions were also audiotaped in order to provide independent raters an opportunity to monitor the content of IPT-M sessions using a psychotherapy rating scale developed especially for this project (Frank 1985). The treatment offered by IPT-M therapists was thus monitored and standardized to a criterion equivalent to those sessions which had been judged acceptable IPT sessions by the Yale University supervisors (Dr. Rounsaville and Ms. Chevron).

Thus, the major requirements for the testing of a psychotherapy in a refined controlled trial methodology were met in the pilot testing of IPT-M. First, the treatments were standardized and monitored both openly (in the group sessions) and independently (by objective raters) to ensure treatment integrity. Treatment sessions were of comparable length (45–50 min) and all patients received the same number of sessions at the same frequency. Therapists were deemed to be both appropriate to the patient population (inasmuch as each had had extensive experience in treating depressed outpatients and had successfully delivered acute IPT treatment to the patients on whom IPT-M was being piloted) and competent in the specific therapy (inasmuch as each therapist had been certified as an IPT therapist and, in addition, was well acquainted with the goals of IPT-M).

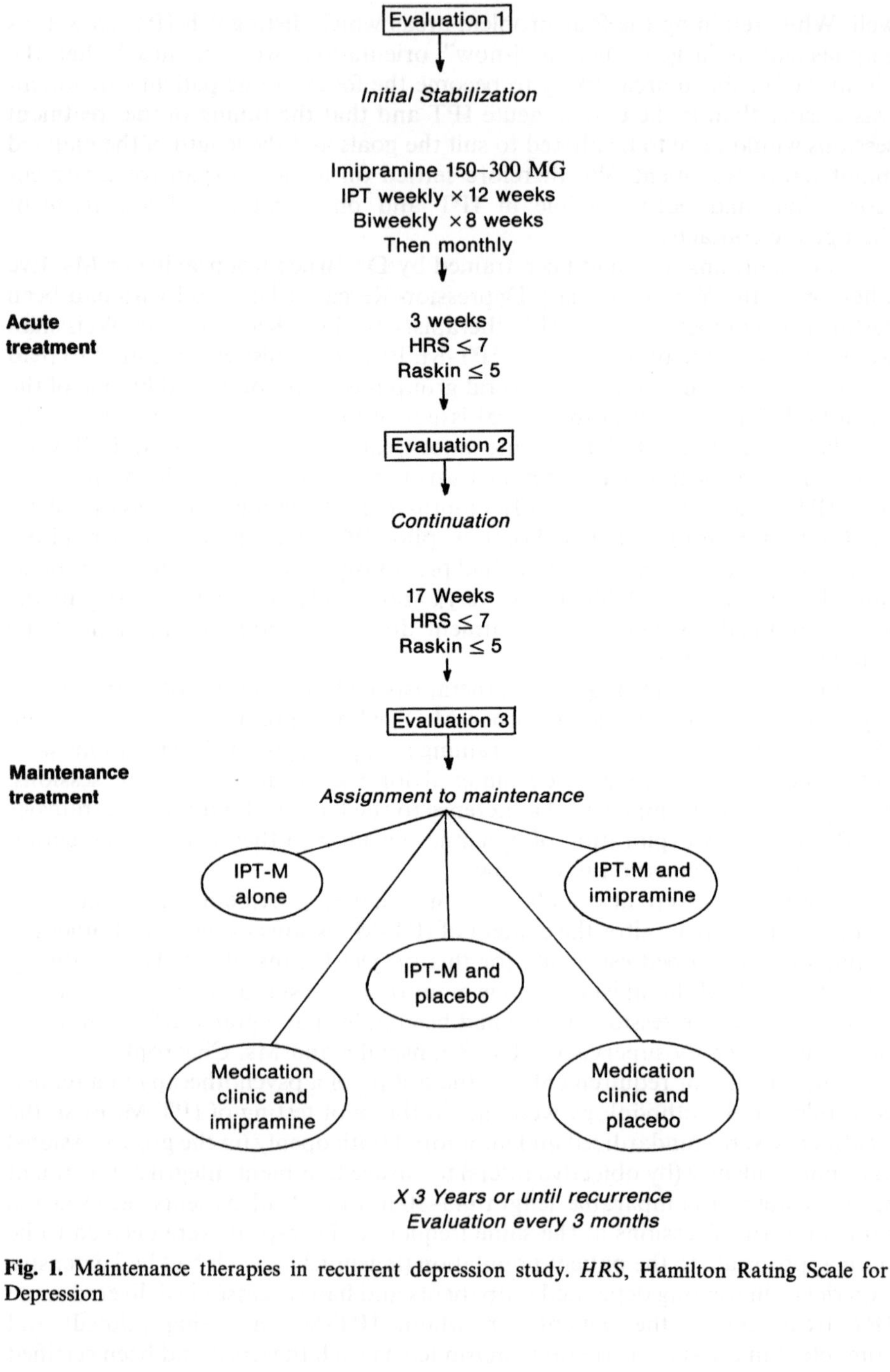

Fig. 1. Maintenance therapies in recurrent depression study. *HRS*, Hamilton Rating Scale for Depression

IPT-M was modified from IPT specifically for use in the Maintenance Therapies in Recurrent Depression protocol (Fig. 1). This protocol, which has been described in detail elsewhere (Frank and Kupfer 1985; Frank et al. 1989), involves acute, continuation, and maintenance treatment of individuals who have had a minimum of three episodes of unipolar depression. Patients are treated acutely with imipramine (150–300 mg per day) and weekly IPT. When a stable remission (HRSD <7, Raskin <5) had been sustained for 20 weeks (during which medication dose is constant, but frequency of psychotherapy sessions is gradually reduced to biweekly and then monthly), patients were randomly assigned to one of five maintenance treatment cells (IPT-M alone, IPT-M with active imipramine, IPT-M with placebo, medication clinic visit with active imipramine, or medication clinic visit with placebo). The description of IPT-M which follows is based on the treatment experience of eight IPT-M therapists with over 90 maintenance treatment cases.

Description of IPT-M

The treatment format of IPT-M draws extensively upon IPT as developed by Klerman and colleagues (Klerman et al. 1984). However, while IPT-M employs all of the strategies of IPT, it differs from IPT in its goals, in the number of problem areas typically addressed with an individual patient and in its timing. In addition, due to the length of treatment, IPT-M therapists, although not attempting to restructure personality in the traditional psychoanalytic sense, often focus on long-standing patterns of interpersonal behavior which appear to be nonadaptive for the patient.

Goals of IPT-M

Since IPT-M begins with patients who are fully remitted, its goal is the maintenance of the remitted state. For this reason, the therapist is vigilant for early signs of interpersonal problems similar to those which the patient and therapist had previously identified as associated with the onset of the patient's most recent depressive episode. The patient and therapist also watch for signs similar to those which preceded earlier episodes of depression. The therapist works towards enhancing those strengths which appear to have been present prior to the patient's illness and/or which began to emerge as the most recent depressive episode remitted. The patient is also encouraged to be on the alert for early warning signs in the noninterpersonal realm. This is accomplished by occasionally focusing discussion on the particular somatic and cognitive symptoms which marked the early stages of prior episodes. When those symptoms are reported to the IPT-M therapist, the therapist and patient together plan strategies for the prevention of the emergence of a new episode, basing those strategies largely in the interpersonal realm and focusing on interpersonal techniques for improving the patient's mood and functioning.

Problem Areas in IPT-M

In IPT, typically only one, or at most, two major problem areas are addressed. In IPT-M, which was designed as a 3-year course of therapy, it is virtually impossible and clearly undesirable to restrict the therapy to a single problem area. During the course of acute treatment, a large number of interpersonal themes emerge which do not become the focus of treatment. The therapist, however, notes these additional themes and reserves them for possible exploration in IPT-M. In almost all instances, IPT-M focuses on a combination of role transitions, role disputes, and interpersonal deficits. As in acute IPT, emphasis is placed on elicitation of feelings and nonjudgemental exploration of the affective quality of relationships.

Individuals faced with *role transitions* are helped to view the new role in the most positive, least restrictive manner. They are encouraged, whenever possible, to see the new role as an opportunity for growth and are helped by the therapist to regain their self-esteem and sense of mastery in relation to the demands of the new role. Patients are guided to a realistic evaluation of what has been lost in the transition and are encouraged to develop a social support system and a repertoire of social skills that can be called upon in the new role.

A majority of the IPT-M patients we have treated needed to address the role transition they made from depressed individual to well individual. For some, this is a relatively easy transition; for others, some of whom may have had many years of recurrent episodes, the experience of remaining consistently well for a long period of time is a new one both for the patient and his or her significant others. Adapting to this new experience, and to the exciting, but often frightening possibilities and responsibilities which go along with being fully well, can require considerable therapeutic work. Long-term commitments which the patient felt uncomfortable making in the past are now possible. Likewise, family members and co-workers may now demand more than the patient can confidently provide.

As we have noted elsewhere (Frank et al. 1987) about one half of the patients reaching the maintenance phase of the Maintenance Therapies protocol, have essentially normal personality profiles when assessed in a remitted state, either by self-report using the Hirschfeld-Klerman Personality Battery (Hirschfeld et al. 1983) or by clinician rating using the Personality Assessment Form developed for the Treatment of Depression Collaborative Research Program (Elkin et al. 1985). The other half of the patient group which enters maintenance treatment displays clinically significant personality pathology, especially avoidant and dependent features. Those individuals who are free of personality pathology have typically viewed themselves (and been viewed by their significant others) at the point of entry into maintenance treatment as "well persons" who occasionally experience episodes of dysfunction. These patients experience no role transition as they move into the maintenance phase of the study. On the other hand, patients with long-standing personality difficulties are likely to find the "well" role more unfamiliar. Their new-found energy and assertiveness often creates a temporary disequilibrium in their interpersonal realm, as does any role transition. This transition then becomes at least a temporary focus of IPT-M.

When *interpersonal disputes* are present, the therapist helps the patient to identify the nature of the dispute, guides him or her in making choices about a plan of action, and encourages the patient to modify maladaptive communication patterns if that is possible. When such modification cannot be accomplished or is not desirable, the patient is encouraged to reassess expectations for the relationship.

Because patients in IPT-M are seen over such a long period of time, interpersonal disputes often develop. These may occur in the context of marriage, family, work, or social settings; however, IPT techniques are easily applied as these interpersonal disputes occur. Our IPT-M experience has indicated that one or two relationships in the patient's life typically emerge as those which are occasionally or chronically fraught with difficulty. Having the opportunity to work with the patient on these relationships over a long period of time enables both the therapist and the patient to recognize characteristic negative, destructive patterns of interaction early in their development, to disrupt those dysfunctional patterns before they become engrained (or, as is often the case, re-engrained), and to try out new patterns of interaction.

For patients whose *interpersonal deficits* do not ameliorate with the resolution of the depressive episode during acute IPT treatment, IPT-M therapists work to reduce patients' social isolation and enhance the quality of any existing relationships. In the acute treatment phase of our study, when there were no current meaningful relationships, the focus of treatment was on past relationships, the relationship with the therapist, and the tentative forming of new relationships. In IPT-M, as in the Stage 2 work described with IPT patients showing interpersonal deficits (Klerman et al. 1984), emphasis is placed on helping the patient apply what is learned in treatment to outside situations in order to facilitate the development of new relationships. Each attempt at a new relationship, successful or not, is analyzed in terms of correctable deficits in the patient's communication skills and interpersonal style.

Although some of the patients treated in the Maintenance Therapies protocol appear to have essentially no interpersonal deficits when they are well, as noted above, many others fall into the avoidant/dependent personality spectrum (Frank et al. 1987). Many of these patients need encouragement to decrease their social isolation, increase their social interaction, and, in general, to pay more attention to their interpersonal needs. Some patients may need to form more independent, self-reliant, styles in order to not feel at the mercy of others in their interpersonal sphere. The long course of IPT-M provides a secure base from which patients can experiment with new interpersonal styles and they can bring their questions and concerns about the success of the experimentation into the therapy.

Grief reactions are rarely a focus in IPT-M unless a death occurs during the course of maintenance treatment. In that event, the strategies employed parallel those used in IPT, with the exception that the therapist emphasizes the normality of the symptoms the patient is experiencing and attempts to clarify distinctions between a normal grief reaction and a depressive episode. As noted above, on rare occasions, a loss during the course of maintenance treatment can reveal unresolved feelings about an earlier death. In this instance, the IPT-M therapist employs the strategies suggested by Klerman et al. (1984) for treatment of unresolved grief reactions.

The Timing of IPT-M

The timing of sessions in IPT-M differs from that in IPT. Because patients are asymptomatic, the projected treatment length is several years, and the goal is the prevention of new episodes rather than remission of current symptoms, IPT-M is scheduled on a once-a-month basis.

We noted two kinds of responses on the part of patients to the once-a-month scheduling. While the majority of patients had a smooth transition from IPT to IPT-M, some patients perceived the decreased contact as a loss and experienced difficulty in moving from the weekly IPT sessions, through the transition period of bi-weekly sessions called for in the study protocol, to a final schedule of monthly sessions. Several patients initially approached the monthly sessions with a defeatist attitude: What can be accomplished when we meet so infrequently? Others were directly or indirectly hostile, expressing anger either at the therapist or at the research protocol for reducing the frequency of visits. In such instances, the patient's discouragement or anger sometimes led to adopting a "reporting" stance in the first few monthly sessions. When this occurred, therapists raised this as a therapeutic issue. Patients ultimately resolved their discomfort in moving to monthly sessions and returned, generally within one to two sessions, to serious therapeutic work.

When, in one of the early monthly sessions, patients return to the therapeutic focus of his or her earlier IPT experience, the therapists reinforces these efforts by commenting that it is to the patient's credit that he or she is independently continuing to work on an issue raised many months earlier. A surprising aspect of the transition from IPT to IPT-M has been the sizable group of patients who made major therapeutic breakthroughs as a result of moving from weekly to monthly contact. These individuals seemed to benefit from the longer distance between therapy sessions and seemed able to bring richer material to the therapy sessions as a direct consequence of having had more time between sessions to think about and observe the interpersonal context of their lives and to experiment with new interpersonal behaviors.

Acceptance of IPT-M

Prior to conducting the Maintenance Therapies protocol, both the investigators and their consultants had some questions as to whether it would be possible to maintain a therapeutic relationship on a once-a-month basis. Both therapists and patients wondered whether the therapy sessions would deteriorate to mere diaries of those events which occurred over the course of the preceding month.

Concerns were also raised as to whether a true therapeutic relationship could be maintained throughout the course of a 3-year, once-a-month protocol. As noted above, one consistent problem focus is neither possible nor sensible in IPT-M; however, patients and therapists can and do maintain a consistent therapeutic relationship on a once-a-month basis. The monthly IPT-M sessions conducted in the maintenance phase of our protocol have the therapeutic intensity of IPT sessions. It is noteworthy, however, that while the typical IPT-M treatment session may seem to "jump" from problem area to problem area, the particular nature of the role transition, role dispute, or interpersonal deficit which is being addressed is consistent from session to session. In other words, several threads may be picked up in a single session; however, because of their long-standing relationship, the patient and therapist communicate easily about these familiar problems without the need for background explanation. It appears to be the nature of this treatment, when offered on a once-a-month basis, that various problem areas emerge and recede over the course of the 3-year treatment period; however, patient and therapist are able to retain a consistent approach to these problem areas throughout that time period.

While therapists had many questions about the therapeutic value of a one session per month format and initially expressed doubts about their ability to offer treatment within such a context, once confronted with the patient population for whom it was intended, (i.e., fully remitted recurrent depressives), they became advocates of IPT-M as a therapeutic modality. The majority of the original group of IPT-M trainees remained with the project throughout its 8-year duration and continued to provide IPT-M to patients in the Maintenance Therapies in Recurrent Depression protocol. These therapists also continued to work actively in group supervision sessions throughout the protocol to improve the quality of the treatment being offered. Finally, many of these therapists volunteered to pilot-test IPT-M with elderly individuals (age 60–80 years) suffering from recurrent depression.

If therapists are accepting IPT-M, patients are as well. Indeed, many patients who were assigned to the control condition (medication clinic visits) expressed disappointment at this assignment. Over the 3 years of maintenance treatment, only 9% of the patients assigned to the three IPT-M cells dropped out or were terminated for noncompliance. It should be noted that attrition from the two medication clinic visit cells was also relatively low (16%).

Efficacy of IPT-M

The following results are summarized from "*Three-Year Outcomes for Maintenance Therapies in Recurrent Depression*" (Frank et al. 1990).

Using the Cox proportional hazards model, the continuation of imipramine throughout the 3-year maintenance protocol was highly significant in delaying recurrence ($p < 0.0001$); IPT-M was also significant ($p = 0.052$) while the drug by IPT-M interaction was not ($p = 0.49$). When groups receiving active medication were omitted from the analysis, IPT-M was significantly related to

Table 1. Survival time in five maintenance treatment conditions for 3 years

Group	Mean survival time in weeks (SE)	Median survival time in weeks
Medication clinic and active imipramine	124 (13)	[a]
IPT-M and active imipramine	131 (10)	[a]
Medication clinic and placebo	45 (11)	21
IPT-M alone	82 (13)	54
IPT-M and placebo	74 (12)	61

[a] Since 50% of the subjects did not have a recurrence, no median can be reported.

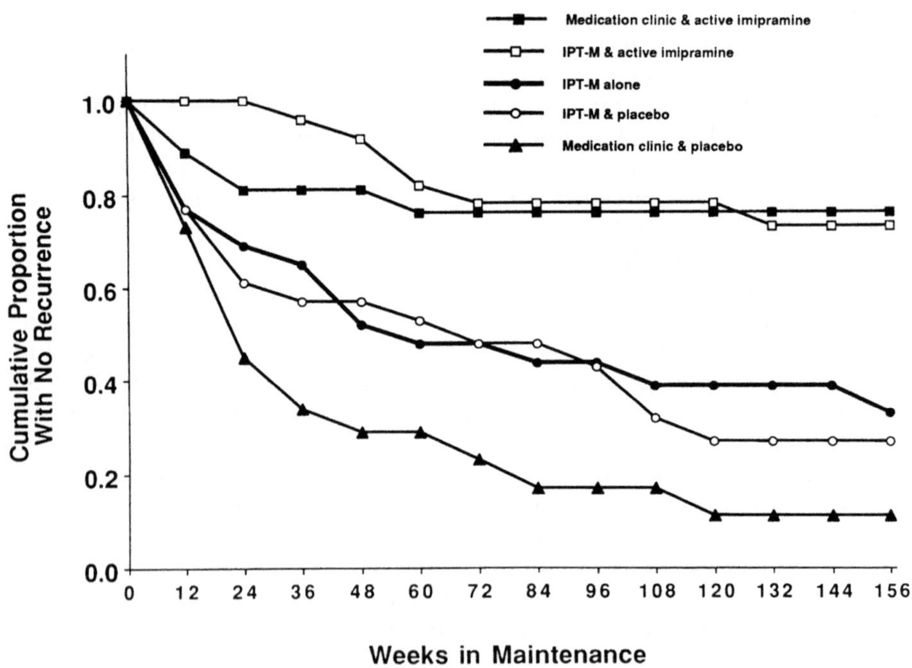

Fig. 2. 3-year survival curves for each of the five treatment conditions

survival with a probability of $p = 0.043$. Using the regression coefficient for imipramine status (1.58 $\pm$ 0.33 SE), the hazard of recurrence when not receiving drug is 4.9 with 95% confidence limits 2.5–9.4, while that associated with not receiving IPT-M (coefficient = 0.5012 $\pm$ 0.2672) was 1.7 with 95% confidence limits of 0.98–2.8.

Mean survival time for the total group of 128 patients was 75.7 weeks $\pm$ 61.8 with a median of 54.4 weeks. Mean survival times for each of the five treatment conditions are displayed in Table 1, while Fig. 2 presents a graphic illustration of the five 3-year survival curves.

Discussion

The first question which this study was designed to address was whether IPT, offered either alone or as an adjunct to pharmacotherapy, had a role to play in the prevention of new episodes of depressive illness in patients with a history of recurrences. A second question of clinical relevance was whether the traditional approach to maintenance pharmacotherapy, (i.e., using approximately half of the patient's acute treatment dose), could be improved upon by treating the acute episode aggressively and then maintaining patients at the acute treatment dose. A third question was whether the addition of psychotherapy, irrespective of its capacity to prevent new episodes of affective illness or extend the well interval, would enhance the interepisode social functioning of patients with recurrent affective disorders. Only, the first two of these questions are addressed in the analyses presented above.

The overall survival analysis provides two important pieces of information with respect to the prophylaxis of new episodes in patients with recurrent unipolar depression. Active imipramine, maintained at an average dose of approximately 200 mg, provided protection against recurrence of illness to a larger proportion of patients over a longer period of time than in any previous study of maintenance therapy of recurrent depression. In contrast, for those patients not maintained on active medication, continued monthly IPT sessions significantly extended survival time, with a median survival time of greater than a year. While the analysis fails to provide evidence for an additive effect for the combination, it also fails to provide evidence against one. The absence of a significant interaction effect in the analysis suggests that IPT-M functioned *similarly* whether used with or without medication, i.e., it extended survival time.

Both the prophylaxis provided by medication and that provided by psychotherapy need to be viewed in the context of the prior illness history of the patients studied in this investigation. One of the key issues in assessing the prophylactic efficacy of a treatment modality is whether it modifies the course of the disorder. In our sample of recurrent depressives, on average patients had been having repeated episodes of depression every 2.17 years for 12.5 years. Consistent with the findings of Angst (1973) and others, in the population studied in this investigation the time between episodes had diminished to the point where individuals were experiencing a new episode every 1–2 years. In our particular population, the period between the end of the previous episode and the beginning of the index episode was a median 25 weeks or approximately one half year. It is interesting to note that the median survival time of the placebo and medication clinic groups as 21 weeks, not dissimilar from the previous well interval of 25 weeks. We would argue that we have increased confidence in characterizing the medication clinic with placebo condition as an appropriate contrast to the remaining conditions since it appears to so closely approximate the natural history of the disorder in this population. Thus, any group that did significantly better than the medication clinic with placebo group was experiencing a level of prophylaxis that went beyond what would have been expected on the basis of natural history. Although the median survival time experienced by the IPT-M alone (54 weeks) and IPT-M with placebo (74 weeks) patients does not approximate that experienced by the patients in the active drug conditions, it substantially improves upon what the patient could have expected on the basis of natural history alone.

When the cost of even a single additional lifetime episode of major depression is considered, both in terms of economic loss and in terms of the suffering experienced by the patient and his or her family members, the public health significance of these findings is clear. While we do not yet know what will happen to such patients beyond the 3-year point, even 3 years of freedom from episodes is a boon to individuals with histories similar to those of the patients in this investigation.

While this investigation would appear to provide some important guidelines for the clinician working with recurrent unipolar patients, it should be noted that the results have limited generalizability. The patients for this study were selected for the relative absence of other Axis I and serious Axis II disorders. All patients were treated initially with a combination of IPT and imipramine hydrochloride. Thus, all of these patients should be considered responders to short-term and continuation *combined* treatment. The study fails to provide information about what might have happened had patients been treated initially only with pharmacotherapy or only with psychotherapy. Furthermore, the study was conducted in a speciality clinic with over a decade of expertise in the treatment of recurrent affective disorders.

Nonetheless, some implications for clinical practice are clear. By drawing comparisons between the earlier investigation of Prien et al. (1984) and the present investigation, it would appear that there is a distinct advantage to maintaining such patients at a dosage in the range of 200 mg, rather than tapering the patient to a "maintenance" dose. Second, it would appear that for the patient who cannot be or chooses not to be continued on pharmacotherapy, even monthly sessions of IPT may be helpful in extending the well interval. This finding is of particular importance in the case of the woman wishing to become pregnant or in the case of the patient who develops a medical condition incompatible with continued tricyclic pharmacotherapy.

The results presented here also lead to a number of additional research questions. First, will patients with a history of multiple previous episodes continue to receive protection beyond the 3-year point if continued on their short-term treatment dose of imipramine? What is the extent to which these results can be generalized to other pharmacologic agents used to treat recurrent mood disorders? Would the results have been similar had we employed another tricyclic antidepressant, a monoamine oxidase inhibitor, or a nontricyclic antidepressant such as fluoxetine? Would those patients who were treated with psychotherapy alone have experienced more extended well intervals had the psychotherapy been offered on a biweekly instead of monthly basis? In this regard, it should be pointed out that while imipramine was given in doses higher than previously used for maintenance treatment, the "dose" of IPT during maintenance was lower than in any previously published studies. We can also ask whether the results would have been similar if a different type of psychotherapy had been employed? Although the "quality" of imipramine therapy can be considered relatively constant throughout the maintenance phase, the "quality" of the psychotherapy is dependent on the extent to which both the patient and the therapist were able to focus on interpersonal concerns throughout the 3-year treatment period. Thus, a remaining question with respect to the psychotherapy is whether higher "quality" IPT-M is associated with more extended well intervals.

Acknowledgements. This work was supported in part by National Institute of Mental Health Grants MH-29618 and MH-30915 and by the John D. and Catherine T. MacArthur Foundation Network on the Psychobiology of Depression and Related Affective Disorders.

References

Angst J (1973) The course of monopolar depression and bipolar psychoses. Psychiatr Neurol Neurochir 76: 489–500

Elkin I, Parloff MB, Hadley SW, Autry JH (1985) NIMH treatment of depression collaborative research program: background and research plan. Arch Gen Psychiatry 42: 305–316

Frank E (1985) Psychotherapeutic approaches to treatment of recurrent unipolar depression: work in progress. Paper presented at the annual meeting of the American College of Neuropsychopharmacology, Maui, Hawaii

Frank E (1991) Interpersonal psychotherapy as a maintenance treatment for patients with recurrent depression. Psychotherapy 28: 259–266

Frank E, Kupfer DJ (1985) Maintenance treatment of recurrent unipolar depression: pharmacology and psychotherapy. In: Kemali D, Racagni G (eds) Chronic treatment in neuropsychiatry. Raven, New York, pp 139–151

Frank E, Kupfer DJ, Jacob M, Jarrett D (1987) Personality features and response to acute treatment in recurrent depression. J Pers Disord 1: 14–26

Frank E, Kupfer DJ, Perel JM (1989) Early recurrence in unipolar depression. Arch Gen Psychiatry 46: 397–400

Frank E, Kupfer DJ, Perel JM, Cornes CL, Jarrett D, Mallinger A, Thase M, McEachran AB, Grochocinski VJ (1990) Three-year outcomes for maintenance therapies in recurrent depression. Arch Gen Psychiatry 47: 1093–1099

Glen AIM, Johnson AL, Shepherd M (1984) Continuation therapy with lithium and amitriptyline in unipolar depressive illness: a randomized, doubleblind, controlled trial. Psychol Med 14: 37–50

Hamilton M (1960) A rating scale for depression. J Neurol Neurosurg Psychiatry 23: 56–62

Hirschfeld RMA, Klerman GL, Clayton PJ, Keller MB, McDonald-Scott P, Larkin BH (1983) Assessing personality: effects of depressive state on trait measurement. Am J Psychiatry 140: 695–699

Keller MB, Shapiro RW, Lavori PW, Wolfe N (1982) Relapse in major depressive disorder: analysis with the life table. Arch Gen Psychiatry 39: 911–915

Klerman GL, Dimascio A, Weissman M, Prusoff B, Paykel ES (1974) Treatment of depression by drugs and psychotherapy. Am J Psychiatry 131/2: 186–191

Klerman GL, Weissman MM, Rounsaville BJ, Chevron RS (eds) (1984a) Interpersonal psychotherapy of depression. Basic Books, New York

Klerman GL, Weissman MN, Rounsaville BJ, Chevron RS (1984b) Interpersonal psychotherapy of depression. Academic, New York

Mindham RH, Howland C, Shepherd M (1973) An evaluation of continuation therapy with tricyclic antidepressants in depressive illness. Psychol Med 5: 5–17
Montgomery SA, Dufour H, Brion S, Gailledreau J, Laqueille X, Ferrey G, Moron P, Parant-Lucena N, Singer L, Danion JM et al. (1988) The prophylactic efficacy of fluoxetine in unipolar depression. Br J Psychiatry 153 [Suppl 3]: 69–76
Prien RF, Kupfer DJ, Mansky PA, Small JG, Tuason VB, Voss CB, Johnson WE (1984) Drug therapy in the prevention of recurrences in unipolar and bipolar affective disorders: a report of the NIMH Collaborative Study Group comparing lithium carbonate, imipramine, and a lithium carbonate-imipramine combination. Arch Gen Psychiatry 41: 1096–1104
Raskin A, Schulterbrandt J, Reatig N, McKeon JJ (1969) Replication of factors of psychopathology in interview, ward behavior, and self-report ratings of hospitalized depressives. J Nerv Ment Dis 148: 87–98
Simons AD, Murphy GE, Levine JL, Wetzel RD (1986) Cognitive therapy and pharmacotherapy for depression: sustained improvement over one year. Arch Gen Psychiatry 43: 43–48
Weissman MM, Klerman GL, Paykel ES, Prusoff B, Hanson B (1974) Treatment effects on the social adjustment of depressed patients. Arch Gen Psychiatry 30: 771–778
Wells KB, Steward A, Hayes RD, Burnam A, Rogers W, Daniels M, Berry S, Greenfield S, Ware J (1989) The functioning and well-being of depressed patients: results from the Medical Outcomes Study. JAMA 262: 914–919

Lithium Treatment: Relationship Between Relapses and Personality Disorders

M. Gasperini, A. Lucca, S. Cogrossi, R. Zanardi, and E. Smeraldi

Lithium has been proved to be the most effective treatment in the prophylaxis of major affective disorders (Abou-Saleh and Ghodse 1983; Bunney and Gurland-Bunney 1987; Coppen and Abou-Saleh 1983; Prien et al. 1984; Smeraldi et al. 1980). An increasing bulk of evidence suggests the possibility that concurrent personality disorders (PD) could negatively affect the outcome and the course of affective disorders (Akiskal 1983; Charney et al. 1981; Johnson 1980; Maj et al. 1985).

In this paper we examined the possible effect of some clinical and biologic factors including the copresence of PD on the course of the illness during lithium prophylaxis.

The great variability of the outcome on lithium has been previously studied from several points of view. Clinical, biologic, and social variables have been focused as possible conditioning predictors of bad/good outcome. However, unequivocal reports failed to be found (Balon 1989; Silverstone and Romans-Clarkson 1989) (Jamison et al. 1979; Jamison and Akiskal 1983).

Our sample included 70 subjects, 29 with a diagnosis of major depression, recurrent (MDR) and 41 with bipolar disorder (BP), all diagnosed according to DSM-III-R (American Psychiatric Association 1987).

All subjects were referred to our Mood Disorder and Lithium Outpatients Unit. Only the patients with a minimum period of 24 months of lithium therapy were included in this study.

Table 1 shows some characteristics of the sample. The mean age of onset was 36 in MDR and 32 in BP ones. The mean current age was 51 in MDR and 36 in BP with an identical mean duration of illness of about 14 years in both the groups.

The rate of relapses from the onset of the illness until the period of beginning lithium treatment was quite similar in MDR and BP patients, i.e., 4.5 and 5.2.

Table 1. Variables of the sample 5(n = 70; female = 51)

	MDR (n = 29)	BP (n = 41)
Age of onset (± SD)	36 ± 12	32 ± 12
Current age (± SD)	51 ± 13.5	46.6 ± 13
Index of relapses before lithium	4.5	5.2
Duration of illness (mean years)	14.6	14.4
Index of with lithium	7.03	5.9

We considered the index of relapses during the lithium prophylaxis measured as the rate of the number of manic and depressive episodes over the duration of lithium maintenance calculated in months. That index was about 7 for MDR and about 6 for BP, and it was considered as a dependent variable of our analysis in the hypothesis that some clinical and biologic variables could condition the variability of relapses on lithium treatment.

The independent variables we considered in the analyses were: the age, the age of onset, the duration of illness, the polarity of the mood disorders, and the index of episodes prior to the start of lithium treatment.

We carried out some logistic analyses using a reglinear model, taking into account the index of relapses during lithium treatment as a dependent variable tested against the other variables. The dependent variable was tested in the group of 70 patients against all variables, except for PD diagnoses which were available only in a subgroup of patients (Stangl et al. 1985).

Table 2 summarizes the results of this analysis performed on the whole sample. The duration of illness appeared to be statistically significant ($t = 2.47$; $P \leq 0.01$) as a condition of the variability of relapse index. In other words, the longer the duration of the illness was, the larger the number of relapses during lithium treatment was.

The sex, the polarity of the form, the index of episodes before lithium, the age of onset, and the current age of the subjects did not show differences in increasing or decreasing the index of relapses during the treatment.

The significant effect of duration of illness could be explained in terms of higher recurrence of episodes as the illness persists. That is in agreement with the clinical findings of the worsening trend of recurrence of major affective disorders along their time course (Goodnick et al. 1987; Goodwin et al. 1984; Post et al. 1984; Prien and Gelenberg 1989). Table 3 shows the results of the analysis on the

Table 2. Results of the statistical analysis in the global sample

	t value	
Sex	0.35	NS
Polarity	0.56	NS
Onset/current age	0.33	NS
Duration	2.47	$P \leq 0.01$
Index of recurrence before lithium	0.63	NS

Table 3. Results of the statistical analysis in the subgroup with a diagnosis on axis II ($n = 37$)

	t-value	
Personality disorders	3.01	$P \leq 0.008$
Polarity	−0.08	NS
Index of recurrence before lithium	−2.83	$P \leq 0.01$
Age	−1.07	NS
Onset	−0.22	NS

sample of 37 subjects when also taking into account the variable absence/presence of PD. As one can see, the presence of PD did systematically increase the index of relapses during lithium treatment and that effect was statistically significant with a probability of .008 ($t = 3.01$). In other words, the relapse index during lithium maintenance was increased in the subjects with any PD, mainly in the subjects with early age of onset. The onset age, however, was not statistically significant in this analysis.

The same higher index of relapses was true for patients with PD vs patients without PD in their period of life without lithium prophylaxis. In fact the variable index before lithium was statistically significant ($t = -2.83$; $P \leq 0.01$) as a condition of the variability of the index for recurrence during lithium treatment.

Higher rates of illness before lithium corresponded to higher rates of recurrence during lithium treatment among subjects with PD. That could confirm the findings of other studies, supporting a worse outcome with pharmacological treatment depending on maladaptative personality traits. This could be explained in terms of poor compliance of these patients, both from the clinical point of view and from the point of view of familial load, in terms of higher morbidity risk in first- and second- degree relatives (Weissman et al. 1984, 1986; Gasperini and Provenza 1987).

The reduced size of our sample did not allow us to analyze extensively which specific traits could increase the liability to fail to successfully respond to treatments. However, we were looking for some indications at least of the specific PD involved by studying the distribution of relapse index in the different PD clusters.

Figure 1 shows the distribution of relapse index according to the clusters subdivision. The first category represents the subjects without any PD and shows the lowest index of relapses during lithium treatment with mean values decreasing from the initial recurrence index before the treatment. That could be due to the role of lithium salts in decreasing the recurrence rate of the illness, one of the major goals of lithium prophylaxis.

Cluster 1 is not represented in the figure because schizotypal, paranoid, and schizoid PD were not diagnosed in our subjects. In the cluster 2 (in which histrionic PD accounted for 15%) the index of relapses during lithium treatment was quite high with respect to the initial recurrence rate both in the group of MDR and BP.

The same trend was observed in subjects belonging to cluster 3, which included mainly dependent (17.5%) and compulsive (7.5%) PD. Therefore, histrionic, dependent, and compulsive PD appeared to be possibly related to predisposing predictors of poor outcome for lithium treatment in our sample. These three PD showed the worst recurrence rates even before lithium.

We could hypothesize that a particular personality pattern can be involved in conditioning a major susceptibility to stressor events interacting with the biologic liability to mood disorders. Alternatively, we could think that the subgroups of mood disorders associated to an axis II concurrent disorder represent a more severe form in affective disease, characterized by early age at onset, higher MR as we found in a previous study (Gasperini and Provenza

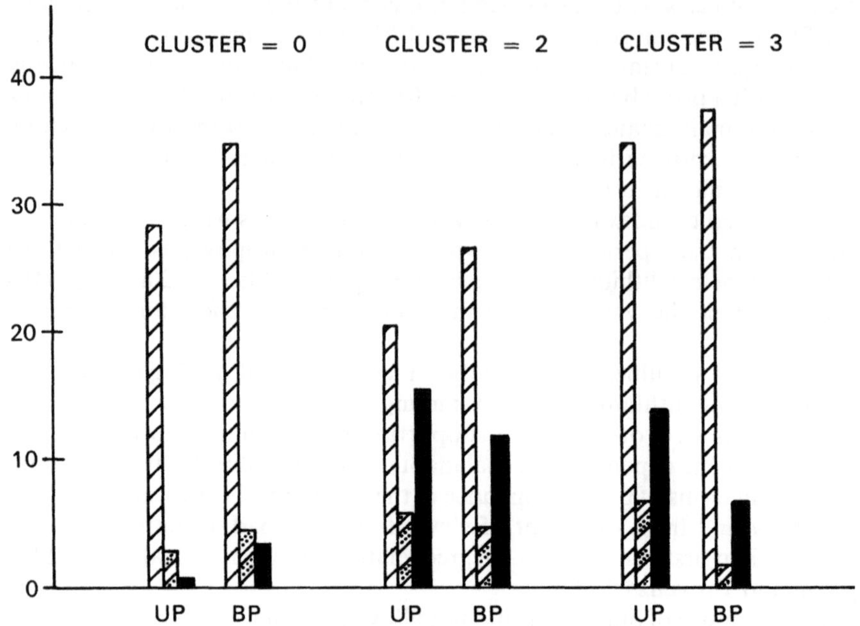

Fig. 1. Index of relapses on lithium treatment in different PD Clusters. *Hatched columns*, Mean age of onset (NS); *half-filled columns*, index of relapses before lithium treatment ($P \leq 0.04$); *solid columns*, index of relapses during lithium treatment (dependent variable); Subdivision according to clusters ($P \leq 0.05$)

1987), and poor outcomes and courses of illness (Akiskal 1983; Charney et al. 1981; Johnson 1980; Maj et al. 1985).

In addition, beyond the categorial classification of PD we are interested in looking for common traits shared by the specific PD which could be related to a possible worsening effect on the illness recurrence.

As our Lithium Unit is growing up, our proposal is to validate the reliability of these preliminary findings in a larger sample size.

References

Abou-Saleh MT, Ghodse AH (1983) Lithium in medical practice. Pharm J 231: 618–621

Akiskal HS (1983) Disthymic disorder: psychopatology of proposed chronic depressive subtypes. Am J Psychiatry 140: 11–20

American Psychiatric Association (1987) Diagnostic and statistical manual of mental disorders, 3rd edn, revised. American Psychiatric Association, Washington DC

Balon R (1989) Biological predictors of antidepressant treatment outcome. Clin Neuropharmacol 3: 195–214

Bunney WE, Gurland-Bunney BL (1987) Mechanisms of action of Lithium in affective illness. In: Meltzer NY (ed) Psycopharmacology: a third generation of progress. Raven, New York, pp 553–565

Charney BS, Nelson CC, Quinlan DM (1981) Personality traits and disorders in depression. Am J Psychiatry 138: 1601–1604
Coppen A, Abou-Saleh MT (1983) Lithium in the prophylaxis of a unipolar depression: a review. J R Soc Med 76: 297–301
Gasperini M, Provenza M (1987) The relationship between affective illness and personality disorders. Preliminary reports. In: Racagni G, Smeraldi E (eds) Anxious depression: assessment and treatment. Raven, New York, pp 81–87
Goodnick PJ, Fieve RR, Schlegel A (1987) Prediction of interepisode symptoms and relapse in affective disorder patients treated with Lithium carbonate. Am J Psychiatry 144: 367–369
Goodwin FK, Jamison KR (1984) The natural course of maniac-depressive illness. In: Post RM, Ballenger JW (eds) The neurobiology of affective disorders. Williams and Wilkins, Baltimore, pp 20–37
Jamison KR, Akiskal HS (1983) Medication compliance in patients with bipolar disorder. Psychiatr Clin North Am 6: 175–192
Jamison KR, Gerner RH, Goodwin JK (1979) Patient and physician attitudes towards Lithium: relation to compliance. Arch Gen Psychiatry 36: 866–869
Johnson FN (1980) Predicting lithium responders and non-responders: psychological indicators. In: Johnson FN (ed) Handbook of lithium therapy. MTP Press, Lancaster
Maj M, Arena F, Lovero N (1985) Factors associated with response to Lithium prophylaxis in DSM-III major depression and bipolar disorder. Pharmacopsychiatry 18: 309–313
Post RM, Rubinow DR, Ballenger JC (1984) Conditioning, sensitization and kindling: implication for the course of affective illness. In: Neurobiology of mood disorder. Williams and Wilkins, Baltimore, pp 432–436
Prien RF, Gelenberg AJ (1989) Alternatives to Lithium for preventive Treatment of bipolar disorder. Am J Psychiatry 146: 840–848
Prien LH, Kupfer DL, Mansky PA (1984) Drug therapy in the prevention of recurrences in unipolar and bipolar affective disorders. Arch Gen Psychiatry 41: 1096–1104
Silverstone T, Romans-Clarkson S (1989) Bipolar affective disorder: causes and prevention of relapse. Br J Psychiatry 154: 321–335
Smeraldi E, Saccheti E, Bellodi L (1980) Uso clinico e modalità d'azione dei sali di litio nei disordini affettivi. In: Smeraldi E, Sacchetti E (eds) La depressione come problema psicobiologico. Edi Ermes, Milano
Stangl D, Pfohl B, Zimmerman M, Bowers W, Carenthal C (1985) Structured interview for DSM-III personality disorder. Arch Gen Psychiatry 42: 591–596
Weissman MM, Wickramaratne P, Merikangas KR (1984) Onset of major depressive in early adulthood. Arch Gen Psychiatry 41: 1136–1143
Weissman MM, Merikangas KR, Wickramaratne P (1986) Understanding clinical heterogeneity of major depression using family data. Arch Gen Psychiatry 46: 430–434.

Effects of Lithium on Information Processing: Evidence from Partial Responders and Nonresponders

F.N. Johnson

Introduction

Attempts have been made for at least 20 years to provide a psychological model for the actions of lithium, and indeed there is a wealth of information about the behavioral and cognitive changes brought about by lithium administration in both humans and animals (Johnson 1984). Despite this, the psychological models which have been proposed have had relatively little impact upon clinical practice, or upon the way in which the therapeutic actions of lithium are conceptualized by psychiatrists. Why should this be so? The answer does not lie in the adequacy of the models themselves: indeed, of all available models of lithium action, those based upon psychological principles are the most complete and should make most direct intuitive appeal to the psychiatrist. In all probability, the failure of psychological models to make an impact is due to the manner in which they have been presented.

Psychological investigations are often highly technical, and employ specialized terminology, and what therefore is needed is a more simple and direct demonstration of psychological principles which will have immediate appeal to psychiatrists and others who are unfamiliar with the jargon of psychology. Recent work in the Department of Psychology and Lancaster University has been designed with this specific need in mind.

A Simplified Psychological Analysis

Figure 1 illustrates a simplified schema for considering the effects of lithium and affect upon psychological processing. Sensory input is first subjected to sensory analysis, after which an appropriate response is selected. Affective dysfunction may affect either sensory analysis or response selection (or, of course, both). Similarly, lithium, administered to treat the affective disorder, may affect sensory analysis, response selection, or both. In addition, the lithium may interact with the mechanisms of affective dysfunction. The situation is thus complex, even on this relatively simple model.

In patients receiving treatment for affective disorders, lithium and affective dysfunction coexist, making their separate investigation difficult. One way of avoiding this problem is to use animal subjects in which the affective dysfunction

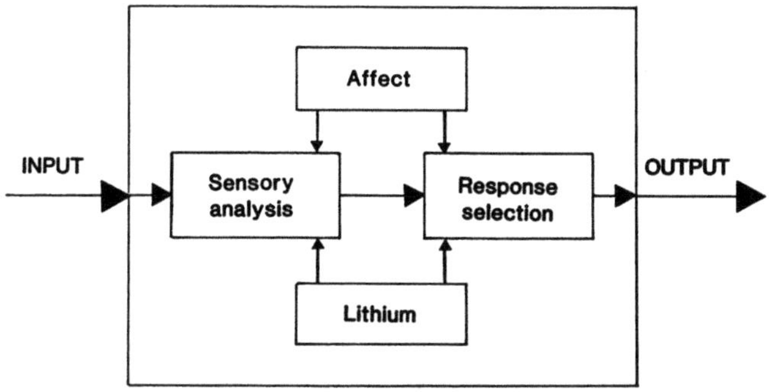

Fig. 1. A simple psychological model of the relationship between lithium treatment in patients with affective disorder

component is absent, allowing lithium levels to be manipulated separately. This is why many of the early psychological investigations were animal based.

From the results of the animal studies it was suggested that lithium acts primarily at the level of sensory processing, leaving response selection untouched. From this, a working model of affective disorders was developed which proposed that mania is a state of stimulus overprocessing, while depression is a state of stimulus underprocessing. The full details of this model, with a full discussion of the evidence, have been presented by Johnson (1984).

Investigations in Patients

To see whether this psychological model, which was derived from animal studies, was applicable to the human clinical context, studies using patients became necessary. However, as noted above, the problem with such studies is that lithium and affective dysfunction occur together in the same patient. If the lithium is clinically effective, there is no variation in affect which can be investigated, but if one examines partial responders or nonresponders there is the possibility of studying both affect and lithium simultaneously, using the techniques of partial correlation analysis to separate the influences of the two factors.

Johnson (1988) applied this technique to a group of partial and nonresponders, using a signal detection analysis paradigm, and adduced evidence which supported the idea that lithium acts to impair sensory analysis, a result which was consonant with a stimulus-processing model of mania and depression.

However, signal detection analysis is not immediately understandable without some detailed knowledge of its theoretical basis, and it therefore becomes necessary to illustrate the psychological models of lithium action and of affective dysfunction in some more direct manner. Accordingly, a technique has been devised which relies upon the phenomenon of "incidental learning" or "incidental memory."

Incidental Learning Task

Ten test sheets were prepared, as shown in Fig. 2, on which there was an array of six-letter, two-syllable words. Each of the ten sheets bore identical words, with the exception of one word which was shown in a box placed centrally on the sheet. There were thus ten different words in boxes, one on each sheet. Each patient was presented with the sheets, one at a time, each one for a 3-s period, and was asked to learn the words in the boxes. No reference was made to the other words surrounding the central word. When all ten sheets had been presented, the patient was asked to recall, in the correct sequence, the ten words which had been in the boxes. Then the procedure was repeated a second and third time.

After the third presentation of the sheets, the subject was not asked about the words in the central boxes, but was instead asked to recall the words which had been presented in a circular array around the boxes (Fig. 3). Since no instructions had been given about learning these words, any recall of them must be regarded as incidental memory based upon incidental learning.

Recall was assessed by asking each patient to complete a score sheet, as shown in Fig. 4. On the score sheet there were 40 words; 20 of these had appeared in a circle around the central box on the test sheets, while 20 had never

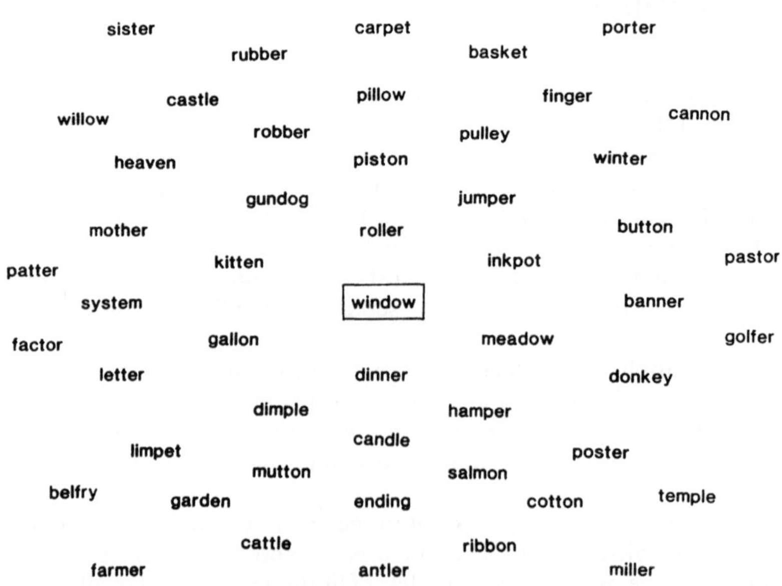

Fig. 2. An example of a test sheet with the target word which is to be learned shown in a central box

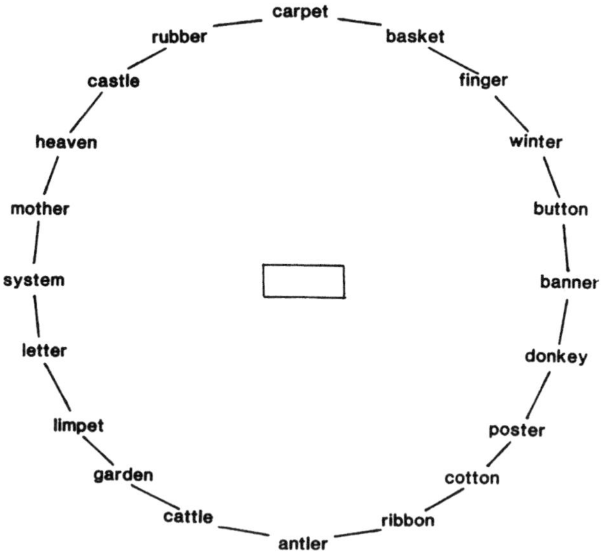

Fig. 3. The circle of 20 words around the central box on the test sheets; these are the words subjected to incidental learning

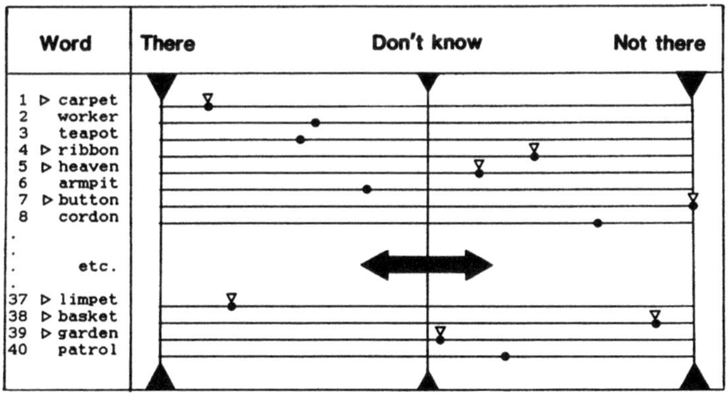

Fig. 4. Representation of the score sheet used for assessing incidental learning. The sheet bears the 20 words present on the test sheets (shown by *triangles* in this figure) and 20 words not present. The patient indicates certainty that the word was or was not present, by placing a mark on the 10-cm line on either side of the "don't know" position

been presented on the test sheets. The patient was asked to indicate, by putting a mark at one end or the other of a 10-cm line, whether the word had or had not been on the test sheet. A mark in the middle of the line indicated "don't know." The patient was also allowed to indicate degrees of confidence in his or her judgment, by placing the mark between one extremity of the line and the "don't know" position.

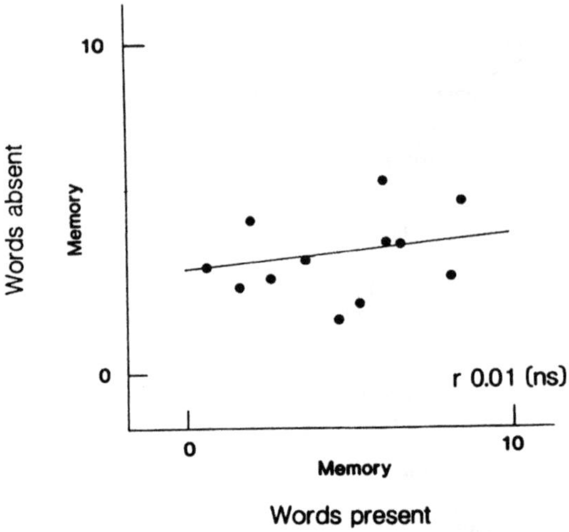

Fig. 5. The lack of a significant correlation between memory for words present and "false" memory for words not present on the test sheet; this indicates that information processing and response readiness are separable psychological functions

The length of the line from the "not there" position to the mark placed by the patient was averaged for each of the 20 words given on the test sheets, and this value was taken as an index of the efficiency of information processing shown by the patient. A value was determined similarly for the 20 words not on the test sheets, and this was taken as representative of the "response readiness" of the patient. It was found that these two measures, i.e., memory based upon stimulus processing (rated 0 to 10) and false memory based upon response readiness (also rated 0 to 10), were not correlated (Fig. 5) and thus represent separate psychological processes. This test is relatively crude and far less sensitive than more sophisticated signal detection test procedures, but it proved adequate to demonstrate the effects of lithium and of affective dysfunction.

Results

It was found that incidental memory based on sensory analysis was less efficient during depressed mood states and more efficient during elevated mood, as shown in Fig. 6. Clinical status was rated on a seven-point scale, based upon a combination of a global psychiatric rating and scores on the Hospital Anxiety and Depression (HAD) Scale; the values ranged from -3 for deep depression to $+3$ for severe mania, though in fact in this study, which involved only 12 patients, none of the patients had a score outside the range of -2 and $+2$, with 0 indicating normothymia.

The positive correlation between incidental memory for words present on the test sheets is in line with the notion that affect is related to information

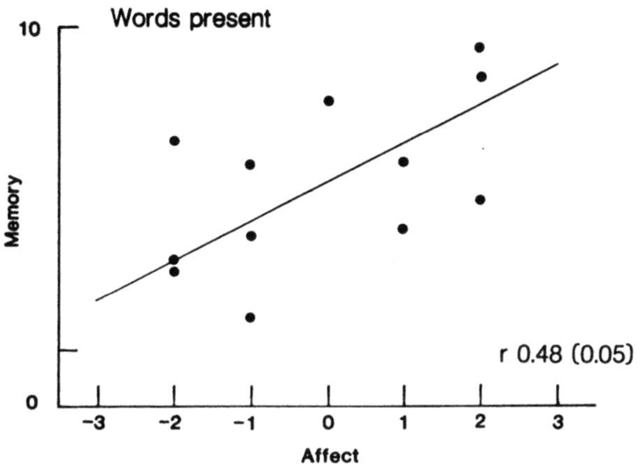

Fig. 6. Correlation between affect rating and information processing (memory for words present)

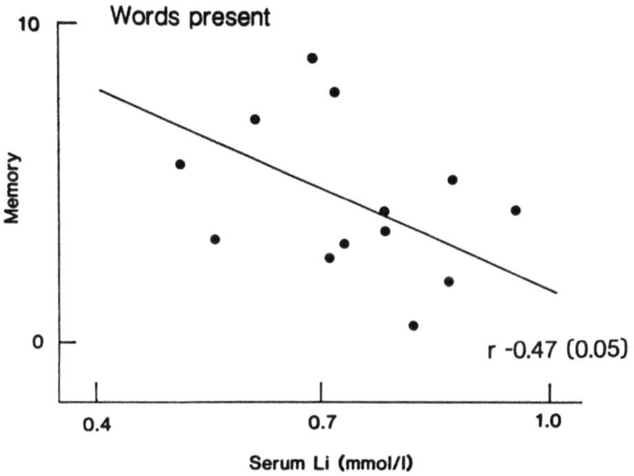

Fig. 7. Correlation between serum lithium level and information processing (words present)

processing. The idea that lithium acts to impair information processing was also supported by this study (Fig. 7), there being a negative correlation between the incidental memory for words present on the sheets and the serum level of lithium.

The correlation coefficients were not high, and there was considerable variability in the data, but given the simple nature of the test and its inherent variability, the demonstration is sufficient to establish the point.

It was also found that there was a correlation between clinical status and lithium serum level ($r = -0.22$). This was statistically nonsignificant, but was nevertheless used to calculate partial correlation coefficients, establishing that there was a significant positive correlation between information processing (incidental memory for words present) and affect, *independent of serum lithium levels*, and a significant negative correlation between information processing (incidental memory for words present) and serum lithium levels, *independent of affect*) .

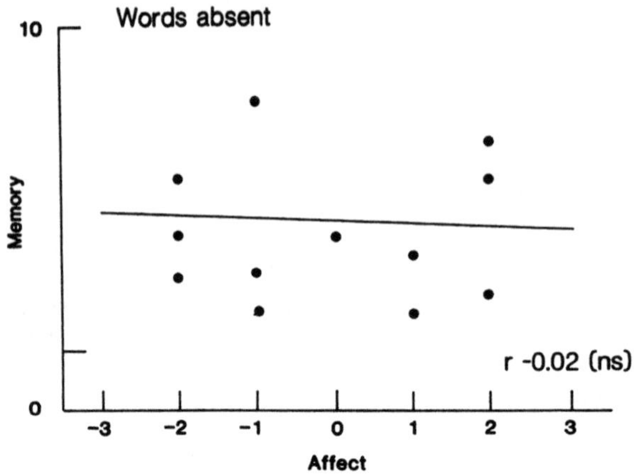

Fig. 8. Correlation between affect rating and response readiness (words absent)

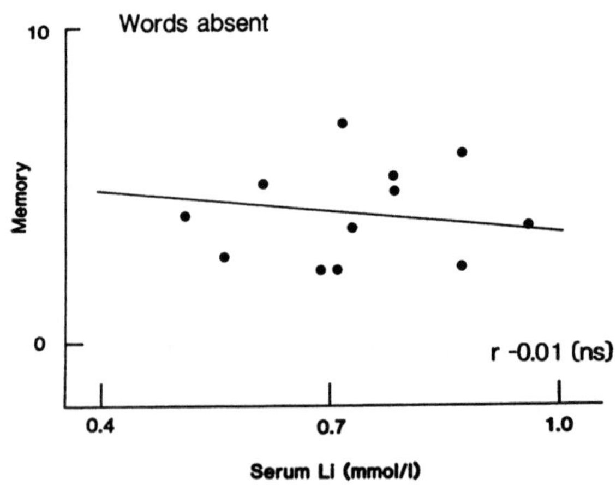

Fig. 9. Correlation between serum lithium level and response readiness (words absent)

When response readiness was examined, by looking at incidental memory for words not present on the test sheets, no correlations were seen with either affect score (Fig. 8) or serum lithium level (Fig. 9). These findings are therefore in conformity with the psychological models of lithium action and affective dysfunction previously presented.

Graphic Representation of Perceptual Fields

At this point in the study, it was decided to try to provide some form of graphic representation of the incidental memory for words which had been present on the test sheets. Accordingly, a circular grid was constructed, 10 cm in radius, with twenty 10-cm lines radiating out from a central point. Each line pointed

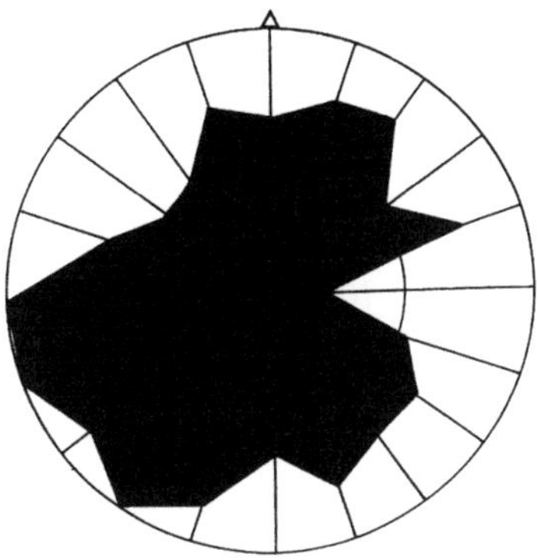

Fig. 10. Perceptual field (attentional, memory field) for a subject with an affect rating of A = 2 (hypomanic) and a serum lithium level of S = 0.58 mmol/liter. The mean memory score, M = 7.1

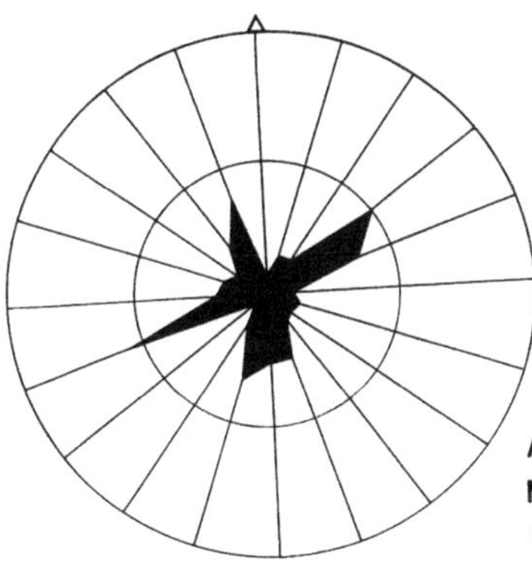

Fig. 11. Perceptual field for a depressed subject

toward one the 20 words which had been arranged around the central box on the test sheet. It was then possible to indicate on each line the memory score for that word, with the central point representing the "not there" decision, and the outermost extremity representing the "there" position, with a point midway between the center and the outer rim representing "don't know." When all the points had been plotted, they could be joined up and the area thus enclosed could be shaded in to represent the "perceptual field" or "incidental memory field" for the patient.

Figure 10 shows such a field for a hypomanic patient, while in Fig. 11 there is the typically contracted perceptual field of a patient in a depressed state. What is particularly curious about the latter is that the depressed patient does not simply record "don't know" responses, but actually errs on the side of *denial*, i.e., making the type I error of saying that a word was not there when it was.

In Fig. 12 the perceptual field of a euthymic patient is shown and in Fig. 13 the perceptual field of another hypomanic patient. What is curious about these two fields, and particularly the second, is that there is a high degree of asymmetry. This was never observed in healthy volunteer subjects who were not taking lithium; in such individuals the perceptual fields were more or less radially symmetrical. It is by no means clear what these findings mean. It may be

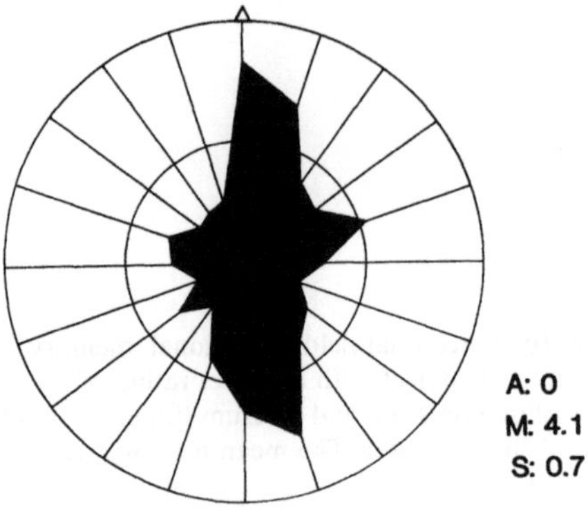

Fig. 12. Perceptual field for a normothymic, lithium-treated subject

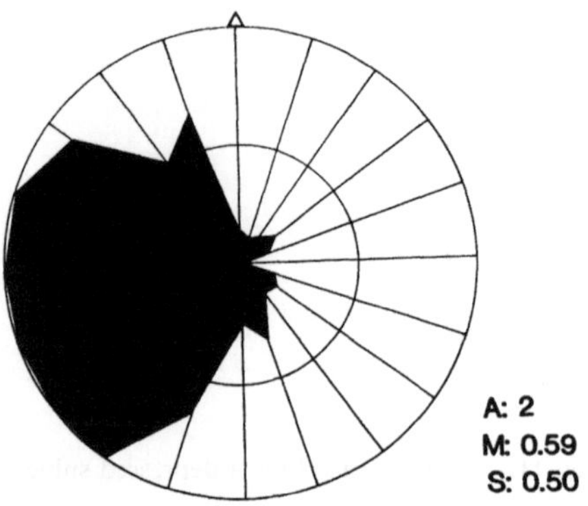

Fig. 13. Perceptual field for a hypomanic subject, showing marked asymmetry

that the asymmetry is a feature of the affective dysfunction, or possibly the lithium is having some distorting effect. The matter is currently under investigation.

These results are shown here for the first time as a further indicator that much remains to be discovered about the psychological processes which underlie lithium action and the symptoms of affective dysfunction.

References

Johnson F.N (ed) (1984) The psychopharmacology of lithium. Macmillan, London

Johnson F.N (1988) Signal detection analysis of information processing in patients receiving prophylactic lithium therapy. Hum Psychopharmacol 3: 95–100

Chronic Lithium Salt Treatment and Calcium Metabolism

M.L. Bianchi, G. Conte, and E. Sacchetti

Introduction: Literature Review

Since the early 1970s, when lithium salts were definitively introduced for the routine prophylaxis of major affective disorders (MAD), their probable negative action on mineral and bone metabolism has represented an important point in the evaluation of side effects. This special interest is also justified by the fact that in patients with manic-depressive disorders inherent derangements of calcium metabolism have been suggested as a primary cause of the disorder itself, at least in some cases (Faragalla and Flach 1970; Mellerup and Rafaelsen 1974; Rafaelsen et al. 1975; Carman et al. 1984).

Both acute and chronic lithium administration seem to affect calcium-phosphate metabolism in some way, although different and even opposite alterations in calcium homeostasis have been found, depending on the short- or long-term use of the drug.

Moreover, there are few findings of obvious pathological modifications: in the majority of cases, derangements of calcium-phosphate metabolism are slight and substantially consist of small differences from the values observed in suitable control groups.

To put it in one sentence, while a number of studies have been published on this subject, the results are not conclusive.

In some of the first animal studies on lithium and calcium-phosphate metabolism, Gotfredson et al. (1969) found an increase in urinary calcium excretion in rats treated acutely with lithium, and Andreoli et al. (1972) reported an increase in both urinary and plasma calcium. Lithium-induced hypercalcemia in rats has also been observed by some authors (Mellerup and Rafaelsen 1974; Mellerup et al. 1973; Birch and Jenner 1973) but, under the same experimental conditions other studies have failed to confirm this change (Henneman and Zimmerberg 1974; Bellwinkel et al. 1975).

However, in human patients treated with lithium, decreased calcium excretion was noticed at the beginning of treatment (Crammer 1975; Bjiorum et al. 1975). This decrease in calcium excretion was probably related to an increase in fractional tubular reabsorption (Nielsen et al. 1977).

Christiansen et al. (1975) reported increased levels of serum calcium in 98 patients chronically treated with lithium salts when compared with a control group of healthy subjects; furthermore, in this study the incidence of hypercalcemia (plasma calcium 2 SD over the mean of controls) was 12% and a correlation between serum calcium levels and duration of lithium therapy and lithium total intake was found. Increased levels of calcemia were subsequently reported by other studies (Feinberg et al. 1979; Christiansen et al. 1980; Colt et al. 1981; Herman 1981; Franks et al. 1982; Mallette et al. 1989; Shen and Sheppard 1982).

The finding of a relationship between lithium salt treatment and an increase in serum calcium levels was the starting point for two complementary types of study: the first aimed at identifying its pathological mechanism, concentrating particularly on the hormonal regulation of calcium metabolism; the second aimed at evaluating the clinical relevance of this derangement.

In the studies concerned with hormonal regulation, special attention was given to calcitonin (CT) and parathyroid hormone (PTH). Feinberg et al. (1979) found increased CT levels in patients treated chronically with lithium salts and suggested that this increase in CT was an indirect consequence of prolonged and constant hypercalcemia. However, opposite results were reported by McEachron et al. (1980) who found lower levels of CT in rats treated with lithium than in control rats, and no correlation between calcium and CT levels. Furthermore, these investigators noted that even when rats were hypercalcemic, the modifications of plasma CT and PTH concentrations were similar to those occurring in hypocalcemic animals. This picture resembles secondary hyperparathyroidism. Therefore, it was hypothesized that lithium could compete with calcium at the level of the parathyroid gland receptors for calcium, thus inducing these hormonal derangements.

Subsequently, some case reports of parathyroid gland adenoma during chronic treatment with lithium were published (Christensson 1976; Garfinkel et al. 1973; McGregor 1977) and acute and transient increases in PTH levels at the beginning of lithium therapy were also reported (Henneman and Zimmerberg 1974; Rothman 1982).

Christiansen et al. (1980) observed a rise in PTH levels associated with hypercalcemia and decreased bone mineral density (BMD) and they concluded that lithium therapy could induce a degree of "mild hyperparathyroidism". Their study, however, was based on only 3 months of treatment.

Davis et al. (1981) found higher than normal PTH levels with normocalcemia and a positive correlation between the serum levels of lithium and calcium. They suggested two possible interpretations of these results: the presence of a "functional hypocalcemia" causes a persistent elevation of PTH levels, or the presence of slight renal damage determines increased levels of PTH, with the same mechanism as that seen in classical secondary hyperparathyroidism. With regard to the first hypothesis they supposed that normal levels of total calcium might not be enough for the biological activity of this ion in the presence of lithium, which antagonizes some calcium-dependent processes. However, no experimental evidence was given to support this hypothesis.

Franks and colleagues (Franks et al. 1982) observed that calcemia and plasma carboxyl-terminal PTH levels were higher in a group of 12 patients treated chronically with lithium than in a matched control group. Using the nomogram developed by Hawker (quoted in Franks et al. 1982), where calcium levels are plotted on one axis and PTH levels on the other, they found that the values observed in their patients clustered in the same area as those observed in subjects affected by mild primary hyperparathyroidism.

In a recent study, Mallette et al. (1989) have noted that short-term lithium treatment causes an increase in serum calcium levels without a reciprocal decrease in intact PTH. This lack of connection between calcium and the PTH could be explained by a lithium-induced shift in the set-point for the inhibition of PTH secretion, requiring higher calcium levels than normal. They suggested that the lower than normal suppression of PTH secretion causes parathyroid enlargement. While this study explains how the continuous parathyroid hyperfunction can lead to a hyperplasia of these glands during long-term lithium treatment, it does not explain the formation of a parathyroid adenoma.

However, Spiegel and colleagues (Spiegel et al. 1976) did not support the hypothesis that clinically relevant concentrations of lithium alter the suppressibility of PTH secretion by calcium; this study, however, was performed in normal men treated with lithium for only 5 days.

In an in vitro study on normal dispersed bovine parathyroid cells, Brown (Brown 1981) observed a slight increase in the concentration of calcium required for the inhibition of half the PTH release, (i.e., the set-point for calcium), after incubation with lithium at concentrations within the therapeutic range for man. This author hypothesized that lithium decreases intracellular calcium at any extracellular calcium concentration. However, direct measurements of cytosolic calcium in parathyroid cells are required to verify this possibility.

In conclusion, some data are available concerning possible lithium interference at the calcium receptor sites of parathyroid gland cells. This could be the pathophysiological mechanism priming hyperparathyroidism. However, even if this hypothesis is accepted, many other findings still need to be explained: for example, why is there adenoma and not hyperplasia of PTH glands (we have not found any histological studies of parathyroid tissue) and why are there no clinical manifestations typical of primary hyperparathyroidism, such as nephrolithiasis, hypertension, etc.

Some authors suggest a different mechanism of action: lithium exerts its effects on the monoaminergic neurotransmitter system in the brain. Recent studies have shown that dopamine increases PTH release and cyclic adenosine monophosphate (cAMP) accumulation in dispersed bovine parathyroid cells (Brown et al. 1977), through the specific activation of a dopamine receptor linked to adenylate cyclase (Attie et al. 1980). These preliminary data seem to indicate that lithium could influence PTH secretion and calcium homeostasis because of an interaction with monoaminergic systems. However, this hypothesis is still under evaluation and no conclusion can be drawn for the moment.

The clinical relevance of the interaction between lithium and calcium metabolism has still not been fully evaluated. Some studies have reported the development of hypercalcemia during long-term lithium treatment, without any of the other manifestations characteristic of prolonged high levels of calcium, such as renal stones or subperiosteal resorption (Christensson 1976). Other studies have referred to some cases of parathyroid adenoma during chronic lithium therapy. However, no evaluation of the incidence of this finding in manic-depressive patients treated with lithium has been made and so it is not possible to make any comparison with the incidence in the normal population. Moreover, it should be underlined that in normal older people, especially women, primary hyperparathyroidism can often clinically appear as mood modification, depression, asthenia, lethargy, body weight loss, and reduction of mental capacity (Kleinfeld et al. 1984).

Long periods of increased serum calcium levels could lead to calcification affecting vascular and soft tissues, could favor the appearance of hypertension and duodenal ulcer, and could induce relapsing renal stones.

At present, there are no longitudinal nor transversal studies on such systemic side effects during the course of lithium therapy.

However, there has been some investigation into the possible influence of prolonged lithium use on bone tissue. In rats, some authors have found decreased calcium (Birch and Jenner 1973) and high lithium concentrations (Birch and Hullin 1972) or a decreased uptake of ^{45}Ca in bone (Mellerup et al. 1970). Therefore, it has been hypothesized that lithium might have replaced the other divalent ion. However, other investigators have been unable to demonstrate significant changes in the calcium content of wet-weight bone of lithium-treated rats (Henneman and Zimmerberg 1974).

Christiansen et al. (1975) measured BMD in 98 patients treated with lithium and found a mean value just below the mean value of a matched control group of healthy subjects (93% of normal BMD). However, they did not observe any correlation between BMD and the length of therapy or the cumulative dose of lithium, and concluded that the observed osteopenia does not seem to be caused by the lithium treatment.

Baastrup et al. (1977) studied 83 manic-depressive patients on long-term lithium therapy, divided into a unipolar and a bipolar group, and found a decrease in BMD values (88% of those of a control group) only in bipolar patients. Since PTH levels were increased in the same way in both groups, they hypothesized a decreased sensitivity of bone tissue to PTH in the unipolar group. However, these data have never been observed by anybody else and this hypothesis has never been confirmed.

In a subsequent longitudinal study, Christiansen et al. (1980) observed a slight decrease in BMD and an increase in calcium and PTH after lithium administration, although basal BMD values were no different from those of controls. However, no firm conclusions could be reached because the observation period was only 3 months and the patient sample was rather small (13 subjects). Finally, Thysell et al. (1981) observed an increase in BMD, despite the presence of the increased calcium and PTH.

As we have tried to show in our survey of recent literature, there are striking discrepancies among the various reports which we think might be accounted for by some not necessarily mutually exclusive factors. For example, none of the studies examined all the main parameters of calcium metabolism simultaneously. This is a very weak point, considering the complexity of calcium homeostasis and the strict interaction of the various factors involved.

Most studies report an increase in calcium and PTH levels, suggesting the presence of primary hyperparathyroidism. However, in the majority of them there was no direct evaluation of any renal damage predisposing the development of secondary hyperparathyroidism; this is especially relevant, since there are reports that the kidneys of lithium-treated patients (Mellerup et al. 1987) show functional alterations and morphological damage.

In many studies, the prescribed lithium dosages were higher than those currently recommended. One is tempted to ask whether the reported alterations in calcium metabolism would be different or less relevant if patients were treated with lower dosages.

The majority of these studies agree on the absence of important clinical effects related to the elevation of calcium and PTH levels, although these and other side effects have not been systematically evaluated. For example, osteopenia (decreased BMD) has been investigated in only a few studies, characterized by cross-sectional analysis and short observation periods.

Vitamin D active metabolite levels have never been evaluated in long-term lithium therapy, despite their central role in the regulation of calcium metabolism. In a very recent study, Rosenblatt et al. (1989) observed a decrease of $1,25(OH)_2D$ during a short period of lithium therapy (1 month) in ten patients. He supposed that lithium may inhibit the activation of the renal hydroxylase involved in the $1,25(OH)_2D$ synthesis.

Finally, almost all studies are cross-sectional, but only an adequate follow-up period can provide significant information about a long-term treatment.

Our Study: Results and Discussion

We undertook a 2-year longitudinal study of a group of 25 patients treated with lithium carbonate for MAD. The diagnosis was made according to DSM III criteria (American Psychiatric Association 1980).

This group of patients included 15 women and 10 men, aged 29–65 years, affected by MAD, either unipolar (8 subjects) or bipolar (17 subjects). None of the patients suffered from any other systemic disease known to influence calcium metabolism. Special attention was paid to the evaluation of renal function, but the results of the appropriate tests were perfectly normal in all of the patients (plasma creatinine, blood urea nitrogen, creatinine clearance, tubular phosphate reabsorption).

All of the patients were treated with lithium carbonate (mean lithium dosage: 824 ± 163 mg/day, range 600–1200 mg/day). We chose patients whose clinical condition was stable and who had been regularly treated for at least 6 months (Table 1). A control group of 25 normal subjects, matched for age and sex, was also studied.

A complete screening of calcium-phosphate metabolism (plasma and urinary calcium and phosphorus, plasma alkaline phosphatase, urinary hydroxyproline, plasma levels of PTH, CT, 25-OHD and $1,25(OH)_2D$) was performed in all subjects on entry to the study and after 2 years. At the same times BMD was also measured in all patients. A full description of laboratory methods can be found in a previous study (Bianchi et al. 1990).

Table 1. General parameters, calcemia, and renal function indexes in patients on chronic lithium treatment at study entry

Indexes	Results
Plasma lithium (mEq/l)	0.23 ± 0.03
Months on lithium therapy	55.30 ± 36.00
Plasma calcium (mg/dl)	8.90 ± 0.28
Plasma creatinine (mg/dl)	0.83 ± 0.04
BUN (mg/dl)	17.10 ± 2.90
Creatinine clearance (ml/min)	114.20 ± 17.70
TmP/GFR (mg/100 ml)	3.50 ± 0.40

BUN, blood urea nitrogen; TmP/GFR, glomerular filtration rate

A cross-sectional study of our patients revealed calcium metabolism parameters substantially within the normal range. A clear increase in PTH levels was found only in two out of 25 patients (8%), but there was no relation between this and plasma lithium carbonate levels or duration of therapy.

Longitudinal study of all of the patients for 24 months showed a significant variation in only one important factor, i.e., a decrease in plasma levels of $1{,}25(OH)_2D$ (Table 2).

We looked for correlation between calcium metabolism parameters and lithium treatment duration, plasma lithium levels, or lithium cumulative dose, but did not find any significant result.

BMD required special evaluation, considering the influence of sex and chronological age on bone mass: for this reason, we considered three subgroups of patients, i.e., men, premenopausal women, and postmenopausal women.

Comparison between the basal BMD levels of our patients and those of matched controls showed normal bone mass in the lithium-treated subjects and no differences were observed (Table 3).

In men and premenopausal women treated with lithium carbonate, BMD was unchanged after 2 years, as was the case with control subjects. We noticed a slight decrease in BMD (−2%) in postmenopausal women, but a comparable decrease was also found in the appropriate control group.

Our data seem to differ in some aspects from other studies, and we think they have raised some new points. First of all, plasma lithium levels in our patients were lower than those commonly suggested in the literature (Baldessarini 1980; Dunner and Clayton 1987) and this could possibly explain the generally lower degree of calcium metabolism derangement.

In particular, the parathyroid glands seem to be less involved in our patients: plasma levels of calcium were well within the normal range, except in two cases who presented calcemia at the lower limits and plasma PTH levels at the higher limits of the normal range. We followed these patients for a long period in order to verify the consequences of chronic lithium therapy.

The decrease in $1{,}25(OH)_2D$ to the lower limits of normal seems to be an aspect never previously reported in long-term lithium therapy. Many studies

Table 2. Calciotropic hormones in 25 patients on chronic lithium treatment at study entry and after 24 months and in a control group

	Controls	Patients	
		0 months	24 months
PTH (pmol/l)	35.2 ± 5.5	33.1 ± 4.1	37.2 ± 4.5
25-OH D (ng/ml)	41.0 ± 4.4	39.9 ± 2.3	40.2 ± 2.5
1,25-$(OH)_2$D (pg/ml)	32.3 ± 4.2	31.5 ± 1.9	26.6 ± 1.6*
CT (pg/ml)	28.6 ± 3.5	27.9 ± 3.2	28.2 ± 3.3

* $p < 0.01$, 0 vs 24 months.

Table 3. Bone mineral density in 25 patients on chronic lithium treatment at study entry and in control groups

	BMD (mg/cm^2)	
	Controls	Patients
Men	694 ± 37	736 ± 75
Premenopausal women	658 ± 39	687 ± 44
Postmenopausal women	602 ± 39	634 ± 51

(Mellerup et al. 1987) are indeed available on the effects of lithium on renal morphology: in particular, lithium induces lesions of cells in different portions of tubules, with no development of renal failure. Such cellular derangements of the proximal tubule could have a negative influence on renal production of 1,25$(OH)_2$D. This most active form of vitamin D, in fact, is synthesized almost exclusively there (Midgett et al. 1973).

In our opinion, the ultrastructural lesion of renal tubular cells could explain the progressive reduction of 1,25$(OH)_2$D levels observed in our patients.

In conclusion, a prominent role in the appearance of calcium metabolism derangements could be assigned to the progressive decrease of 1,25$(OH)_2$D. This reduction of 1,25$(OH)_2$D could determine an abnormal stimulation of parathyroid glands to secrete PTH, either by direct action at 1,25$(OH)_2$D-specific receptors, or indirectly because of the decrease in calcium levels.

Our patients presented only subtle biochemical and hormonal alterations, with no clinical evidence of calcium metabolism alteration. We paid particular attention to bone mass: the separate study of male and female patients, and for women, of pre- and post-menopausal subjects is mandatory in order to correctly evaluate BMD (Nilas and Christiansen 1987; Gensens et al. 1986). It is now universally accepted that these are the main factors influencing both the peak and the loss of bone mineral mass.

In our study, the comparison of lithium-treated patients with healthy subjects matched for age, sex, and menopause revealed a conserved bone mass in lithium patients. A decrease of BMD was found only in postmenopausal women, both lithium-treated and healthy controls. In our opinion, such a decrease is no proof of any direct effect of lithium therapy on bone, but is a normal physiological event related to the decrease in sexual hormone production common to all postmenopausal women.

Acknowledgements. The authors are grateful to Dr. Flavia Campanini and Dr. Maria Jannetta for radioimmunological assays and thank Mr. Kevin Smart for his revision of the English text.

References

American Psychiatric Association, Committee on Nomenclature and Statistics (1980) Diagnostic and statistical manual of mental disorders, 3rd edn. American Psychiatric Association, Washington

Andreoli VM, Villani F, Brambilla G (1972) Increased calcium and magnesium excretion by lithium carbonate. Psychopharmacology 25: 77–85

Attie MF, Brown EM, Gardner DG, Spiegel AM, Aurbach GD (1980) Characterization of the dopamine-responsive adenylate cyclase of bovine parathyroid cells and its relationship to parathyroid hormone secretion. Endocrinology 107: 1776–1781

Baastrup PC, Christiansen C, Transbol I (1977) Calcium metabolism in lithium-treated patients. Relation to uni-bipolar dichotomy. Acta Psychiatr Scand 57: 124–128

Baldessarini RJ (1980) Drugs and the treatment of psychiatric disorders. In: Goodman LS, Gilman A (eds) The pharmacological basis of therapeutics. McMillan, New York, pp 391–447

Bellwinkel S, Schafer A, Minne H, Ziegler R (1975) The effect of chronic lithium application on the mineral content of rat bone and soft tissue. Int Pharmachopsychiatry 10: 9–16

Bianchi ML, Bardare M, Caraceni MP, Cohen E, Falvella G, Borzani M, DeGaspari MG (1990) Bone metabolism in juvenile rheumatoid arthritis. Bone Miner 9: 153–162

Birch NJ, Hullin RP (1972) The distribution and binding of lithium following its long-term administration. Life Sci 11: 1095–1099

Birch NJ, Jenner FA (1973) The distribution of lithium and its effects on the distribution and excretion of other ions in the rat. Br J Pharmacol 47: 586–594

Bjorum N, Hornum I, Mellerup ET, Plenge PK, Rafaelson OJ (1975) Lithium, calcium and phosphate. Lancet i: 1243

Brown EM (1981) Lithium induces abnormal calcium-regulated PTH release in dispersed bovine parathyroid cells. J Clin Endocrinol Metab 52: 1046–1048

Brown EM, Carrol RJ, Aurbach GD (1977) Dopaminergic stimulation of cyclic AMP accumulation and parathyroid hormone release from dispersed bovine parathyroid cells. Proc Natl Acad Sci USA 74: 4210–4213

Carman JS, Wyatt ES, Smith W, Post RM, Ballenger JC (1984) Calcium and calcitonin in bipolar affective disorder. In: Post RM, Ballenger JC (eds) Neurobiology of mood disorders. Williams and Wilkins, Baltimore, pp 340–345

Christensson TAT (1976) Lithium, hypercalcemia and hyperparathyroidism. Lancet ii: 144

Christiansen C, Baastrup PC, Transbol I (1975) Osteopenia and dysregulation of divalent cations in lithium-treated patients. Neuropsychobiology 1: 344–354

Christiansen C, Baastrup PC, Lindgreen P, Transbol I (1978) Endocrine effects of lithium: II. 'Primary' hyperparathyroidism. Acta Endocrinol (Copenh) 88: 528–534

Christiansen C, Baastrup PC, Transbol I (1980) Development of 'primary' hyperparathyroidism during lithium therapy: longitudinal study. Neuropsychobiology 6: 280–283

Colt EWD, Kimbrell D, Fieve RR (1981) Renal impairment, hypercalcemia, and lithium therapy. Am J Psychiatry 138: 106–108

Crammer J (1975) Lithium, calcium and mental illness. Lancet i: 215–216

Davis BM, Pfefferbaum A, Krutzik S, Davis KL (1981) Lithium's effect on parathyroid hormone. Am J Psychiatry 138: 489–492

Dunner DL, Clayton PJ (1987) Drug treatment of bipolar disorders. In: Meltzer HY (ed) Psychopharmacology. The third generation of progress. Raven, New York, pp 1077–1083

Faragalla FF, Flach FF (1970) Studies of mineral metabolism in mental depression. J Nerv Ment Dis 151: 120–129

Feinberg M, Steiner M, Carrol BJ (1979) Effects of long-term lithium treatment on serum calcium, magnesium, and calcitonin. Psychopharmacol Bull 15: 81–84

Franks RD, Dubovsky SL, Lifshitz M, Coen P, Subryan V, Walker SH (1982) Long-term lithium carbonate therapy causes hyperparathyroidism. Arch Gen Psychiatry 39: 1074–1077

Garfinkel PE, Ezrin C, Stancer HC (1973) Hypothyroidism and hyperparathyroidism associated with lithium. Lancet ii: 331–332

Gensens P, Dequeker J, Verstraeten A, Nijs J (1986) Age-, sex-, and menopause-related changes of vertebral and peripheral bone: population study using dual and single photon absorptiometry and radiogrammetry. J Nucl Med 27: 1540–1549

Gotfredson CP, Mellerup ET, Rafaelsen OJ (1969) In: Abstracts of the 2nd international meeting of the International Society of Neurochemistry, p 169

Henneman D, Zimmerberg JJ (1974) Lack of effect of chronic lithium chloride on bone composition and metabolism. Endocrinology 94: 915–917

Herman SP (1981) Lithium, hypercalcemia, and hyperparathyroidism. Biol Psychiatry 16: 593–595

Kleinfeld M, Sebastian P, Gilbert G (1984) Delirium as the predominant manifestation of hyperparathyroidism: reversal after parathyroidectomy. J Am Geriatr Soc 32: 689–693

Mallette LE, Khouri K, Zengotita H, Hollis BW, Malini S (1989) Lithium treatment increases intact and midregion parathyroid hormone and parathyroid volume. J Clin Endocrinol Metab 68: 654–660

McEachron DL, Kripke DF, Eaves M, Lenhard L, Pavlinac D, Deftos L (1980) The interaction of lithium and time-of-day on calcium, magnesium, parathyroid hormone, and calcitonin in rats. Psychiatry Res 7: 121–131

McGregor GA (1977) Hyperthyroidism and parathyroid adenoma complicating lithium treatment. Lancet ii: 1129–1130

Mellerup ET, Rafaelsen OJ (1974) Heterogeneity and biochemical findings in manic-melancholic disorders. Acta Psychiatr Scand 50: 104–111

Mellerup ET, Plenge R, Ziegler R, Rafaelsen OJ (1970) Lithium effects on calcium metabolism in rats. Int Pharmachopsychiatry 5: 258–264

Mellerup ET, Plenge P, Rafaelsen OJ (1973) Lithium effects on magnesium metabolism in rats. Int Pharmachopsychiatry 8: 178–183

Mellerup ET, Plenge P, Rafaelsen OJ (1987) Renal and other controversial effects of lithium. In: Meltzer HY (ed) Psychopharmacology: the third generation of progress. Raven, New York, pp 1443–1448

Midgett RJ, Spielvogel AM, Coburn JW, Norman AW (1973) Studies on calciferol metabolism. The renal production of the biologically active form of vitamin D, 1,25-dihydroxycholecalciferol: species, tissue and subcellular distribution. J Clin Endocrinol Metab 36: 1153–1161

Nielsen JL, Pedersen EB, Amidsen A, Darling S (1977) Reduced renal calcium excretion during lithium therapy. Psychopharmacology 54: 101–103

Nilas L, Christiansen C (1987) Bone mass and its relationship to age and the menopause. J Clin Endocrinol Metab 65: 697–702

Rafaelsen OJ, Mellerup ET, Shapiro RW (1975) Lithium research: does it lead to an integrative hypothesis for the manic-melancholic disorders? Psychopharmac Commun 1: 611–618

Rosenblatt S, Chanley JD, Segal RL (1989) The effect of lithium on vitamin D metabolism. Biol Psychiatry 26: 206–208

Rothman M (1982) Acute hyperparathyroidism in a patient after initiation of lithium therapy. Am J Psychiatry 139: 362–363

Shen FH, Sheppard DJ (1982) Lithium-induced hyperparathyroidism. An alteration of the 'set-point'. Ann Intern Medicine 96: 63–65

Spiegel AM, Gerner RH, Murphy DL, Aurbach GD (1976) Lithium does not inhibit the parathyroid hormone-mediated rise in urinary cyclic AMP and phosphate in humans. J Clin Endocrinol Metab 43: 1390–1393

Thysell H, Brante G, Sjostedt L, Lindegard B, Lindholm T, Franzen G, Rorsman B (1981) Glomerular filtration rate and calcium metabolism in long-term lithium treatment. Neuropsychobiology 7: 105–111

Amiloride and Severe Lithium-Induced Nephrogenic Diabetes Insipidus

M. Tuoni, M. Taddei, C. Pasquini, M. Bertoli, M. Meschi, A. Bionda, S. Battini and G.F. Placidi

Introduction

Lithium (Li) has been and continues to be a linking force in biomedical science generally, creating an area of interest for specialists in different scientific disciplines, even if the field of most common application is psychiatry. In current psychiatric practice Li represents the therapy of choice in treatment-resistant depression. The special physical characteristics of the Li ion, combined with its chemical relationship with sodium, mean that it penetrates into a wide variety of physiological systems. There is competition with sodium transport in the distal tubule and inhibition of renal sodium appears to be antidiuretic hormone (ADH)-mediated, although it has not been demonstrated in man.

The renal effects of Li salts have interested investigators and clinicians for several years (Singer 1981); Li therapy and kidney function are associated, and sometimes permanent renal damage may result (Alexander and Martin 1980; Bucht and Wahlin 1980). The most well known side effect is the impairment of urine-concentrating capacity, which becomes less severe after an interruption in therapy (Alexander and Martin 1980; Bucht and Wahlin 1980; De Paulo et al. 1981; Singer 1981). The treatment of Li-induced polyuria is therefore problematic; thiazide diuretics are sometimes used to reduce excessive urine output in patients receiving Li (Himmelhoch et al. 1977a, b). Such a reduction causes a compensatory increase in sodium and Li reabsorption in the proximal nephron which results in raised plasma Li levels with the potential risk of toxicity (Himmelhoch et al. 1977b; Petersen et al. 1974). Amiloride markedly improves the deficiency in free-water reabsorption caused by Li in experimental animals (Martinez-Maldonado and Opava-Stitzer 1977; Mehta et al. 1979; Webb et al. 1975) which led us to investigate the therapeutic effect of amiloride in polyuric patients who were receiving chronic Li therapy; amiloride, a potassium-sparing diuretic, seems to correct the development of hypokalemia, which is Li-induced also.

The widespread use of Li salts in mania treatment has produced nephrogenic diabetes insipidus in approximately 20%–70% of patients undergoing chronic Li therapy, even if plasma Li levels are within the therapeutic range, so that it is the most common cause of polyuria today. Because the diuretic amiloride (*N*-amidino-3,5-diamino-6-chloropyrazine-carboxamide) impairs mucosal entry of Li in ADH-responsive epithelia and reduces Li-induced antagonism to ADH in animal studies, we have investigated the action of this potassium-sparing diuretic on Li-induced polyuria in manic patients subjected to continuous Li treatment. The diuresis and urinary osmolality variations have been evaluated; renal function and Na^+–K^+ plasma and urinary concentrations have been monitored.

Materials and Methods

We have evaluated the effect of amiloride on Li-induced polyuria in 12 patients treated at the Clinical Psychiatry Institute, University of Pisa, Italy (8 women and 4 men with a mean age of 54 ± 11 years).

The patients were affected by manic depression and were undergoing different long-term Li therapies: 6 months (three patients), 1 year (two patients), 2 years (four patients), 4 years (one patient), and 6 years (two patients), and taking different daily doses of Li carbonate (from 600 to 1200 mg).

The criteria for admission to the study were:excessive total urinary volume (more than 3 l/day) and thirst; the patients had been kept on normal caloric uptake and known amounts of dietary sodium and potassium (60 mEq/day) and received 28 days of additional therapy with amiloride (5 mg three times a day).

Before and after amiloride administration, osmolality and urine volume were controlled, the following chemical plasma and urine analyses were performed: creatinine clearance, Na^+, K^+ as well as Li plasma concentration.

Urine was collected for 24 h and Na^+–K^+, creatinine, and Li in plasma and urine were assayed by means of atomic absorption spectrophotometry.

Results

The clinical and biochemical characteristics of each patient are shown in Table 1, in which Li plasma, urine volume, urine osmolality, creatinine clearance, and plasma and urine Na^+–K^+ are reported before and after amiloride therapy was combined with Li therapy.

The data were processed as mean ± standard deviation ($\bar{M}$ ± SD) for each parameter. Graphic representations of the data ($\bar{M}$ ± SD) are given in Fig. 1 (creatinine clearance, urine osmolality, and urine volume) and Fig. 2 (plasma and urine Na^+–K^+).

The administration of amiloride resulted in a significant reduction in urine volume (mean value of 5400 vs 2783 ml/24 h) and an increase in urine osmolality (mean value of 238 vs 360 mOsm/kg). Despite a decrease in urine volume no significant changes in plasma levels of Li (mean value of 0.7 vs 0.7 mmol/l), sodium (mean value of 140 vs 138 mEq/l), or potassium (mean value of 4.2 vs 4.3 mEq/l) were observed.

A reduced creatinine clearance (mean value of 124 vs 102 ml/min) and a significant increase in urinary sodium excretion (a mean value of 129 vs

Table 1. Clinical and biochemical characteristics of 12 patients receiving long-term lithium therapy with induced polyuria before and after amiloride administration

Patients and therapy	Age yr	Sex	Plasma lithium mmol/l	Urine volume L/24 h	Urine osmolality MOSM/kg	Creatinine clearance ml/min	Plasma NA mEq/L	Urine NA mEq/L	Plasma K mEq/L	Urine K mEq/L
1) LI	70	M	0.35	5700	250	95	140	145	4.9	53
LI + A			0.20	2300	410	99	140	96	4.4	91
2) LI	58	F	0.50	5450	220	86	151	154	4.1	69
LI + A			0.80	2550	380	88	142	141	3.7	35
3) LI	72	F	0.65	4600	260	152	139	85	4.3	45
LI + A			0.70	4000	380	130	137	135	4.4	21
4) LI	52	F	0.85	5000	218	121	144	90	4.7	69
LI + A			0.80	3000	400	80	141	106	4.8	23
5) LI	54	F	0.70	5500	226	157	139	136	4.5	21
LI + A			0.80	2450	365	120	137	139	4.5	56
6) LI	48	F	0.65	4500	233	126	143	163	4.9	80
LI + A			0.95	4100	280	102	141	179	4.7	88
7) LI	58	M	1.05	5750	250	68	149	135	3.9	42
LI + A			0.70	2600	395	86	134	152	3.8	61
8) LI	46	M	0.70	5800	260	144	134	140	4.0	54
LI + A			–	2700	380	–	–	–	–	–
9) LI	34	F	0.70	5900	236	168	135	110	4.6	36
LI + A			0.70	2450	285	108	137	130	4.7	44
10) LI	40	F	0.85	5700	214	146	138	135	4.1	41
LI + A			0.80	2500	340	103	135	132	3.9	53
11) LI	52	M	0.70	5300	245	110	137	150	4.3	45
LI + A			0.75	2550	340	118	138	152	3.7	38
12) LI	68	F	0.90	5600	234	115	137	110	3.9	42
LI + A			0.70	2200	370	98	140	198	5.2	28
M ± SD	54 ± 11	LI	0.7 ± 0.18	5400 ± 460	238 ± 22	124 ± 30	140 ± 5	129 ± 25	4.2 ± 0.3	49 ± 16
		LI + A	0.7 ± 0.19	2783 ± 624	360 ± 42	102 ± 15	138 ± 2	142 ± 29·	4.3 ± 0.5	48 ± 23
					(NR500–800)	(NR80–120)	(NR136–145)	(NR80–180)	(NR3.4–4.5)	(NR25–100)

Li + A, lithium plus amiloride; NR, normal range

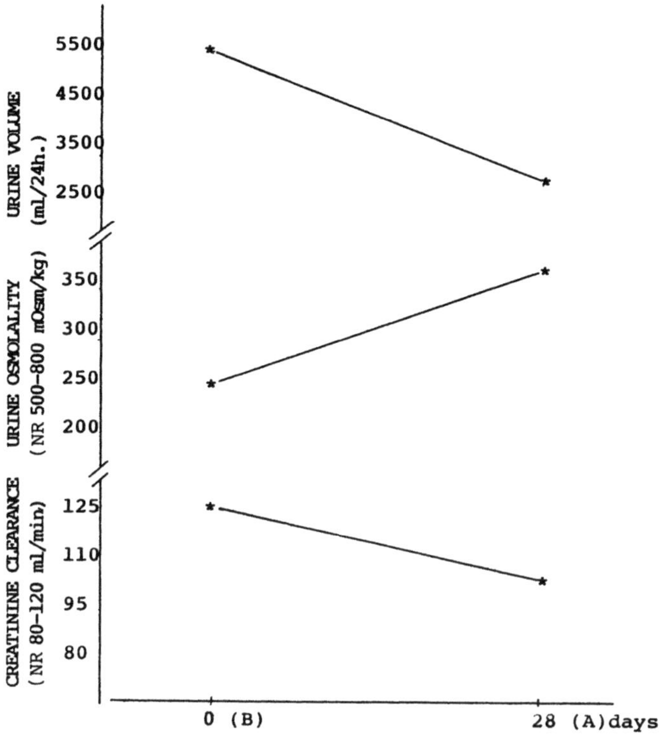

Fig. 1. Creatinine clearance, urine osmolality, and urine volume ($\bar{M} \pm SD$) before and after amiloride administration. (*B*), before amiloride administration; (*A*), after amiloride administration; *NR*, normal range

142 mEq/l), were noted, even though these variations have to be considered as being within the normal range.

Conclusions

The addition of amiloride to the Li therapy resulted in a significant reduction in urine volume and an increase in urine osmolality; the effect of amiloride on Li handling is safe and differs from that produced during thiazide administration (no hypokalemia was observed and its prevention is also desirable, because hypokalemia in itself may decrease the urinary-concentrating capacity). In our patients polyuria was reduced in 83% of cases so that amiloride appears to be the initial treatment of choice for Li-induced polyuria even if further studies are necessary in order to explore this hypothesis.

These findings were associated with subjective decreases in thirst and urinary frequency. The amiloride reduces urinary volume without decreasing Li

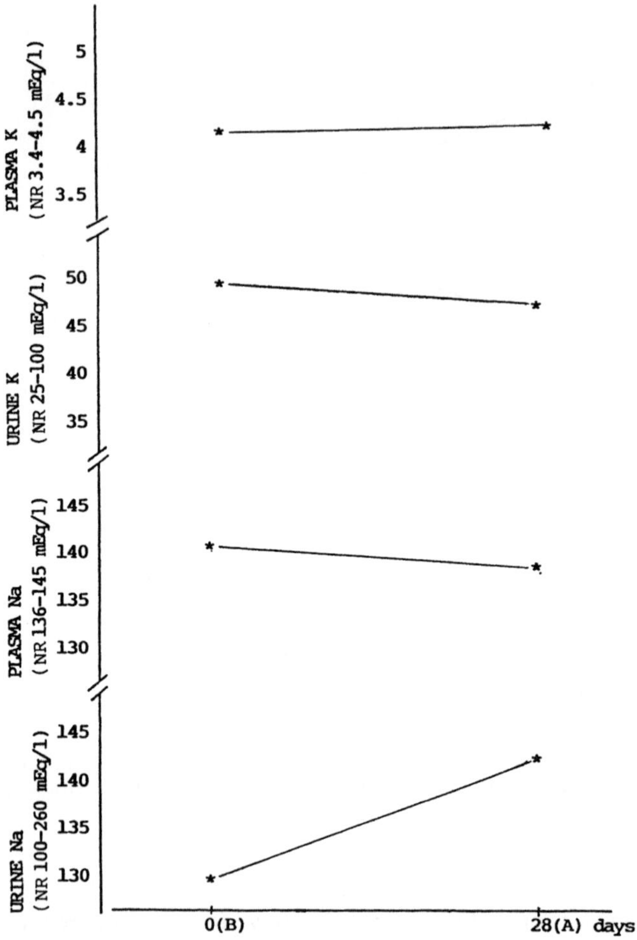

Fig. 2. Na^+ and K^+ (plasma–urine) before and after amiloride administration ($\bar{M} \pm SD$). (*B*), before amiloride administration; (*A*), after amiloride administration; *NR*, normal range

clearance (no Li plasma concentration differences have been noted during the amiloride therapy: 0.7 mmol/l before and 0.7 mmol/l after amiloride).

We conclude that a large number of patients may benefit from this method of treatment.

References

Alexander F, Martin J (1980) Lithium and nephrotic syndrome. Lab Invest 42: 97–99
Baylis PH, Heath DA (1978) Water disturbances in patients treated with oral lithium carbonate. Ann Intern Med 88: 607–609
Battle D, Gaviria M, Grupp M, Arruda JAL, Wynn J, Kurtzman NA (1982) Distal nephron function in patients receiving chronic lithium therapy. Kidney Int. 21: 477–485.
Bucht G, Wahlin A (1980) Renal concentrating capacity in long-term lithium treatment and after withdrawal of lithium. Acta Med. Scand. 207: 309–314.
De Paulo R, Correa ET, Saphir DG (1981) Renal toxicity of lithium and its implications. Johns Hopkins Med J. 149: 15–21.
Forrest JN Jr, Cohen AD, Torretti J, Himmelhoch JM, Epstein FH (1974) On the mechanism of lithium-induced diabetes insipidus in man and rat. J Clin Invest 53: 1115–1123.
Himmelhoch JM, Forrest J, Neil JF, Detre TP (1977a) Thiazide lithium synergy in refractory mood swings. Am J Psychiatry 134: 149–152.
Himmelhoch JM, Poust RI, Mallinger AG, Hanin I, Neil JF (1977b) Adjustment of lithium dose during lithium chlorothiazide therapy. Clin Pharmacol Ther 22: 225–227.
Kosten TR, Forrest JN Jr (1982) Treatment of severe lithium-induced nephrogenic diabetes insipidus with amiloride. Clin Res 30: 540A
Martinez-Maldonado M, Opava-Stitzer S (1977) Distal nephron function of the rat during lithium chloride infusion. Kidney Int 12: 17–22.
Mehta PK, Sodhi B, Arruda JAL, Kurtzman NA (1979) Interaction of amiloride and lithium on distal urinary acidification. J Lab Clin Med 93: 983–994.
Petersen V, Hvidt S, Thomsen K, Schou M (1974) Effect of prolonged thiazide treatment on renal lithium clearance. Br Med J 3: 143–145
Shou M (1958) Lithium studies. Acta Pharmacol Toxicol 15: 85–124.
Singer I (1981) Nephrology forum: lithium and kidney. Kidney Int 19: 374–387.
Webb RK, Woodhall PB, Tisher CC, Robinson RR (1975) Acute effects of lithium on the renal concentrating mechanism in a primate. Am J Physiol 228: 909–914.

New Pharmacological Aspects of Rubidium Salts

F. Vaglini, M. Petrini, and G.U. Corsini

Introduction

Rubidium (Rb) is an alkaline metal that was discovered by Bunsen and Kirchoff in 1861. Botkin was the first to describe the effects of bradycardia and hypertension induced by Rb (Botkin 1888). For 30 years Rb has been employed as a drug useful in cardiology, neurology, and for the therapy of syphilis. After this period its use decreased; it has only recently been reintroduced in therapy.

Rubidium (Rb) salts exert several pharmacological effects on the central nervous system; most of these are directed on neurotransmitters, specifically norepinephrine (NE) (Stolk et al. 1970). Rb enhances the turnover of NE in rats and modifies the lithium-induced increase of NE into synaptosomes.

More recently one of the most interesting aspects of the pharmacology of Rb regards its action on hematologic cells. It is known that lithium (Li) salts induce the maturation of bone marrow cells (Joyce 1984; De Vries et al. 1983), although uncertainties still exist about the exact mechanism of action and type of target cells. Its clinical use is thus justified in patients affected by leukopenia, in spite of certain limitations deriving from the demonstration that this metal is able to induce the proliferation of leukemic cells (Doukas et al. 1985). Lithium moreover inhibits some functions of neutrophil granulocyte such as adherence and bactericidal activity.

Recently Rb has been evaluated in leukocyte functions by means of chemotaxis under agarose and the nitroblue tetrazolium (NBT) reduction test, and it has been found to enhance several of these leukocyte functions (Azzara et al. 1986). These results have been indirectly confirmed by chemoluminescence assay, which indicated that Rb significantly increases, in a dose-dependent fashion, the chemoluminescence induced in leukocytes by opsonized zymosan. These considerations prompted us to study whether Rb could play any role in leukocyte differentiation and proliferation. With this aim, culture tests were carried out in vitro to evaluate whether Rb could act on hematologic precursors.

Materials and Methods

Bone Marrow Cultures

Bone marrow cultures were performed in accordance with previous methods with only slight modifications (Metcalf 1977). To summarize, bone marrow cells were obtained from patients while undergoing surgery on the thorax which were then centrifuged on a Ficoll-Hypaque density gradient at 1800 rpm for 30 min at room temperature. Mononuclear cells were washed twice and resuspended in α-medium (Gibco) supplemented with 20% of fetal calf serum (FCS) (Eurobio) and 10% of glutamine (Eurobio), then 2×10^5 were plated in 0.3% agar (Difco) with optimal concentrations of commercially conditioned medium. The concentrations of RbCl (Sigma) added to medium ranged from 0 to 1.5 mEq/liter. Cells were cultured in duplicate in 5% CO_2 humid atmosphere at 37 °C for 14–16 days and examined using an Olympus inverted microscope. Cell aggregates counting more than 50 cells were counted as colonies. Counting was performed blind.

HL 60 Cultures

HL 60 cells, a human bipotential cell line, were kept in Dulbecco's modified Eagle's medium (Grand Island Biological Co), containing 20% of FCS (Flow Laboratories), 10% of trypticase soy broth (BBL Microbiological System, Becton-Dickinson), and antibiotics (medium A) (Sambuy et al. 1985). By substituting the culture medium with RPMI 1640 supplemented with 20% of FCS (Eurobio lot. no. 756729), 10% glutamine, and 20% hepes (Eurobio) (medium B), with or without 1 mEq/liter of RbCl (Sigma), differentiation of these cells was achieved.

Cell typing was performed by immunofluorescence as previously described (Petrini et al. 1983). Briefly, monoclonal antibodies anti-Dr (Becton-Dickinson) and CD11b (Coulter) were used as a first layer. A FITC antiserum antimouse immunoglobulin as a second layer was employed. Appropriate controls were performed. A Leitz Ortholux microscope was used to examine flourescent cells. Cytochemical typing was performed on cytocentrifuged cells to put into evidence the positive myeloperoxidase or α-naphthyl butyrate esterase cells (Petrini et al. 1986). Experiments were performed in triplicate. By adding $10^{-8} M$ $1.25(OH)_2D_3$ to the culture medium, monocyte differentiation of the line was obtained.

In Vivo Administration

RbCl (180 mg × 3/day) was administered to two patients affected by chronic myeloid leukemia during a blast crisis. They were unresponsive to any conventional therapy.

Results

Bone Marrow Cultures

Bone marrow mononuclear cells from 12 donors produced 172 (range 112–284) clusters plus colonies. No significant modification of this figure was induced by the addition of Rb to the culture medium ($\bar{x} = 236$; range 90–528). Nevertheless

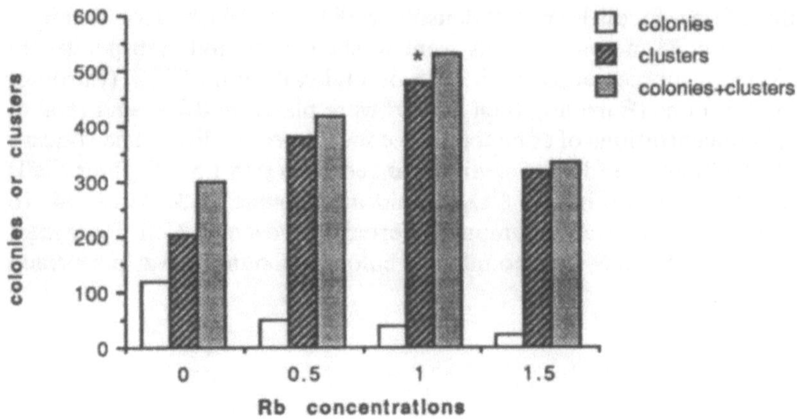

Fig. 1. Dose-response activity of different concentrations of Rb on colonies, clusters, and clusters plus colonies. *$p < 0.05$ compared with controls

by evaluating separately the numbers of colonies and clusters, the latter increased significantly in the presence of Rb ($\bar{x} = 332$; range 144–227; $n = 6$; $P < 0.05$ Wilcoxon's test). The colonies decreased at the same time (Rb $\bar{x} = 34$, range 16–92; controls 64, range 32–98). When the commercial conditioned medium was substituted by the supernatant of lymphocyte cultures, similar results were obtained. When the cells were cultured without any conditioned medium, no effects of the metal were seen. In a dose-response curve, Rb from the dose of 0 to 1 Eq/liter increased the cluster number. Higher concentrations caused a decrease of the clusters (Fig. 1).

Conditioned media from PHA-activated lymphocytes cultured both with or without 1 mEq/liter of Rb did not differ in their ability to induce colony or cluster proliferation (colonies plus clusters $\bar{x} = 255$; range·200–310).

HL 60 Cultures

HL 60 cells were continuously cultured in medium A in 5% CO_2 humidified atmosphere at 37 °C. The cells were diluted and every 3 days the medium was changed. This line was < 5% reactive for HLA Dr though not for CD11b. Less than 5% of the cells were myeloperoxidase positive. When 1 mEq/liter of Rb was added to the medium A, no difference was found in this pattern. A fast myeloid differentiation was achieved when the HL 60 cells were cultured in medium B: after 6 days the cells were clearly Dr + (56%) and 70% peroxidase + cells were found. After 9 days the cells were Dr + 90%, CD11b + 30%, and 90% intensively reactive to myeloperoxidase. The morphological analysis indicated that the cells were intensively granulated, showing less stained nucleoli, and rare granulocytes were found between them. The differentiation became faster by adding Rb to the medium B, and after 3 days 12% Dr + and 12%

Table 1. Modification of the HL 60 line induced by a differentiating medium with (+Rb) or without (−Rb) 1 mEq/liter RbCl after different periods

	Day 0		Day 6			
	Medium A	Medium B	Medium A		Medium B	
			−Rb	+Rb	−Rb	+Rb
HLA Dr	<5%	<5%	<5%	<5%	56%	60%
CD 11b	neg	neg	neg	neg	neg	20%
Px	<5%	<5%	<5%	<5%	70%	90%
	+ − −	+ − −	+ − −	+ − −	+ + −	+ + +

CD11b and HLA Dr, surface markers evaluated by monoclonal antibody, Px, myeloperoxidase reaction: − negative; + positive; + rare positive granules; + + many positive granules; + + + cytoplasm filled with positive granules.

CD11b + cells, after 6 days 60% Dr + and 20% CD11b + cells, and after 9 days 90% Dr + and 60% CD11b + cells. A faster differentation was confirmed by morphological examinations of the cells. After 6 days almost all the cells were peroxidase + (Table 1). The appearance of a 10% α-napthyl butyrate positive cells was induced by the use of $1.25(OH)_2D_3$, but not with Rb. Cell counts were not different in samples with or without Rb.

In Vivo Administration

The administration of Rb to the first patient did not modify the peripheral blood cell count that was about $100 \times 10^9/mm^3$ with 98% of blast cells. However, after 3 days of treatment, marked morphological modifications of the blasts occurred. More interestingly, the interruption of the therapy with Rb was followed by an increase of peripheral leukocytes, and their morphological characteristics were the same as those of the blasts before the therapy. Rb was administered again to the same patient, and after 10 days, the peripheral blood cell number decreased to $74 \times 10^9/mm^3$ cells.

Rb was administered to the second patient with the same schedule. We observed a reduction of the leukocyte figure from 62×10^9 (100% blasts) to $16 \times 10^9/mm^3$ during the administration time.

After these treatments, both patients returned to a previous stage of the disease. Subsequently further blast crisis was fatal in both patients.

Discussion

Many studies have indicated that Rb plays an anti-Li activity in different biologic systems, including leukocytes. A preliminary report from our laboratory indicated that Rb, opposite to Li, induced a high number of peroxidase positive cells and a low figure of α-naphthyl butyrate positive cells in culturing mononuclear cells from healthy donors (Petrini et al. 1986). This experiment suggested that Rb may have a differentiating activity on circulating leukocyte cells. The present study confirmed this suggestion, indicating specifically that Rb reduces the number of colonies whereas it increases the number of clusters in a dose-dependent fashion. Rb may act by stimulating more mature progenitors which form clusters and, on the contrary, suppressing immature progenitors which form colonies. An alternative interpretation consists of the inability of colonies to grow to a full extent in the presence of Rb which might result in the formation of clusters. We have excluded a possible cytotoxic or nonspecific antiproliferative activity of Rb by evaluating its action on the incorporation of H^3 thymidine in lymphocytes stimulated with optimal doses of different mitogens (data not shown). Rb did not affect the number of HL 60 cells cultured from 3 to 9 days. Rb may act by enhancing the activity of factors present in the culture medium, which contains a specific conditioned medium. However, Rb is not able to induce the production of CSF from lymphocytes as evaluated by substituting the conditioned medium from the supernatant of lymphocytes cultured with the metal. Experiments with HL 60 have indirectly confirmed that Rb has an activity on leukocyte differentiation. When cultured in the medium B, enriched with FCS Eurobio (lot no. 756729), HL 60 cells were able to differentiate toward granulocytes. Although it seems that FCS was responsible for the differentiating activity, we cannot exclude that other components may play a role. Rb was able to facilitate the differentiation promoted by this medium. No differentiating activity was obtained on this line continuously cultured in the regular medium that does not induce differentiation. It has been shown that Rb modifies the contents of second messengers of different cells (Geisler et al. 1984). This biochemical modification, after receptor activation by soluble factors, present in the medium, could account for our results.

The modifications of number and morphology of circulating blasts found in the patients treated with Rb salt are in agreement with an in vivo differentiating activity. This effect must be further confirmed, and it could be useful in the management of leukemic patients.

References

Azzara A, Petrini M, Carulli G, Polidori R, Vaglini F, Trombi L, Mian M, Bertėlli A, Ambrogi F (1986) The effects of lithium and rubidium on human leukocyes functions. Int J Immunother II(3): 233–238

Botkin SS (1888) The influence of the salts of rubidium and cesium upon the heart and circulation in connection with the laws of physiological action of alkali metals (doctoral dissertation). St Petersburg Military Academy, St Petersburg

De Vries EG, Van Luyn MJ, Mulder NH, Bins M, Haile MR (1983) In vitro effects of lithium on granulocyte colony formation in normal men, in haematological disorders and in small-cell carcinoma of the lung. Acta Haematol 70: 97–107

Doukas MA, Niskanen EO, Quesenberry PJ (1985) Lithium stimulation of granulopoiesis in diffusion chambers – a model of a humoral, indirect stimulation of stem cell proliferation. Blood 65: 163–168

Geisler A, Klynser R, Andersen PH (1984) Opposite effects of Li and Rb on neurohormone-stimulated cyclic AMP accumulation in brain. In: Corsini (ed) Current trends in lithium and rubidium therapy. MTP Press, Boston, pp 37–57
Joyce RA (1984) Sequential effects of lithium on haematopoiesis. Br J Haematol 56: 307–321
Metcalf D (1977) Hematopoietic colonies. In: In vitro cloning of normal and leukemic cells, vol 1. Berlin: Springer, Berlin Heidelberg New York, pp 225–235
Petrini M, Emerson DL, Galbraith RM (1983) Linkage between immunoglobulin and cytoskeleton of B lymphocytes may involve Gc protein. Nature 306: 73–75
Petrini M, La Gioia A, Lofaro A, Dastoli G, Ambrogi F, Spremolla G (1986a) A case of idiopathic myelofibrosis with poorly differentiated circulating blast. The role of the fixative in the peroxidase reaction. Haematologica 71: 411–416
Petrini M, Vaglini F, Carulli G, Azzara A, Ambrogi F, Bertelli A (1986b) Effects of lithium and rubidium on the differentiation of mononuclear cells. Int J Tissue React 7: 391–392
Rossini D, Petrini M, Vaglini F, Bertelli A (1987) Lithium versus rubidium in chemiluminescence. Acta Haematol 77: 241–242
Sambuy Y, Spagnoli LG, Vigneti E, Revoltella RP (1985) Ultrastructural studies of spontaneous in vitro transformation of cultured marrow monocyte-macrophage cells from a patient with congenital hypoplastic anemia. Cancer Res 45: 1392–1401
Stolk JM, Nowack WJ, Barrhas JD (1970) Brain norepinephrine: enhanced turnover after rubidium treatment. Science 168: 501–503

Rubidium – 20 Years On

S.R. Platman

Introduction

Rubidium (Rb) from the Latin word "rubidus" (darkest red) was discovered by Bunsen and Kirchoff in 1861. It is one of the Group IA alkali metals. This is the same periodic series to which lithium, sodium, potassium, francium, and cesium belong. Rubidium, like potassium, is concentrated intracellularly by most living tissue. It is found in all foods and the average person contains 4.2 mEq (0.36 g) of rubidium as compared with 3200 mEq of potassium. Physiologically, it most resembles potassium but also shares properties with cesium. Rubidium is rapidly and completely absorbed, reaching maximum plasma levels within 60–90 min. Once absorbed it is widely distributed to all tissues and is primarily found in erythrocytes, platelets, brain, kidney, and liver. In the brain it is highest in the basal ganglia and has been found to decrease with increasing age. In contrast to humans, rubidium is relatively lacking in the brain and CSF of animals. In general there is a tendency for rubidium to have higher intracellular to extracellular ratios than potassium; however, one exception appears in brain tissue, which prefers potassium to rubidium.

The first documented use of rubidium in human treatment was in 1877 for acute cardiovascular disease. It was noted that most subjects showed an improvement in their subjective sense of well-being. Botkin, a student of Pavlov, performed this work in Leningrad, then St. Petersburg, and he administered rubidium chloride orally in daily doses of approximately 1.6 g, up to a total of 300 mEq. This is a total dose of 25.7 G and modern studies have only recently treated patients with equivalent amounts. It was noted that the pulse slowed and the blood pressure increased (Botkin 1888). Fieve et al. noted in 1973 that in their survey of the entire foreign literature no one ever died from taking rubidium; and, as reported by its users, it produced no surprising or irreversible side effects. They also noted that the 1940 edition of The Merck Manual listed rubidium compounds in recommended dosages for use as an antiepileptic, as a hypnotic, for nervous afflictions, and for external use in optic neuritis and conjunctivitis. Certainly this history documents rubidium as having a long clinical history, and its use has not been associated with any major toxic side effects.

A Relook at Rubidium in the United States

In the 1960s I was fortunate to be working at Columbia University with Ronald Fieve, Herbert Meltzer, and others in research involving the alkali metals. At that time we were comfortable with the fact that lithium was an impressive agent for the treatment and prevention of manic episodes in many individuals with affective disorders. However, we were less convinced of its therapeutic effect on the treatment or prevention of depression. It is of interest that even today, the 1990 United States Physician's Desk Reference (PDR) only recommends lithium for the treatment of the "manic episode of manic depressive illness and maintenance therapy to prevent or diminish the intensity of subsequent episodes in those manic-depressive patients with a history of mania". Although it is probably true that lithium may be valuable in some patients with depression, this is still a controversial subject. Yet depression is a much commoner problem than mania and creates an enormous economic and human burden. More than 6% of the general population of the United States meet primary diagnostic criteria for affective disorder, according to the NIMH Epidemiological Catchment Area Study assessing the incidence of various forms of psychopathology. This total does not include those individuals who are dually diagnosed and whose depression is considered secondary to another psychiatric condition. The 6-month prevalence rates for subtypes of affective disorders are: bipolar disorder, 0.5%; major depression, 3%; and dysthymia (depressive neurosis), 3.3%. Only one-third of those suffering from primary affective disorder are currently receiving any form of treatment. Depression has many consequences; the most serious is suicide. Therefore, our interest was turned to the possibility of using an alkali metal for the treatment of depression.

At that time we had a belief – probably wrong – that total body changes of potassium were related to depression and sodium to mania. The interrelationship between sodium and lithium led us to look at the known relationship between potassium and rubidium. Herbert Meltzer, who was part of our team at Columbia University, had shown that rubidium had an opposite effect to lithium in vitro on strandin constrained in an artificial membrane (Meltzer 1966). We then attempted to show that this opposite effect might be observed in vivo in animals by changes in overall behavior and in the EEG. Our 1969 article in *Nature* (Meltzer et al. 1969) showed that rubidium in macacus rhesus monkeys produced a shift in the EEG to a preponderance of higher frequencies (alerting response) and also an increase in alertness and activity. In contrast, we had shown that lithium tends to slow the EEG and reduce hyperactive behavior and excessive affect in humans (Platman and Fieve 1969). This exciting finding was followed by Stolk's study published in *Science* examining the effects of rubidium on the metabolism of brain catecholamines in rats (Stolk et al. 1970). It was found that again lithium and rubidium had opposite effects on catecholamine metabolism and suggested that studies needed to be performed with rubidium to evaluate its possible use in depressive states. One year later Stolk showed that daily doses of rubidium increased the level of shock-elicited aggressive behavior in rats in contrast to the effect of lithium (Stolk et al. 1971).

At the same time (1971) Carroll and Sharp in Australia showed that rubidium potentiated morphine activation in mice like that of antidepressant drugs such as imipramine and pargyline. Lithium and other antimanic drugs had the opposite effect.

These findings on behavior, amines, and EEG led to the consideration that rubidium might have a therapeutic effect on depression as lithium had a therapeutic effect on mania. Proving this was more difficult. In addition, it was known that rapid intravenous use in animals was lethal and that the biologic half-life was 50-60 days. Human clinical studies were initiated in Italy and the United States. Fieve et al. (1971) performed acute loading studies using doses of 0.5–1.0 g of rubidium chloride. They also performed chronic loading studies on depressed patients and reached a maximum plasma level of 0.30 mEq/liter. No consistent side effects or behavioral effects were noted on the patients. It was confirmed that by using total body potassium measures, potassium is replaced by rubidium approximately milliequivalent for milliequivalent when the latter is ingested orally. The authors warned that any studies using rubidium should assure adequate potassium intake and balance and that caution should be observed if the cumulative retained milliequivalent of rubidium exceeds 10% of the estimated milliequivalent of total body potassium. More recently, Meltzer (1990) has found that the replacement of 30% of intracellular potassium is a toxic threshold level. This would suggest that maintaining rubidium/potassium intake ratio at or below 1/5 would prevent potential toxicity.

Table 1. The "opposites" (modified from Williams and Sky-Peck 1986)

Rubidium	Lithium
Antagonizes alcohol-induced narcosis	Augments alcohol-induced narcosis
Potentiates morphine-induced hyperactivity	Antagonizes morphine-induced hyperactivity
Prolongs refractory periods of all nerve fibers	Prolongs only the longer refractory periods of nerve fibers
Increases turnover of NE	Increases uptake of NE
Catecholamine metabolism directed toward O-methylation pathway	Catecholamine metabolism directed toward deamination pathway
Increases dopamine-sensitive adenylate cyclase	Decreases dopamine-sensitive adenylate cyclase
Major physiological effect on potassium metabolism	Major physiological effect on sodium metabolism
Decreases activity of ATPase	Increases activity of ATPase
Increased activity of NE-stimulated adenyl cyclase	Decreases activity of NE-stimulated adenyl cyclase
Increases spontaneous motor activity	Decreases spontaneous motor activity
Increases shock-elicited aggressive behavior	Decreases shock-elicited aggressive behavior
Increases EEG activity	Decreases EEG activity
Predominantly antidepressant	Predominantly antimanic
May cause mania	May cause depression

In 1972 the National Institute of Mental Health held a workshop entitled "Rubidium: Safety and Potential as an Antidepressant." At this meeting Gershon (1974) wisely noted that much of the data presented was based on the hypothesis of opposites (Table 1). By this Gershon meant that the value of rubidium was based on the premise that lithium and rubidium should have opposite effects. As a criticism of this simplistic concept, he noted that lithium was useful in treating mania but it might also be useful in treating depression and therefore the "opposite hypothesis" should not be the single criterion for developing research paradigms. In addition other possible criticisms of the value of rubidium was the lack of a uniform, simple animal model for depression and that behavioral changes that are found may not be related to changes in amine metabolism. However, this concept of "opposites" has continued, and Geisler et al. (1990) now suggest that rubidium may be a lithium antagonist.

In 1975 Meltzer and Fieve wrote an overview of the use of rubidium in psychiatry and medicine, in which they discussed the effects of chronic administration to 15 affectively ill patients. They noted that when patients retained more than 200 mEq of rubidium and attained peak levels greater than 0.25 mEq/liter, mood was noted to improve. In addition, their study showed that lithium increased the excretion of rubidium. Thus, at this time these authors had basically repeated and gone beyond the 1877 study of Botkin. They had used a dose of rubidium up to 1 g three times a day without significant side effects and with apparent improvement in mood.

More Recent Clinical Studies

Since these early findings a number of clinical studies have been performed predominantly in Italy. It should be noted that many of the earlier studies are of limited value as they were of an open design and utilized clinical populations lacking in any rigid selection of patients with affective disorders. They have gradually improved in their quality and sophistication.

The first systematic clinical report (Carolei et al.) appeared in 1975 (in Italian) and compared rubidium to imipramine in a single blind study. I reviewed an English translation of Carolei's paper, which was a randomized open study comparison of 15 patients treated with rubidium and 15 with imipramine. Those treated with rubidium received increasing doses from 180 mg to 540 mg over the first 7 days and those with imipramine were increased from 45 mg to 200 mg for the first 7 days and both groups were treated for 3 weeks. All patients requested and received benzodiazepines. Improvement was basically comparable in the two groups although rubidium appeared to be somewhat more effective with psychomotor retardation. Thirty-three percent showed very good results and 33% showed good results. Rubidium appeared endowed with more specific activating properties. Results were better in endogenous depression. In three cases treated with rubidium there was transitory but not significant increase of anxiety and restlessness. Rubidium levels in total blood after the 1st week averaged 0.31 and at the end of treatment was 1.22 mEq/liter. There was no relationship between improvement, dose, and blood level. Peak improvement was noted at 10 days for rubidium.

In 1980 Calandra and Nicolosi (in Italian) reported a double-blind study in which rubidium appeared superior to clomipramine. Twenty-eight depressed patients received rubidium chloride at a dose of 540 mg daily or chlorimpramine at 100 mg/day for a total of 30 days. No particular side effects were reported and the therapeutic effect was best at plasma levels of rubidium ranging from 0.10 to 0.32 mEq/liter.

In 1981 G.U. Corsini et al. (Preliminary Results with Rubidium in Depressed Patients, unpublished work) from the University of Cagliari in Italy reported in an open study the results of rubidium treatment of ten patients with a range of affective disorders treated for 4 weeks. Dose ranged from 180 to 540 mg and lorazepam was allowed. Six patients did well. Side effects were minimal.

In 1984 Sarteschi et al. studied 21 female depressed patients and used standardized measures to record improvement on rubidium 180–540 mg/day for 3 weeks. A net improvement of 61.9% was noted and there was no improvement in five patients. Two patients were withdrawn from the study, one because of diarrhea and one because of an increase in liver enzymes due to prior chronic hepatitis. A mild well-tolerated bradycardic effect was noted in six patients.

In 1988 Placidi et al. published an open study at the University of Pisa. All 31 patients had been previously treated with various antidepressant modalities and none had been found to be resistant to such treatment. There was a washout period of 1 week, and each patient received a flexible dosage varying from 180 mg to 720 mg daily over a 3-week period. Average dose over the 3-week period was 370–407 mg. The rubidium blood level was between 0.15 and 0.37 mEq/liter, and no significant correlation was found between blood concentration and clinical improvement. Lorazepam was given as needed as the authors felt rubidium possessed activating and disinhibiting properties. The mean age of the patients was 56 and age of onset was 39. Eighteen of the patients were thought to have a major depression, single or recurrent. Of the 16 that completed the trial, 70% showed a significant improvement that appeared greatest during the 2nd week. Terminations were due to adverse reactions (2), inefficacy (7), mania (1), and 5 as they had improved significantly prior to the end of the study. Individuals with chronic mood disorders as opposed to episodic disorders accounted for most terminations. Pulse rate decreased. The most common reactions that necessitated downward adjustment of dosage or interruption of treatment included diarrhea, polyuria, confusional state, and/or excitement. Twelve responders elected to continue the drug after the completion of the 3-week trial. At 8 weeks most continued to improve. It was noted that response was predicted by a retarded depressive profile, and the authors interpret that this may mean that its therapeutic action may be limited to bipolar depressives. They also reported a case of combined lithium and rubidium without side effects.

Two recently published papers in Italian (Bonelli et al. 1989; Calandra et al. 1989) showed similar rapid improvement utilizing a dose up to 900 mg daily and noted similar side effects.

Chronic studies have been performed but only with a limited number of patients. In 1976 Fieve reported that bipolar patients showed a decrease in both the duration and severity of depressive episodes and prolongation of manic episodes. In 1978 Paschalis et al. reported in five rapid cycling patients resistant to other therapy that rubidium decreases the duration and severity of dysthymic phases but prolongs manic episodes. No side effects were noted. In 1983 Jenner et al. studied five patients suffering from periodic affective disorders with short mood cycles and treated with rubidium chloride producing peak erythrocyte concentrations between 9 and 13 mmol/liter. Loading caused decreased total body potassium but erythrocyte potassium was unchanged. Mood cycling was disturbed as well as the usual weight changes.

There has been limited use of rubidium in clinical states other than the affective disorders. However, there have been studies in Canada in patients with schizophrenia and some consideration of its use in alcoholism. In 1977 Chouinard and Annable studied the use of rubidium in individuals with chronic schizophrenia. They added a single dose of rubidium chloride at each of four dose levels (0.5 g, 1 g, 1.5 g, 2 g) to the regular neuroleptic medication of 18 chronic schizophrenic patients in a double-blind, placebo-controlled study lasting 56 days. A dose-related response suggested that rubidium increased the affectivity of these patients. The maximum therapeutic effect appeared to occur 3 weeks after ingestion. However, individuals on the highest dose also showed an increase in hostile suspiciousness and anxious depression, and this was assumed to be due to an excess of cerebral norepinephrine. At a later date, Chouinard and Annable (1983) presented at the May 1983 APA meeting an extension of a prior double-blind study, in which he had shown that giving 1 G of rubidium monthly to 24 hospitalized chronic schizophrenic patients led to a gradual improvement of function over 12 weeks. This improvement appeared to correlate with the serum concentration. In contrast to a rapid improvement in negative symptoms, positive symptom improvement was delayed in response, and this suggested that rubidium desensitized the supersensitive dopamine neurons responsible for positive symptoms. This study was now extended to 24 weeks and the neuroleptics were partially reduced by 26% of their dose. The patients treated with rubidium required little "as needed" chlorpromazine as compared with the placebo group. Rubidium tended to exacerbate the extrapyramidal symptoms of the neuroleptics, and it should be recalled that rubidium is at maximum brain concentration in the basal ganglia. There were no other toxic side effects. Rubidium serum levels at 6 months varied between 0.0–0.13 and 0.023 mEq/liter and in red cells between 0.218 and 0.452 mEq/liter.

There have been studies (Messiha 1978, 1984; D'Amato and Feis 1990; Demmel et al. 1984) showing that rubidium is helpful in the treatment of alcoholism by reducing the central depressant effect of alcohol. A study of patients with alcoholism suffering from Wernicke-Korsakoff syndrome showed diminished values of rubidium in nearly all analyzed studies of cerebral nuclei. It is of interest that in this clinical situation, rubidium may have a similar therapeutic action to lithium although even the reported lithium studies have not been validated.

Discussion

In the United States in spite of our early interest and work with rubidium, there has been little progress since the early 1970s. Of course this does not reflect a lack of interest but is related to the conservative stance of the FDA and the fact that development of this substance as a therapeutic agent has not been of interest to the pharmaceutical industry.

This is unfortunate as depression is all too common a problem and many patients are still not responsive to the present antidepressant agents available. They all have potentially serious side effects. Their effectiveness is real but limited. In controlled trials 60%–70% of patients improve substantially but the placebo response is 20%–40%. Regardless of what antidepressant and dose is used, there is a resistant group of patients. In addition, there is a substantial number of patients that will not take the existing medications due to the presence of unacceptable side effects or from the fear of ingesting a nonnatural substance. ECT may be of value for some of these failures but in the United States its use is becoming increasingly burdensome. Mood stabilizing agents such as lithium or carbamazepine (Tegretol) may be helpful in some patients but often do not help individuals with depression.

It is evident that rubidium has the potential to be an additional therapeutic agent in this spectrum of approaches for depressed patients (Table 2). However, existing studies have been limited in numbers and design. An excellent recent review was published in 1988 by Angelis et al. and in this research review, they noted that a major trial is taking place at the University of Siena. In this study a total of 400 patients are being given 180 mg three times a day for a period of 1 month. However, the dose utilized in this study appears to be below that which will give rise to maximum therapeutic effect even though side effects at the present dosage regimen are minimal. Improvement, in those patients who improve, is rapid and it appears especially beneficial for those patients who appear depressed and withdrawn.

Table 2. Clinical aspects of rubidium

A 60%–75% improvement in depressed patients
Comparable effect to TCAs
Maximal action in 1–2 weeks
Best in individuals with retarded symptoms
Present dose uses from 180–900 mg/daily
Period of treatment usually up to 4 weeks
Maximum plasma levels obtained to date are 0.35–0.5 mEq/liter

Table 3. Side effects of rubidium

None serious to date with oral dose
Agitation
Anxiety
Mania
Confusion
Dry mouth
Nausea/vomiting
Diarrhea
Polyurea
Bradycardia
Exacerbates EPS from neuroleptics

Rubinorm (rubidium chloride) has now been released to patients in Italy for approximately 2 years. It is stated that over 5000 patients have received rubidium for depression in Italy without any major toxic problems and no mortality (Table 3). This release was expedited by a report at the 37th National Congress held in Rome in February 1989. This report was based on a multicenter study held by ten centers including four university centers and six psychiatric centers (Dell'Osso et al. 1989): 87 of the patients were hospitalized, 5 were in a day hospital, and 61 were outpatients. The commonest diagnosis was recurrent depression. The study included 154 individuals. The usual dose of rubidium chloride was 540 mg daily although the maximum dose used was 900 mg daily. Benzodiazepines could be used. The study was finished by 122 and 13 stopped because of side effects. Of those who finished the 28-day study, 73% improved, 20% were unchanged, and 7% were worse at the end of 4 weeks. Improvement began in 1 week. In addition there were two reports of randomly assigned studies comparing rubidium with Elavil (amitriptylene) and Tofranil (imipramine). The rubidium dose was 540–720 mg daily and the TCAs were used with a dose of 75–100 mg daily. Rubidium and the TCAs were equal in their effectiveness. Side effects noted included agitation, confusion, mouth dryness, skin rashes, stomach pain, nausea, and vomiting.

Apparently there are problems in getting physicians in Italy to prescribe Rubinorm. Physicians fear its side effects and diarrhea has proved a problem. Its long half-life worries many physicians and there is a fear that once ingested, toxicity cannot be easily countered. Most patients have only been treated with a maximum dose of 540 mg daily and its effect at this level is not outstanding. Activity is not impressive until a dose of 720 mg daily is reached and it is stated to be even better at 900 mg daily. Of great interest is its rapid onset of action. Maximum effect is often in the first 10 days and this is superior to many other antidepressants. It certainly would appear that rubidium is suffering problems similar to the use of lithium in its early modern clinical history. It took a number of years for lithium to become an acceptable treatment.

I would suggest that rubidium is at the beginning of a treatment learning curve and a comfort factor will only become established as:

1. Improved controlled studies are used
2. Rubidium is matched against the more modern antidepressants
3. Higher doses of rubidium are tried
4. When physicians feel there is a relatively simple way to deal with or prevent toxicity

It is evident that these approaches are now beginning to happen. I believe that like lithium, rubidium will prove to be a valuable therapeutic agent and also a substance that will teach us more about affective disorders.

References

Angelis I et al. (1988) Rubidium chloride: current status of the present research. Drugs Today 24: 733–741

Bonelli G et al. (1989) Trattamento dei disturbi depressivi con rubidio cloruro. Recenta Med 28: 19–34.

Botkin SS (1888) The influence of the salts of rubidium and cesium upon the heart and circulation in connection with the laws of physiological action of alkali metals (doctoral dissertation). St Petersburg Military Academy, St Petersburg

Calandra C et al. (1989) Valutazione clinica dell'efficacia terapeutica del rubidio cloruro nel trattamento di pazienti depressi. Recenta Med 28: 99–108

Calandri C, Nicolosi M (1980) Confronto fra due farmaci ad azione antidepressiva: rubidio cloruro ed Clormipramina. Proceedings of 34th congress of Italian Society of Psychiatry, Catania, Italy

Carolei et al. (1975) Azione farmacologica del cloruro di Rubidio. Effeto antidepressive: confronto con l'Imipramina. Clin Ter 5: 469–478

Carroll BJ, Sharp PT (1971) Rubidium and lithium: opposite effects on amine-mediated excitement. Science 172: 1355–1357

Chouinard G, Annable L (1977) The effect of rubidium in schizophrenia. Commun Psychopharmacol 1: 373–383

Chouinard G, Annable L (1983) Effect of rubidium chloride on the course of schizophrenia during partial withdrawal of neuroleptics. Presented at APA meeting

D'Amato F, Feis P (1990) Lithium and rubidium in the prevention of alcoholism. International symposium on recurrent mood disorders, Monaco, 23–24 March, 1990

Dell'Osso L et al. (1989) Sali di rubidio nel trattamento della depressione: contributo clinico, XXXVII Congresso Nazionale SIP, Roma, 6–11 feboraro, 1989

Demmel U et al. (1984) Trace elements in brains of patients with alcohol abuse, endogenous psychosis and schizophrenia. Sci Total Environ 38: 69–77

Fieve RR et al. (1973) Rubidium: biochemical, behavioral and metabolic studies in humans. Am J Psychiatry 130(1): 55–61

Fieve RR (1976) Therapeutic uses of lithium and rubidium. In: Simpson LL (ed) Drug treatment of mental disorders. Raven, New York, pp 193–208

Fieve RR, Meltzer HL, Taylor RT (1971) Rubidium chloride ingestion by volunteer subjects: initial experience. Psychopharmacologia 20: 307–314

Geisler A, Mork A, Klysner R (1990) Influence of lithium and rubidium on adenylate cyclase activity in rat brain. International symposium on recurrent mood disorders, Monaco, 23–25 March, 1990

Gershon S (1974) Rubidium: safety and potential as an antidepressant – abridged proceedings of a workshop. Psychopharmacology 10(1): 26–50

Jenner FA et al. (1983) Electrolyte metabolism in patients with periodic affective disorders during treatment with rubidium. Psychopharmacology 81: 301–309

Meltzer HL (1966) J Neurochem 13: 423

Meltzer HL (1990) Biochemical and physiological guidelines for long term rubidium therapy. Presented at the international symposium on recurrent mood disorders, Monaco, 23–25 March, 1990

Meltzer HL, Fieve RR (1975) Rubidium in psychiatry and medicine - an overview. Curr Dev Psychopharmacol 1(VI): 205–242

Meltzer HL et al. (1969) Rubidium: a potential modifier of affect and behavior. Nature 223: 321–322

Merck Manual (1940) 7th edn. Merck & Co, Inc. Rahway, NJ, USA

Messiha FS (1978) Pharmacol Biochem Behav 9: 647

Messiha FS (1984) Pharmacol Biochem Behav 21 [Suppl 1]: 87

Paschalis C, Jenner FA, Lee CR (1978) Effects of rubidium chloride on the course of manic-depressive illness. J R Soc Med 71: 343–352

Physician Desk Reference (1990) 44th edn. Medical Economics Data, at Montuale, NJ 07645, USA

Placidi G et al. (1988) Exploration of the clinical profile of rubidium chloride in depression: a systematic open trial. J Clin Psychopharmacol 8: 184–188

Platman SR, Fieve RR (1969) The effect of lithium carbonate on the electroencephalogram on patients with affective disorders. Br J Psychiatry 115: 1185–1188

Sarteschi P et al. (1984) Rubidium salts in depressed patients. An open pilot study using standardized techniques. In: Corsini GU (ed) Current trends on lithium and rubidium therapy. MTP Press, Boston, pp 225–247

Stolk JM et al. (1970) Brain norepinephrine: enhanced turnover after rubidium treatment. Science 168: 501–503

Stolk JM, Conner RL, Barchas JD (1971) Rubidium-induced increase in shock-elicited aggression in rats. Psychopharmacologica 22: 250–260

Williams RH, Sky-Peck HH (1986) Newer understanding of rubidium metabolism. Intern Med 7(1): 184–196

Biochemical and Physiological Guidelines for Long-Term Rubidium Therapy

H.L. Meltzer

Recent reports of the antidepressive effects of short-term rubidium chloride therapy may be the prelude to a more extended clinical application for this substance. If that occurs, the safety concerns arising from long-term therapy must be met by establishing some guidelines which will help to distinguish safe from unsafe dose levels. Because the biologic half-life of the rubidium ion is much longer than that of any other accepted psychopharmacological agent, there is an understandable hesitation to administer a substance which cannot be withdrawn promptly should undesirable side effects suddenly occur. It is therefore necessary to develop some predictive criteria which will give early warning of the occurrence of potentially undesirable changes in the biochemical or physiological systems which are utilized by rubidium. The following discussion will first summarize what we already know about rubidium metabolism and physiology, and then attempt to use certain aspects of that body of knowledge to specify properties which are expected to be constant. A change in any of the specified properties during the course of long-term rubidium therapy would be an indication that we have entered an unknown and potentially hazardous region.

Rubidium, a group one cation with extensive similarities to potassium, is distributed in the body in much the same way as is potassium. Thus, in both animal and human experiments, it has been found that rubidium distributes preferentially into the intracellular space by utilizing the same membrane channels that are available to potassium. Rubidium has been successfully used in many experiments as a tracer of potassium. From this fact alone, it is possible to predict that rubidium has a long biologic half-life. For example, if rubidium were exactly equivalent to potassium in its distribution, considering that the potassium content of a 70-kg man is about 3000 mEq and that the average daily urinary excretion of potassium during potassium balance is 50–60 mEq, the half-life would be calculated (Fig. 1) as 41–34 days. The reports, both with tracer and with therapeutic doses of rubidium, that its biologic half-life is in the range of 50–60 days is consistent with the observation that rubidium moves more slowly than does potassium through plasma membrane potassium channels.

In a large number of animal experiments in which rubidium was administered chronically, toxicity occurred when more than 40% of total body potassium was replaced by rubidium; toxicity never occurred when the replacement value was less than 30% (Meltzer and Lieberman 1971). In an extension of these studies, it has been found (Meltzer 1974) that nonlethal doses of rubidium in rats were characterized by replacement values of 25%–29% in brain and muscle,

$C = C_o \times e^{-kt}$
$k = (l/t) \times ln(C_o/C_1)$
$t_{1/2} = 0.693/k$
$k = ln\ (3000/2950) = 0.0168$ or $ln\ (3000/2940) = 0.0202$
$t_{1/2} = 0.693/0.0168 = 41$ or $0.693/0.0202 = 34$

Fig. 1. Calculation of half-life

while lethal doses increased muscle replacement to 51% without altering the replacement value in the brain. This result suggests that a metabolic transformation, specific to muscle cells, occurred when the cumulative dose reached the toxic level. It thus appears that at least one goal of safe therapy should be to limit potassium replacement by rubidium to less than the 30%–40% threshold value. Up to the present time, the maximum replacement of whole body potassium (determined by counting 40-K with a whole body counter) by rubidium during therapy has been 12% (Gwirtzman et al. 1980). A useful estimate of the extent of intracellular replacement of potassium by rubidium can also be obtained by measuring both of these elements in erythrocytes.

However, it would be more practical if we could predict potential toxicity from plasma rubidium measurements alone. The basis for this approach is as follows. There is an extensive body of data that demonstrates quantitative correspondence between the metabolic parameters obtained from tracer doses and therapeutic doses of rubidium. Because rubidium metabolism is apparently constant over a 100-fold concentration range, a change in some of these parameters during chronic rubidium administration would not be expected. If any of the parameters did change and were reflected in plasma rubidium levels, it would point to a significant and potentially harmful alteration in the underlying biochemical control mechanisms of rubidium metabolism. These aspects of rubidium metabolism are summarized in Fig. 2.

It is known (Burch et al. 1955) that plasma rubidium rapidly reaches a steady-state distribution with other extracellular space; the half-time for this process is about 5 min. However, rubidium distributes slowly between plasma and intraerythrocyte space; the steady-state ratio of about 30 is larger than that of potassium, indicating either that rubidium flows out of red cells at a lower rate than potassium or that it is pumped into these cells at a higher rate. Since tracer experiments (Love and Burch 1953) show no difference between the rate of entry of rubidium and potassium, it is probable that the efflux rate of rubidium is slower than that of potassium. The time required to attain steady-state levels in vivo, which is about 3 days, indicates that rubidium is also taken up slowly from the extracellular space by other intracellular compartments. Indirect evidence of this slow uptake is available from the fraction of a dose excreted in the urine for the first several days after an oral dose; 2%–4% is excreted during the 1st day, while after the 3rd day only about 1% of the remaining dose is found in the urine each day, as more rubidium leaves the extracellular space and enters the intracellular space.

Urinary excretion of rubidium can be modified by lithium. We have found (Meltzer and Fieve 1975) that the urinary ratio of endogenous rubidium to potassium was increased during a brief period of lithium administration to

1. Distribution between intra- and extracellular space (rbc/plasma): K = 30
2. Time to reach steady-state distribution: 3 days after a single dose
3. Urinary excretion 24 h following a single dose: 2%–4% of the dose
4. Urinary excretion for 1-day periods at least 3 days after a single dose: 1%
5. Maximum percent replacement of intracellular potassium during Rb therapy: 12%
6. Threshold replacement of intracellular potassium for toxicity (animals): 30%–40%

Fig. 2. Characteristics of rubidium metabolism

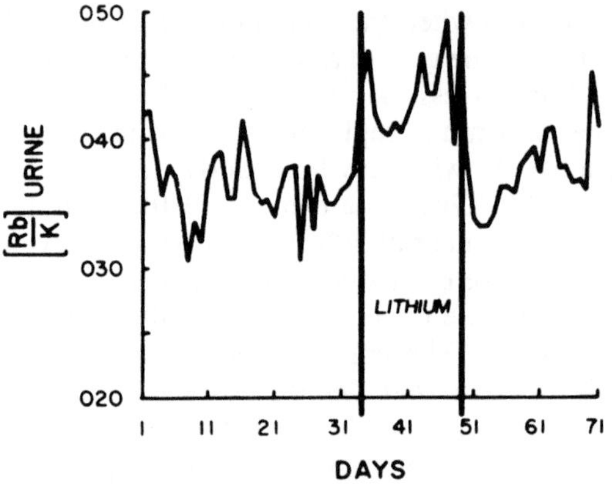

Fig. 3. Effect of lithium therapy on urinary Rb/K. The daily urinary excretion of rubidium occurring naturally in the body, corrected for potassium excretion, is shown for a single subject over an extended period. During the indicated times this bipolar subject received lithium carbonate. The increase in the average Rb/K ratio during this time was reversed promptly when lithium carbonate was withdrawn. (From Meltzer and Fieve 1975)

human subjects (Fig. 3). The rubidium/potassium ratio was also increased when lithium was given at the close of an experimental trial of rubidium (Fig. 4). Since there was no change in the average amount of potassium excreted each day, these observations indicate that the rate of efflux of rubidium from peripheral tissues was increased by lithium. One possible mechanism for this involves the calcium-gated potassium channel in the plasma membrane of many cells. When intracellular free calcium is increased above its resting level, this channel is opened and potassium and rubidium flow through it rapidly to the region of lower concentration in the extracellular space. I have previously postulated (Meltzer 1986) that lithium acts as a calcium surrogate in many neurochemical systems and that its psychotropic actions depend on this property. A similar action at the calcium-gated potassium channel would lead to more rapid rubidium excretion. If this interpretation is correct, the selective increase in rubidium efflux suggests that rubidium efflux through this channel is less sensitive to intracellular calcium than is potassium efflux and that the slower efflux of rubidium referred to above relates to the average level of free intracellular calcium. The observation that lithium protects rats against toxic doses of rubidium (Meltzer and Fieve 1975) suggests that lithium limits intracellular accumulation of rubidium, perhaps by the same mechanism.

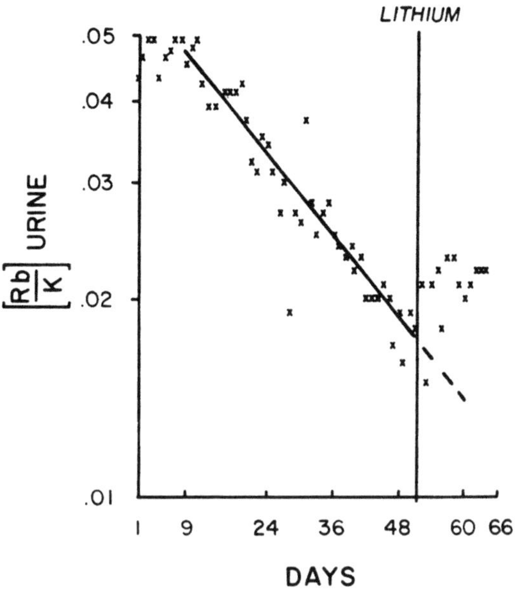

Fig. 4. Lithium administration was begun on the day indicated, following a period of excretion of rubidium administered for therapeutic purposes. (The decline in the urinary Rb/K ratio reflects the loss of rubidium from the body). The increased rate of loss following lithium is due to movement of rubidium from intracellular to extracellular space. See text. (From Meltzer and Fieve 1975)

With this information at hand, I will now turn to the problem of utilizing data from plasma rubidium measurements to detect potentially undesirable changes in its metabolic parameters during the course of therapy. This is essentially a problem in the pharmacokinetics of multiple and variable doses and is best done by modeling the system under study (Fig. 5). A three-compartment model is chosen because this is the simplest one that represents the measurable parameters. Although a separate intracellular compartment can be assigned to each tissue, in practice the model uses only one intracellular compartment which should be thought of as the resultant of all real physiological compartments. It is assumed that there is only one effective extracellular space. The quantity transferred into each compartment per unit time is obtained from the rubidium concentration in its precursor compartment multiplied by a specific rate constant. Thus, the extracellular fluid gains rubidium both from the intestine with the rate constant k_a, and from the intracellular fluid, with the rate constant k_o. It loses rubidium to the intracellular fluid with a rate constant k_i, and to the urine with a rate constant k_e.

The rate of change of rubidium concentration in each of the three compartments can be described by a sequence of differential equations (Table 1). Unidirectional rate constants define transfers between the compartments. A computer solution of these equations can be used to calculate the concentration in each compartment as a function of time after each dose. To use these

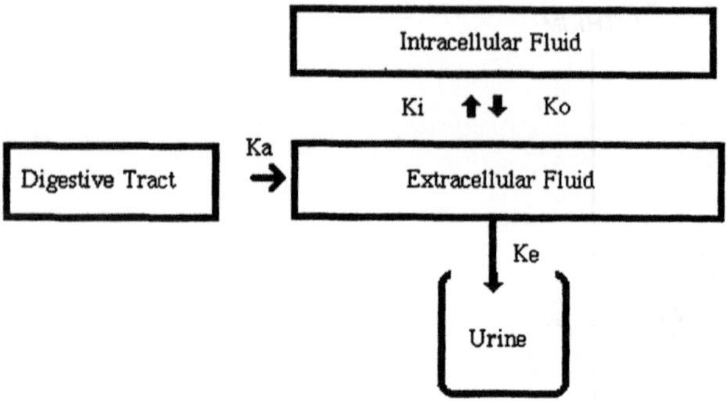

Fig. 5. Minimal model for rubidium pharmokinetics

Table 1. Equations for a pharmacokinetic model

Differential equations

1. $C_g = C_g - [K_a \times C_g] \times dt$
2. $C_e = C_e + [K_a \times C_g + K_o \times C_i - K_e \times C_e] \times dt$
3. $C_i = C_i + [K_i \times C_e - K_o^* C_i] \times dt$
4. $C_u = D_t - [C_e + C_i + C_g]$

C_g = quantity in intestine; C_e = quantity in extracellular fluid; C_i = quantity in intracellular fluid; C_u = quantity in urine; D_t = cumulative dose

equations a differential time interval is selected which is a hundredth of the unit time scale desired, which in the following examples is 1 day. Then the change in concentration described by the first equation is calculated for 0.01 days, and the new concentration is applied to the second equation, which is again recalculated for 0.01 days. The process is extended to the other equations and then recycled back to the first equation. At the end of each cycle, the new concentrations appearing in plasma and intracellular fluid are displayed on the graph as single points. The cumulative effects of new doses introduced at any specified time are apparent from the complete graph. Thus, given appropriate rate constants, this model will predict plasma levels after dose schedules which may be complicated by varying doses at varying intervals.

To use this model it is necessary by trial and error to select rate constants which give curves that match the available experimental data for the initial response to a single dose. The criteria chosen are the time at which rubidium peaks in the plasma, the time required for the intraerythrocyte rubidium/potassium ratio to reach a peak value, the steady-state value of that ratio, and the biologic half-life calculated from rubidium excretion into the urine. To test this approach the rate constants were varied until the values shown in Table 2, which are data obtained from initial experiments with rubidium, matched the computer-generated data for a unit-dose administered for 1 day. The actual mat-

Table 2. Parameters for a single dose of rubidium

Observed values	Patient data	Computer data
Time for peak plasma [Rb]	60–90 min	89 min
Time for steady-state erythrocyte [Rb]	2–3 days	2.58 days
$[Rb]_{red\ cells}/[Rb]_{plasma}$ at steady state	28–32	30.3
Urinary half-life after 10th day	50 days	50.2 days
Parameter description	**Symbol**	**Value**
Absorbtion from intestines	K_a	1.9
Influx into intracellular space	K_i	45
Efflux from intracellular space	K_o	1.5
Excretion into urine	K_e	0.42

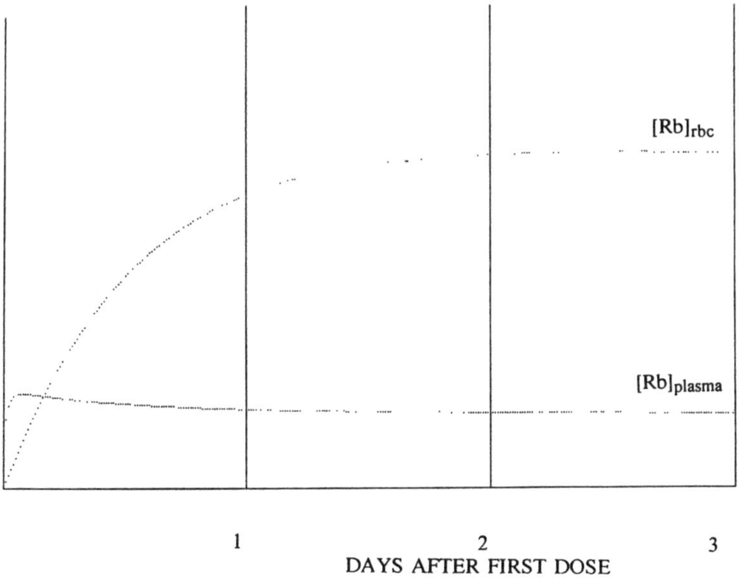

Fig. 6. Plasma and erythrocyte rubidium, calculated from the model as a fraction of a unit dose administered at time 0, is shown for a 3-day period. Plasma rubidium reached a peak value 89 min after a simulated oral dose. The scale for the plasma values is enlarged fivefold with respect to the scale for the erythrocyte values so that the final rbc/plasma ratio is about 30

ching values as well as the selected rate constants are also shown in the table. Computed curves over a 3-day period for intracellular and extracellular rubidium distribution following a single unit dose of rubidium are shown in Fig. 6. It should be noted that the scale for the plasma values is five times greater than the scale for the red cell values and that the values plotted represent fractional distribution of a unit dose into each of these compartments at the indicated times after the dose. The concentration in the extracellular fluid, which is equal

Table 3. Calculation of plasma rubidium from model data

Experimental data: Subject	Dose (mmols)	Peak plasma concentration (m*M*)	
		Measured	Calculated[a]
1	4.1	0.007	0.011
2	6.2	0.018	0.016

[a] Calculations: Predicted fraction of unit dose (1.0 mmol) in extracellular fluid = 0.039. Assumption: extracellular fluid = 15 liters (20% of body weight).
For subject #1:
mmol in ECF = [4.1/1.0] × 0.039 = 0.16
Concentration = 0.16 mmol/15 liters = 0.011
For subject #2:
mmol in ECF = [6.2/1.0] × 0.039 = 0.242
Concentration = 0.242 mmol/15 liters = 0.016

to the concentration in the plasma because of the rapid rate of equilibration between them, can be estimated as illustrated in Table 3. The calculated peak plasma concentrations for two subjects, assuming that rubidium was distributed into 15 liters of extracellular fluid in each subject, shows a reasonable resemblance to the observed values. Since these calculated values were obtained from equations which made no a priori assumptions about concentrations, the results indicate that the model realistically represents the underlying biologic phenomena.

Having established the validity of the model, it is useful to examine some of its more versatile applications. One of these is the ability to predict plasma levels during an intermittent dosage schedule. Figure 7 shows values for extracellular and intracellular distribution over a 10-day period when unit doses of rubidium are given for 3 days, followed by a dose-free interval of 2 days, 2 more dosage days, and a dose-free interval of 3 days. Another application concerns the dose schedule needed to maintain a steady level after a desired response is obtained. This is illustrated in Fig. 8. Suppose a unit dose has been given for each of the first 40 days, and depressive behavior was alleviated at day 30, and it was assumed that the plasma and/or intracellular rubidium levels which occurred at that time were responsible for the therapeutic effect. As is shown in the figure, the desired levels can be maintained by giving a unit dose for 3 consecutive days each week.

The final application concerns the ability to recognize when a physiological change has occurred, from the plasma data alone. Figure 9 shows, on an enlarged scale, plasma levels when a unit dose is given for 60 days, followed by 40 days without dosage. It is assumed that at day 30 the ability to accumulate rubidium intracellularly has changed due to a 20% increase in the influx rate constant. This event could indicate potential hazard, since it would indicate that membrane transport systems had been altered and also lead to an increase in the intracellular Rb/K ratio. A significant drop in expected plasma levels is apparent

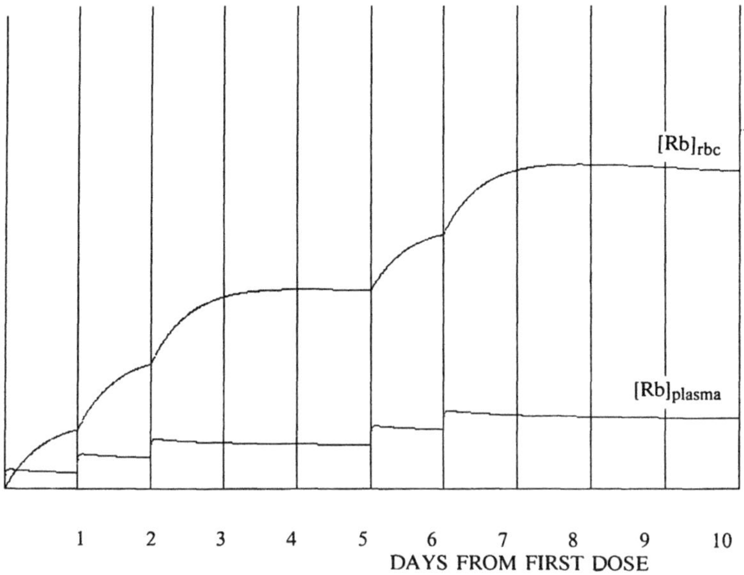

Fig. 7. Unit doses were given at the beginning of the 1st, 2nd, 3rd, 5th, and 6th days. Cumulative values for erythrocytes and plasma are shown. See also the legend to Fig. 6

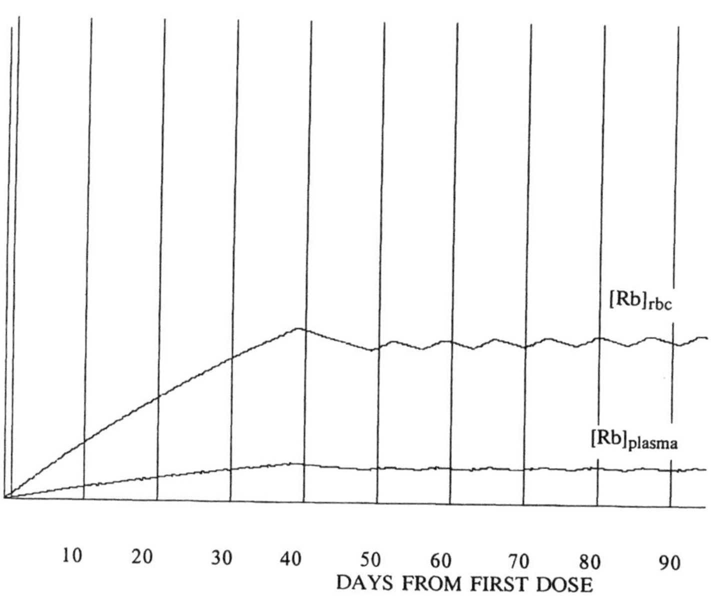

Fig. 8. At the end of a 40-day period during which unit dosages are given each day, rubidium is withheld for the next 10 days and then readministered as a unit dose for the first 3 days of each week. Erythrocyte and plasma levels are stabilized by this dosage schedule. See also the legend to Fig. 6

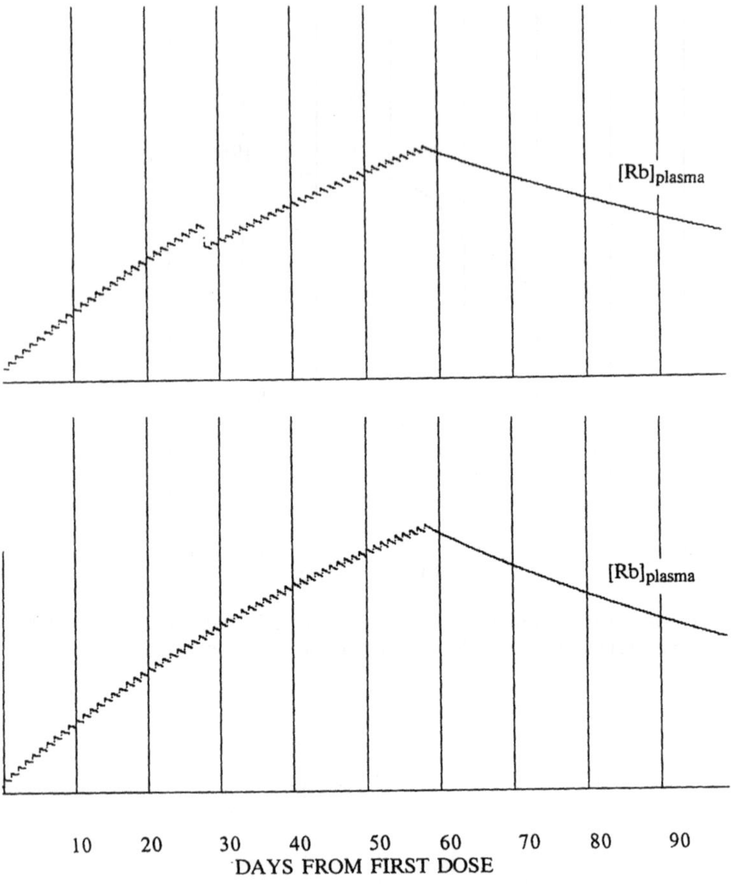

Fig. 9. The *upper portion* shows the change in plasma rubidium when the influx rate constant is increased by 20% at the 30th day. The *lower portion* shows plasma rubidium when the influx rate constant is unaltered throughout the 60 days of rubidium administration. See also the legend to Fig. 6

by comparing the upper portion of the slide with the unaltered flux data in the lower portion. This effect is even detectable at only a 5% increase in the influx rate constant (Fig. 10). Observed plasma levels vary from the predicted levels in the opposite direction when the efflux rate constant is changed. There is no effect on plasma levels of 10% changes in absorption or excretion rate constants. In interpreting plasma levels, it would be important to avoid overinterpretation, i.e., a few lower than expected values, followed by a few values at the expected level, probably indicate laboratory variability, rather than physiological change. However, a period of 10 or more days in which the plasma rubidium level is consistently either lower or higher than the expected level would be a strong signal that a physiological change had occurred and that further dosage might not be desirable.

In summary, the pharmacokinetic model presented here may have particular application to extended dosage schedules with rubidium. Potentially undesir-

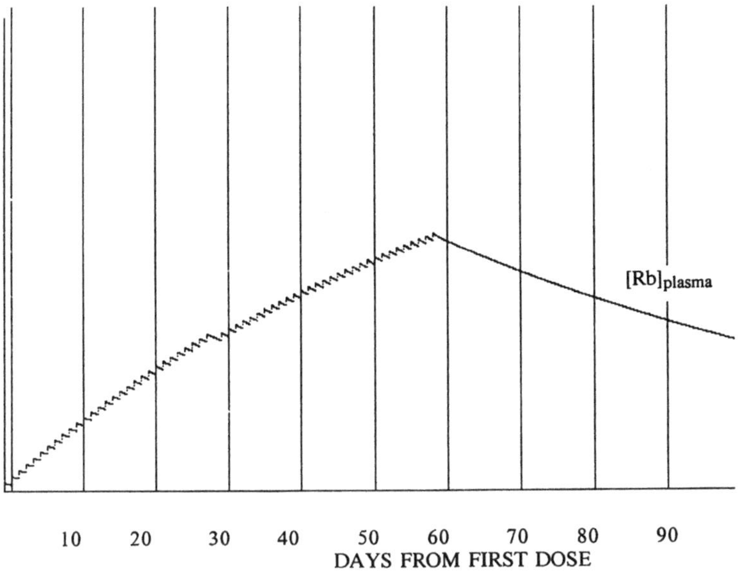

Fig. 10. The influx rate constant is increased by 5% at the 30th day. See also the legend to Fig. 6

able physiological changes can be detected by extended changes in plasma rubidium levels alone. It should be emphasized, however, that the predicted plasma levels depend on assumptions about the exact values of several unidirectional rate constants. These are essentially average values, based on previous experience. If needed, exact predictions for a specific subject can be obtained as follows. It is possible to modify the computer program so as to generate the appropriate rate constants for any individual based on initial data with that individual. Thus, to apply this model rigorously to patients for whom an extended dosage schedule is contemplated, it would be helpful to give each such patient a single unit dose, measure the plasma rubidium concentration at 30-min intervals for 2 h after ingestion of the dose, collect the urine over a 24-h period beginning at the 3rd day, and measure the ratio of rubidium in the red cells and plasma during the 4th day. Appropriate individualized rate constants calculated from this data could be used for predictions of relative plasma levels specific to that subject. However, it should be reemphasized that the principal contribution of the model is the prediction that a sustained change in the plasma rubidium level provides the desired early warning system.

References

Burch GE, Threefoot SA, Ray CT (1955) The rate of disappearance of Rb^{86} from the plasma, the biological decay rates of Rb^{86}, and the applicability of Rb^{86} as a tracer of potassium in man with and without congestive heart failure. J Lab Clin Med 45: 371–393

Gwirtzman HE, Meltzer HL, Dunner DL, Fieve RR, Pierson RN Jr (1980) Rubidium replacement of total body potassium in humans. Horm Metab Res 12: 175

Love WD, Burch GE (1953) A comparison of potassium^{42}, rubidium^{86}, and cesium^{134} as tracers of potassium in the study of cation metabolism of human erythrocytes in vitro. J Lab Clin Med 41: 351–362

Meltzer HL (1974) Human and animal metabolism of rubidium. Psychopharmacol Bull 10: 43–50

Meltzer HL (1986) Lithium mechanisms in bipolar illness and altered intracellular calcium functions. Biol Psychiatry 21: 492–510

Meltzer HL, Fieve RR (1975) Rubidium in psychiatry and medicine. In: Essman WB, Valzelli L (eds) Current developments in psychopharmacology, vol 1. Spectrum, New York, pp 205–242

Meltzer HL, Lieberman KW (1971) Chronic ingestion of rubidium without toxicity: implications for human therapy. Experentia 27: 672–674

Rubidium Shows Different Effects from Lithium on Phosphatidylinositol Metabolism in a Cell Line of Human Neuroblastoma*

A. Spinedi, L. Pacini, P. Luly, and G. Nisticò

Introduction

Rubidium (Rb^+) has been used for many years in the control of endogenous depression (Meltzer et al. 1969; Fieve et al. 1971; Fieve and Meltzer 1974; Sarteschi et al. 1984), despite the fact that its mechanism of action is still unknown. In fact, it has been found to produce therapeutic effect in 65% of patients with endogenous depression (Carolei et al. 1975); also in bipolar patients Rb^+ was shown to decrease both the duration and severity of depressive episodes (Fieve 1976).

In addition, in a double-blind study Rb^+ was reported to be more effective than chlorimipramine (Calandra and Nicolosi 1980). The antidepressant activity of Rb^+ was recently confirmed in a systematic open trial in 31 patients by following the amelioration of clinical symptoms by standard rating scales (Placidi et al. 1988). Like many antidepressants, Rb^+ increases noradrenergic and dopaminergic transmission, but does not affect MAO and COMT enzymatic activities, nor does it possess primary action on catecholaminergic, serotoninergic, GABAergic, or cholinergic receptors (Stolk et al. 1970; Eichelman et al. 1973). In contrast, lithium (Li^+) inhibits noradrenaline transmission by increasing its reuptake into nerve terminals (Colburn et al. 1967) and by increasing the intraneuronal metabolism of noradrenaline as reflected by an increase in both deaminated and deaminated-methylated metabolites (Schildkraut et al. 1966, 1969).

Opposite effects were also observed with Rb^+ and Li^+ as far as the behavioral and EEG changes are concerned; Rb^+ increases locomotor activity and elicits EEG desynchronization and behavioral alertness (Meltzer et al. 1969), whereas Li^+ induces EEG synchronization in manic and nonmanic patients (Mayfield and Brown 1966; Platman and Fieve 1969). Moreover, rats treated with daily doses of Rb^+ chloride show an increase in shock-elicited aggressive behavior (Stolk et al. 1971), whereas Li^+ inhibits this behavior (Sheard 1970).

* The present research was partially supported by the Italian Ministry of University and Scientific-Technological Research (40% and 60% funds).

It has also been reported that Li^+ reduces brain adenylate cyclase activity (Forn and Valdecasas 1971; Palmer et al. 1972) and in the case of noradrenaline-sensitive adenylate cyclase, the inhibition is maintained during chronic treatment (Ebstein et al. 1980). Rubidium, on the contrary, possesses an opposite effect, i.e., enhances adenylate cyclase activity in some brain areas (Geisler et al. 1990).

On the other hand, in recent years evidence has accumulated in favor of an action of Li^+ on the phosphatidylinositol (PI) cycle in the neuronal membranes leading to a decrease in the production of second messengers for those neurotransmitter receptors coupled to phosphatidylinositol-4,5-bisphosphate (PIP_2) metabolism. In fact, the therapeutic effectiveness of Li^+ is observed with serum concentrations (0.5–1 m*M*) that effectively inhibit inositol-1-phosphatase (Naccarato et al. 1974; Hallcher and Sherman 1980) with a consequent decrease in rat brain inositol levels (Allison et al. 1976) and impairment of PIP_2 turnover (Berridge et al. 1982; Berridge 1984; Berridge and Irvine 1984; Drummond et al. 1987). Thus, in cerebral cortex slices, acute treatment with Li^+ results in a reduction in the accumulation of labeled inositol phosphates after stimulation of muscarinic receptors, histamine H_1 receptors, and serotonin receptors. Also, a chronic (2-week) treatment with Li^+ maintained the reduced phosphoinositide response to receptor agonists. On the contrary, when rats were withdrawn from chronic treatment for 18 h, responses to carbachol were significantly enhanced with respect to untreated controls (Kendall and Nahorski 1987).

Recently, it has been reported that in mice following chronic treatment with Li^+, there is a significant increase in the production of IP_3, both in resting conditions and after stimulation with carbachol of muscarinic receptors (Whitworth et al. 1989). This, in contrast to the effectiveness of acute administration of Li^+ in manic states, could explain the activity of chronic Li^+ in the prophylaxis of endogenous depression since, with this modality of treatment, there is a potentiation of the receptors linked to phospholipid metabolism in neuronal membranes.

Taken together, these data strongly support the idea that the antimanic effect of Li^+ is due to a decreased effectiveness of phosphoinositide hydrolysis-signaling pathway with a consequent decrease in activity of those neurotransmitter receptors abnormally stimulated during manic states and which are coupled to inositol lipid metabolism.

The different therapeutic profile of Rb^+, which in contrast to Li^+ antimanic effects, is only provided with an antidepressive activity, and the opposite effects on adenylate cyclase activity prompted us to study Rb^+ effects on phosphoinositide metabolism in a cell line (SK-N-BE) of human neuroblastoma. In particular, the present study was aimed at investigating the effects of Rb^+ on intracellular accumulation of inositol phosphates both under steady-state conditions and after phosphoinositide turnover stimulation; the question addressed was whether any common biochemical property was shared by Rb^+ and Li^+. The results of the present experiments could also provide new insight into the therapeutic action of Rb^+ and eventually explain the different mechanism of action in comparison with Li^+.

Materials and Methods

The SK-N-BE human neuroblastoma cell line was obtained through the courtesy of Dr. Lawrence Helson, Memorial Sloane-Kettering Hospital, New York. Cells were grown at 37 °C in RPMI-1640 medium supplemented with 10% (v/v) heat inactivated fetal calf serum (FCS, 2 m*M* L-glutamine, 100 IU/ml penicillin and streptomicin, 2.0 g/liter bicarbonate and 10 m*M* HEPES in a humidified atmosphere with 5% (v/v) CO_2.

For radioactive labeling, 12.5 μCi of [^{3}H]-myo-inositol (Amersham) were mixed with 2.5 ml of MEM supplemented with 10% FCS and the mixture was added to cells (9×10^4 cells/cm^2) grown in 25-cm^2 flasks. Labeling was carried out for 24 h; when the effect of Rb^+ on labeling of inositol phosphates was to be evaluated, 1 or 10 m*M* Rb^+ was added to the culture medium from a 1 *M* stock solution in MEM. To study the effect of Rb^+ and Li^+ on carbamoylcholine-stimulated inositol phosphate production, cells were prelabeled with [^{3}H]-myo-inositol for 24 h as described above, gently washed with RPMI-1640, and incubated for an additional hour in RPMI-1640 in the presence of 10 m*M* Rb^+ or Li^+, or in the absence of both ions. Cells were then stimulated by addition of carbamoylcholine directly into the incubation medium (1 m*M* final concentration), from a 1 *M* freshly prepared stock solution in RPMI. For inositol phosphate extraction and quantitation cells were scraped off from the flask in 3.0 ml 10% TCA. After centrifugation the supernatant was washed three times with 3 volumes of water-saturated diethyl ether and neutralized with $NaHCO_3$. Inositol phosphates were separated by anion-exchange chromatography on Dowex-1 chloride (8% cross-linked 200–400 mesh, Sigma) as described by Berridge et al. (1983) and radioactivity in the individual fractions determined by a Packard Tricarb 1500 scintillation counter, after additions of columm eluate aliquots into counting vials, using Optifluor (Packard) as scintillation fluid.

Results

The SK-N-BE human neuroblastoma cell line was chosen as the model system for our study since on this line we have observed that: (a) carbamoylcholine stimulates phospholipase C-mediated phosphoinositide hydrolysis and (b) Li^+ affects inositol phosphate levels after cell stimulation with carbamoylcholine, through an inhibitory action on phosphatases (results to be published).

Cell labeling for 24 h with [^{3}H]-myo-inositol under our experimental conditions resulted in about 1×10^3 dpm incorporation per nmol of total phospholipids; over 93% of the incorporated radioactivity was found in phosphatidylinositol, the remainder being divided almost in equimolar amounts between phosphatidylinositol-4-phosphate and phosphatidylinositol-4,5-bisphosphate (phosphoinositide extraction and separation performed according to Creba et al. 1983). Substantial amounts of radioactivity were also found in

Table 1. Effect of Rb^+ on basal levels of [^{3}H]-inositol phosphates in human neuroblastoma SK-N-BE cells

	dpm × 10^{-3}/mg cell protein		
[Rb^+](m*M*)	0	1	10
IP	7.0 ± 0.5	8.0 ± 0.7	7.9 ± 0.6
IP_2	2.3 ± 0.2	3.1 ± 0.4*	3.5 ± 0.4*
IP_3	1.8 ± 0.2	1.9 ± 0.3	2.1 ± 0.3
IP_4	2.2 ± 0.3	2.3 ± 0.2	2.5 ± 0.5

* $p < 0.01$ as from Student's *t* test ($n = 4$).
Cells were incubated for 24 h in the presence of [^{3}H]-myo-inositol (5 μCi/ml) and of the indicated Rb^+ concentrations. At the end of the incubation period, inositol phosphates were extracted and radioactivity determined as described in materials and methods.

Table 2. Effect of Rb^+ and Li^+ on the accumulation of [^{3}H]-inositol phosphates in human neuroblastoma SK-N-BE cells upon stimulation for 6 min with 1 m*M* carbamoylcholine (cch)

	[^{3}H]-inositol phosphate accumulation (folds over basal levels)		
	1 m*M* cch	1 m*M* cch + 10 m*M* Rb^+	1 m*M* cch + 10 m*M* Li^+
IP	2.7 ± 0.7	3.1 ± 0.3	7.4 ± 0.9*
IP_2	2.7 ± 0.9	2.8 ± 0.6	9.6 ± 2.8*
IP_3	1.5 ± 0.3	1.9 ± 0.5	1.5 ± 0.4
IP_4	1.5 ± 0.3	1.8 ± 0.5	1.9 ± 0.4

* $p < 0.001$ as from Student's *t* test ($n = 4$).
Cells were labeled for 24 h with [^{3}H]-myo-inositol (5 μCi/ml), reincubated for 1 h in label-free medium in the presence of 10 m*M* Rb^+ or 10 m*M* Li^+ or in the absence of both ions and stimulated for 6 min with 1 m*M* carbamoylcholine. At the end of stimulation, inositol phosphates were extracted and radioactivity determined as described in materials and methods.

inositol phosphates (as shown in Table 1); labeling values did not change significantly after 3 h of additional incubation and likely this reflects inositol phosphate equilibrium levels due to steady-state phosphoinositide turnover in growing cells. Table 1 shows that the presence of Rb^+ in the medium significantly affects inositol bisphosphate (IP_2) labeling; after 24 h of incubation in the presence of 1 and 10 m*M* Rb^+, IP_2 labeling was significantly increased by 35% and 52%, respectively; labeling of other inositol phosphates was apparently not affected. The possibility that Rb^+ could affect inositol phosphate labeling by an inhibitory action on phosphatases was considered. Table 2 shows the Rb^+ effect on carbamoylcholine-stimulated inositol phosphate accumulation; the effect of Li^+ is also reported. It can be seen that at variance with Li^+, which dramatically enhances inositol monophosphate and IP_2 accumulation in carbamoylcholine-stimulated cells, Rb^+ does not affect to a significant extent inositol phosphate accumulation in the same experimental conditions.

The main indication which can be drawn from the data reported is that Rb^+ does not share a major pharmacological property of Li^+, i.e., it is not an inhibitor of inositol-l-phosphatase; hence, its mechanism of action in the nervous system does not reasonably involve impairment of inositol synthesis. The question still holds as to how IP_2 basal labeling is increased after long-term cell incubation in the presence of Rb^+; among the various possibilities it should also be considered that this circumstance may reflect a new steady-state equilibrium due to an increased phosphoinositide turnover.

Discussion

The present experiments show that Rb^+ in concentrations similar to those achieved therapeutically seems to affect PI turnover, as shown by a significant increase in the formation of IPs. This effect is the opposite to that observed after Li^+ treatment since with the latter cation inhibition of inositol-l-phosphatase occurs with a consequent depletion of the cellular inositol pool in neurons, whose PIP_2 hydrolyzing receptors are being intensely stimulated (Berridge et al. 1982; Drummond 1987; Downes 1988).

The inositol phospholipid-dependent signal transduction pathway is now considered to play an important role in controlling the functions of a variety of cell types within the CNS. In fact, the hydrolysis of PI is an integral part of those receptors (e.g., muscarinic, H_1-histaminergic, α_1-adrenergic, V_1-vasopressin, and NMDA excitatory amino acid receptors) that function through Ca^{2+} (see Berridge et al. 1982; Nicoletti et al. 1986; Cotman and Iversen 1987).

The pathogenesis of endogenous depression is not known at the present time. However, one of the most accredited theories is the monoaminergic hypothesis according to which, in this condition, there is a decrease in the activity of catecholamines and/or serotonin in those areas of the brain (limbic system, neocortex) involved in mood control. Thus, drugs enhancing monoaminergic transmission in the brain by inhibiting monoamine reuptake or by inhibiting MAO are currently used as antidepressant drugs (see refs. in Nisticò 1990).

In addition, more recently, it has been suggested that during endogenous depression and as a consequence of a decreased catecholamine biosynthesis and release there is a supersensitivity at the postsynaptic β-adrenoceptors in the limbic system and frontal cortex (see refs. in Sulser et al. 1978). This could also explain the 2- to 3-week latency period before obtaining a good therapeutic response in patients, which seems to be due to the time required by the increased catecholamine concentration, after tricyclic antidepressants or MAO inhibitors, to reduce β-adrenoceptor supersensitivity ("down regulation"). Therefore, according to this hypothesis, the pathophysiological feature of depression is represented by a receptor alteration. In any case (monoamine deficit or

β-adrenoceptor supersensitivity), it is possible that neurotransmission can be altered at the neuronal membrane level and, in particular, in the mechanisms coupling neurotransmitter receptors to second messengers.

The present experiments show that Rb^+ exerts a different alteration in inositol metabolism compared with Li^+. In fact, we confirmed that Li^+, in contrast to Rb^+, inhibits the conversion of inositol-l-phosphate into inositol by the enzyme inositol-l-phosphatase (Naccarato et al. 1974; Hallcher and Sherman 1980). On the other hand, Rb^+, in comparison with controls and in contrast to Li^+, produced a significant increase in the IP_2 levels, suggesting an increased turnover of inositol metabolism at the membrane level.

Further experiments are now being carried out to assess whether Rb^+ is able to increase PIP_2 turnover, by measuring its second messengers (IP_3 and DAG concentration) both in resting conditions and after stimulation with various neurotransmitters.

Acknowledgments. Our thanks to IFI, Pharmaceutical Co., Rome for their generous supply of Rb^+ chloride and to Mrs. Tiziana Macrì and Marika Nisticò for excellent typing of the manuscript.

References

Allison JH, Blisner ME, Holland WH, Hipps PP, Sherman WR (1976) Increased brain myo-inositol-l-phosphate in lithium treated rats. Biochem Biophys Res Commun 71: 664–670
Berridge MJ (1984) Inositol and diacylglycerol as second messengers. Biochem J 220: 345–360
Berridge MJ, Irvine RF (1984) Inositol triphosphate, a novel second messenger in cellular signal transduction. Nature 312: 315–321
Berridge MJ, Downes CP, Hanley MR (1982) Lithium amplifies agonist-dependent phosphatidylinositol responses in brain and salivary glands. Biochem J 206: 587–595
Berridge MJ, Dawson RMC, Downes CP, Heslop JP, Irvine RF (1983) Changes in the levels of inositol phosphates after agonist-dependent hydrolysis of membrane phosphoinositides. Biochem J 212: 473–482
Calandra C, Nicolosi M (1980) Confronto tra due farmaci ad azione antidepressiva: rubidio cloruro e clorimipramina. In: XXXIV Congr Soc It Psichiatria, Catania, 24–29 Apr, pp 1–45
Carolei A, Sonsini U, Casacchia M, Agnoli A, Fazio C (1975) Azione farmacologica del cloruro di rubidio. Effetto antidepressivo: confronto con l'imipramina. Clin Ter 75: 469–478
Colburn R, Goodwin F, Bunney WE Jr (1967) Effects of lithium on the uptake of noradrenaline by synaptosomes. Nature 215: 1395–1397
Cotman CW, Iversen LL (1987) Excitatory aminoacids in the brain. Focus on NMDA receptors. Trends Neurol Sci 10: 263–265
Creba JA, Downes CP, Hawkins PT, Brewster G, Michell RH, Kirk CJ (1983) Rapid breakdown of phosphatidylinositol 4-phosphate and phosphatidylinositol 4,5-biphosphate in rat hepatocytes stimulated by vasopressin and other Ca^{2+}-mobilizing hormones. Biochem J 212: 733–747
Downes CP (1988) Inositol phosphates: a family of signal molecules? Trends Neurol Sci 11: 336–338
Drummond AL (1987) Lithium and inositol lipid-linked signalling mechanisms. Trends Pharmacol Sci 8: 129–133
Drummond AH, Joels LA, Hughes PJ (1987) The interaction of lithium ions inositol lipid signalling system. Biochem Soc Trans 15: 32–35
Ebstein RP, Hermoni M, Belmaker RH (1980) The effect of lithium on noradrenaline-induced cAMP accumulation in rat brain. Inhibition after chronic treatment and the absence of supersensitivity. J Pharmacol Exp Ther 213: 161–167

Eichelman B, Thoa NB, Perez-Cruet J (1973) Alkali metal cations: effects on aggression and adrenal enzymes. Pharmacol Biochem Behav 1: 121
Fieve RR (1976) Therapeutic uses of lithium and rubidium. In: Simpson LL (ed) Drug treatment of mental disorders. Raven, New York, pp 193–208
Fieve RR, Meltzer HL (1974) Is there clinical evidence that rubidium exerts an antidepressant action? J Pharmacol 1 [Suppl]: 80
Fieve RR, Meltzer HL, Taylor RM (1971) Rubidium chloride ingestion by volunteer subjects: initial experience. Psychopharmacologia 20: 307–314
Forn J, Valdecasas FG (1971) Effects of lithium on brain adenylate activity. Biochem Pharmacol 20: 2773–2779
Geisler A, Mork A, Klysner R (1990) Influence of lithium and rubidium on adenylate cyclase in rat brain. Comm int symposium on recurrent mood disorders. Montecarlo, 23–25 March, 1990. Abstract Book, p 25
Hallcher LM, Sherman WR (1980) The effects of lithium ion and other agents on the activity of myo-inositol-l-phosphate phosphatase from bovine brain. J Biol Chem 255: 10896–10901
Kendall DA, Nahorski SR (1987) Acute and chronic lithium treatments influence agonist and depolarization-stimulated inositol phospholipid hydrolysis in rat cerebral cortex. J Pharmacol Exp Ther 241: 1023–1027
Mayfield D, Brown RG (1966) The clinical, laboratory and encephalographic effects of lithium. J Psychiatr Res 4: 207–219
Meltzer HL, Taylor RM, Platman SR, Fieve RR (1969) Rubidium a potential modifier of affect and behaviour. Nature 223: 321–322
Naccarato WF, Ray RE, Wells WW (1974) Biosynthesis of myo-inositol in rat mammary gland. Isolation and properties of the enzymes. Arch Biochem Biophys 164: 194–201
Nicoletti F, Wroblewski JT, Novelli A, Guidotti A, Costa E (1986) Excitatory aminoacid signal transduction in cerebellar cell cultures. Funct Neurol 4: 345–349
Nisticò G (1990) Neuropsicofarmacologia sperimentale e clinica. Pythagora, Roma-Milan
Palmer GC, Robinson GA, Manian AA, Sulser F (1972) Modification by psychotropic drugs of the cyclic AMP response to norepinephrine in the rat brain *in vitro*. Psychopharmacology 23: 201–211
Placidi G, Lenzi A, Lazzerini F, Dell'Osso L, Cassano GB, Akiskal HS (1988) Exploration of the clinical profile of rubidium chloride in depression: a systematic open trial. J Clin Psychopharmacol 8: 184–188
Platman SR, Fieve RR (1969) The effects of lithium carbonate on the electroencephalogram of patients with affective disorders. Br J Psychiatry 115: 1185–1188
Sarteschi P, Placidi GF, Lenzi A, Rampello E, Cassano GB (1984) Rubidium salts in depressant patients. An open pilot study using standardized techniques. In: Corsini GU (ed) Current trends in lithium and rubidium therapy. MTP Press, Lancaster, pp 225–259
Schildkraut JJ, Schanberg SM, Kopin IJ (1966) The effects of the lithium ion on H-norepinephrine in brain. Life Sci 5: 1479–1483
Schildkraut JJ, Logue MA, Dodge GA (1969) The effects of lithium salts on the turnover and metabolism of norepinephrine in rat brain. Psychopharmacologia 14: 135–141
Sheard HH (1970) Effects of lithium on food shock aggression in rats. Nature 228: 284–285
Stolk JM, Nowak WJ, Barchas JD (1970) Brain norepinephrine enhanced turnover after rubidium treatment. Science, 168: 501–503
Stolk JM, Conner RL, Barchas JD (1971) Rubidium-induced increase in shock-elicited aggression in rats. Psychopharmacologia 22: 250–260
Sulser F, Vetulani J, Mobley PL (1978) Mode of action of antidepressant drugs. Biochem Pharmacol 27: 257
Whitworth P, Heal DJ, Kendall DA (1989) Chronic lithium treatment enhances inositol polyphosphate formation in mouse brain *in vivo*. Br J Pharmacol 99: 834P

Influences of Rubidium and Lithium on Cyclic AMP Formation in Rat Brain

A. Geisler and A. Mørk

Introduction

Substantial evidence has shown that lithium exerts an antimanic effect, a prophylactic effect against recurrent mood alterations in bipolar and unipolar affective disorders, and possibly, an antidepressive effect (Rosenthal and Goodwin 1982). However, it is unclear how lithium exerts these therapeutic actions. In this context it is of interest that another monovalent ion rubidium seems to be an antidepressant agent (Meltzer and Fieve 1975; Placidi et al. 1988). Further, Paschalis et al. (1978) has observed that rubidium can prolong the period of mania and increase its severity. Thus, it has been demonstrated that rubidium and lithium influence human mood. This is of experimental interest since it has been reported that rubidium exerts "opposite" neurochemical effects to those of lithium (Fieve et al. 1973).

Several studies suggest that alterations of one or more cerebral adenylate cyclases may have relevance for the neuropharmacological effects of mood-modulating drugs (Ebstein et al. 1989).

Structure and Regulation of Adenylate Cyclase

The enzyme adenylate cyclase is a transmembranous enzyme system consisting of five subunits (Fig. 1). Neurohormones stimulate or inhibit the cyclic AMP formation through stimulatory or inhibitory receptors, respectively. The structure and the amino acid sequence are known for certain receptors, e.g., dopamine D_2 and β_2-adrenergic receptors. These receptors are transmembrane proteins, and it is likely that other neurotransmitter receptors also span the membrane. The agonist binding site of neurotransmitter receptors is located at the outer site of the cell membrane. For example, dopamine activates or inhibits the enzyme activity by an interaction with D_1 receptors or D_2 receptors, respectively. Similarly, norephinephrine and serotonin stimulate or inhibit this enzyme activity by binding to specific receptors. Some neurotransmitters, e.g., the enkephalins, are only inhibitory. The neurotransmitter receptor signal is transferred to the catalytic subunit by guanine nucleotide binding proteins, named G proteins. The functions of the G proteins are modulated by endogenous GTP. Two proteins, G_s and G_i, interact with the stimulatory and inhibitory

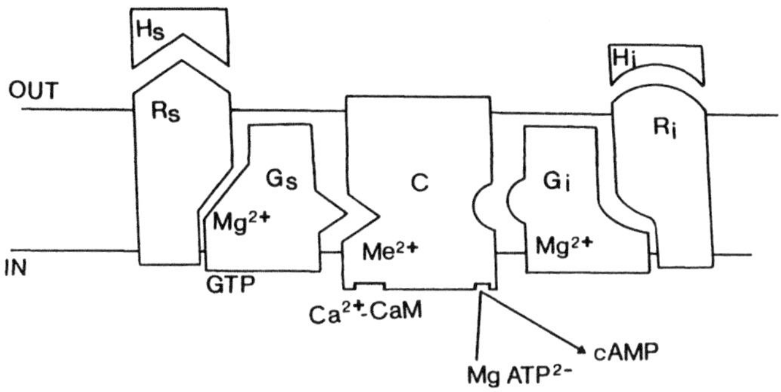

Fig. 1. Schematic outline of the adenylate cyclase system showing its protein components and endogenous regulators. H_s and H_i, stimulatory and inhibitory neurohormones; R_s and R_i, receptors mediating stimulation and inhibition; G_s and G_i, stimulatory and inhibitory GTP sensitive proteins; *C*, catalytic subunit; Me^{2+}, metal ion site sensitive to magnesium and calcium; $Ca^{2+} - CaM$, calcium–calmodulin

receptors, respectively (Gilman 1989). The catalytic subunit, which is a single transmembrane protein having the substrate site at the inner surface of the membrane, converts Mg-ATP to cyclic AMP. This second messenger molecule exerts its influence on cellular processes by an interaction with protein kinases.

The activity of the enzyme is dependent on the divalent cations calcium and magnesium. Magnesium regulates the activity of the G proteins, the catalytic subunit, and complexes with ATP to form the substrate. The effect of magnesium on these processes is stimulatory. On the other hand, calcium regulates the activity of the catalytic subunit. Interestingly, calcium has an activating effect in lower concentrations (submicromolar) while this ion inhibits the activity in higher concentrations.

In addition, it should be mentioned that the catalytic subunit can be activated experimentally by the diterpene forskolin. Possibly, forskolin may influence the activity of the stimulated G_s protein.

Influence of Lithium on Cerebral Adenylate Cyclase

Several studies have clearly shown that lithium in vitro and ex vivo, i.e., after chronic treatment, inhibits the adenylate cyclase activity. Consistently, it has been observed that lithium has no effect on the unstimulated enzyme but modifies its stimulated activity. Lithium decreases the function of β-adrenergic receptors by interacting with the associated adenylate cyclase. Activation of the enzyme by GTP alone is unaffected by lithium ex vivo, but neurotransmitter-induced GTP activation is inhibited (Mørk and Geisler 1989a). This observation is supported by Avissar and Schreiber (1989) who showed that lithium treatment decreased neurotransmitter-induced GTP binding in rat brain. Furthermore, lithium in vitro as well as ex vivo impairs the activity of the catalytic subunit stimulated by calcium-calmodulin or forskolin (Mørk and Geisler 1987; Mørk and Geisler 1989b, c). The in vitro effects of lithium seem to be due to a competition between lithium and intracellular magnesium (Mørk and Geisler 1987; Newman and Belmaker 1987). However, lithium may have a more complex effect on the adenylate cyclase during chronic lithium treatment. Thus, our studies on rat brain adenylate cyclase do suggest that the inhibitory actions of lithium in vitro and ex vivo on the enzyme activity differ (Mørk and Geisler 1989b). The mechanisms by which lithium exerts its ex vivo effects are unknown, but lithium may modify the fluidity of the cell membrane or influence protein kinases which modulate the adenylate cyclase activity by phosphorylating the proteins of the enzyme. The effects of lithium on second messenger systems in the brain have recently been reviewed by Mørk (1990).

Studies on cerebral adrenergic receptors have been contradictory. Presumably, lithium has no effect on either the number of adrenergic receptors or the binding affinity to adrenergic receptors (Gross et al. 1988). Furthermore, it has been observed that lithium can increase the release of norepinephrine by an interaction with presynaptic α-adrenergic receptors (Spengler et al. 1986). However, others have not been able to confirm this observation (Gross and Hanft 1990). Lithium ex vivo reduces the density of pre- and postsynaptic 5-HT receptors without changing their affinities (Mizuta and Segawa 1989). In addition, it has been observed that chronic lithium treatment enhances the presynaptic release of 5-HT by intervening with 5-HT autoreceptors (Friedman and Wang 1988). In spite of a decreased number of 5-HT receptors, it has been shown that lithium treatment enhances 5-HT-stimulated adenylate cyclase activity in rat hippocampus (Hotta and Yamawaki 1986; Mørk and Geisler 1989a). In accordance, electrophysiological studies have demonstrated that short-term lithium treatment enhances serotonergic activity in the rat brain (Blier et al. 1987). This enhancement of serotonergic processes may be involved in the therapeutic action of lithium, since an enhanced serotonergic function may also influence the adrenergic receptor activity. In fact, it has been demonstrated that drug-induced downregulation of β-adrenergic receptors depends on an intact serotonergic function (Brunello et al. 1982; Janowsky et al. 1982).

It is unknown whether the actions of lithium on the cyclic AMP formation are related to its therapeutic properties, but some antipsychotics, antidepressants, and ECS also affect the activity of cerebral adenylate cyclase.

Interactions Between Rubidium and Lithium

Various studies have shown that rubidium and lithium have opposite effects on some physiological processes. This is of interest since rubidium and lithium have diverging effects on mood regulation also. For example, it has been shown that rubidium and lithium have opposite effects on the circadian rhythm of locomotor activity in the cockroach (Engelmann and Casper 1984). Similarly, it has been shown that lithium attenuates while rubidium increases shock-induced changes in open-field activity of rats (Hines 1986). Furthermore, it has been shown that rats consume significantly more alcohol when treated with rubidium while lithium treatment significantly reduces the intake of alcohol (Alexander and Alexander 1978). Also, at the molecular level, lithium and rubidium can have opposing effects. Thus, we have observed that the two ions have different effects in vitro on norepinephrine-induced cyclic AMP formation in cortical slices from the rat brain. In this tissue preparation 2 m*M* of rubidium increased the hormone-induced cyclic AMP formation, while 2 m*M* lithium inhibited the cyclic AMP accumulation. Combination of the two ions neutralized the mentioned effects. On the other hand, neither rubidium nor lithium influenced the basal activity of the enzyme. Furthermore, it was observed, using dose-response curves, that lithium inhibited the enzyme in a noncompetitive manner, while rubidium had a potentiating effect over the whole concentration range of added norepinephrine (10^{-7}–10^{-3} *M*); even at maximal concentrations of norepinephrine rubidium enhanced the formation of cyclic AMP (Geisler et al. 1984). In recent experiments, we have observed that 2 m*M* lithium inhibits the β-adrenergic agonist isoproterenol stimulation of cyclic AMP formation in cortical slices. In accordance with our previous results, it was observed that 2 m*M* rubidium enhanced the isoproterenol-stimulated cyclic AMP accumulation. Further, it was shown that 2 m*M* cesium, which may influence human mood (Messiha 1985), had a similar effect to that of rubidium on the cyclic AMP

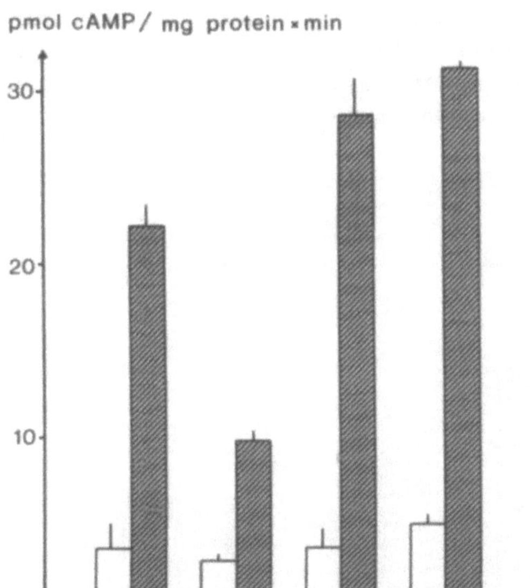

Fig. 2. Influence of NaCl, LiCl, RbCl, and CsCl in vitro on unstimulated (*open bars*) and isoproterenol (10^{-4} *M*)-stimulated (*hatched bars*) cyclic AMP formation in rat brain cortical slices. The results are given as means ±SD, $n = 3$. The cyclic AMP formation was assayed as previously described. (Mørk et al. 1988)

formation (Fig. 2). In contrast, it was observed that adenylate cyclase stimulated by GTP with and without isoproterenol was not influenced by rubidium in rat brain cortical membranes even in high concentrations. In contrast, lithium inhibited these enzyme activities in this membrane preparation. When the two agents were combined, the enzyme activities were similar to those of lithium alone (Fig. 3).

Chronic influence of rubidium on isoproterenol-stimulated cyclic AMP formation in rat brain cortical slices was studied by giving the rats tap water containing rubidium chloride (40 mM) for 14 days. This treatment showed that chronic rubidium administration had no effect on the basal activity of the enzyme while the isoproterenol-stimulated cyclic AMP formation was significantly reduced (Fig. 4).

Rubidium in vitro had no effect on adenylate cyclase activity in cell-free systems. Thus, rubidium does not seem to interact directly with the adenylate cyclase. In intact tissue, rubidium had no effect on the unstimulated activity of the enzyme but enhanced the isoproterenol-stimulated cyclic AMP formation. However, rubidium also increased forskolin-stimulated cyclic AMP accumulation in rat brain cortical slices (results not shown). These results show that rubidium potentiation can also be observed even when the enzyme is stimulated beyond the receptor. Thus, the effect of rubidium in vitro on the adenylate cyclase seems to require an intact cell and may be exerted by an effect independent of the receptor stimulation. After chronic treatment with rubidium, a decreased isoproterenol-stimulated cyclic AMP formation was observed. This may be explained by a rubidium-induced release of norepinephrine from presynaptic terminals (Stolk et al. 1970). However, this conclusion does not correspond with the fact that rubidium in vitro has no effect on the unstimulated cyclic AMP formation in rat brain cortical slices and enhances the enzyme

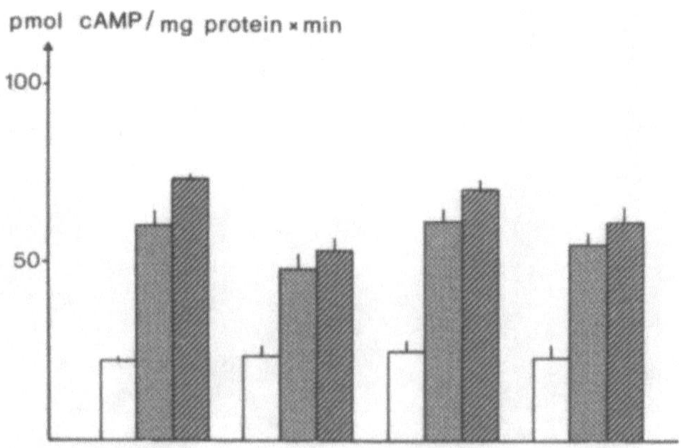

Fig. 3. Influence of NaCl, LiCl, and RbCl in vitro on unstimulated (*open bars*), GTP (10^{-5} M) (*dotted bars*), and GTP (10^{-5} M) + isoproterenol (10^{-5} M) (*hatched bars*) in rat brain cortical membranes. The results are given as means ±SD, $n = 3$. The adenylate cyclase activity was assayed as previously described. (Mørk and Geisler 1989c)

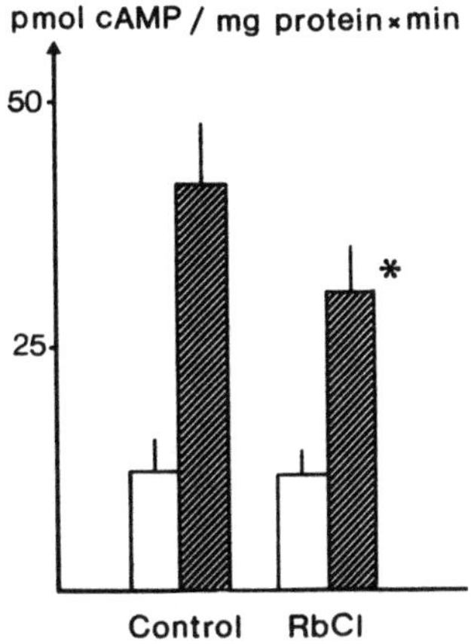

Fig. 4. Effect of chronic rubidium treatment on unstimulated (*open bars*) and isoproterenol (10^{-4} *M*) -stimulated cyclic AMP formation in rat brain cortical slices. Animals were treated for 14 days with rubidium chloride (40 m*M*) given in tap water. The results represent the means ± SD of five animals in each group. **P* < 0.025 significantly different from controls. The cyclic AMP formation was assayed as previously described. (Mørk et al. 1988)

activity fully activated with maximal concentrations of norepinephrine. Thus, further studies are necessary to clarify the molecular mechanism(s) by which rubidium modulates cyclic AMP formation in brain.

Conclusion

Several studies have aimed at elucidating the influence of mood-modifying drugs on cerebral adenylate cyclase. We have found it interesting to compare the actions of lithium and rubidium which seem to have opposite effects on the human mood. As regards lithium, this ion in vitro as well as ex vivo inhibits the cyclic AMP formation in the brain by intervening with the adenylate cyclase, possibly by two different mechanisms (Mørk 1990). The in vitro effect of lithium on the adenylate cyclase seems to be an antagonism between lithium and magnesium. However, the ex vivo effect of lithium on neurohormone-stimulated adenylate cyclase may be due to an interaction with the mechanism(s) by which neurohormones activate the G proteins. Rubidium in vitro increases cyclic AMP formation in intact cell preparations but not in membrane preparations. On the other hand, chronic treatment with rubidium reduces the cyclic AMP production in intact cells.

These effects of rubidium and lithium on the cyclic AMP synthesis lend some support to the assumption that the adenylate cyclase system may be involved in the neurobiologic disturbances underlying the abnormal mood swings of manic-depressive disorder or the pharmacodynamic effects of the drugs used against these emotional disturbances.

References

Alexander GJ, Alexander RB (1978) Alcohol consumption in rat treated with lithium carbonate and rubidium chloride. Pharmacol Biochem Behav 8: 533–536

Avissar S, Schreiber G (1989) Muscarinic receptor subclassification and G-proteins: significance for lithium action in affective disorders and the treatment of the extrapyramidal side effects of neuroleptics. Biol Psychiatry 26: 113–130

Blier P, de Montigny C, Tardif D (1987) Short-term lithium treatment enhances responsiveness of postsynaptic 5-HT_{1A} receptors without altering 5-HT autoreceptor sensitivity: an electrophysiological study in the rat. Synapse 1: 225–232

Brunello N, Barbaccia ML, Chuang D-M, Costa E (1982) Down-regulation of beta-adrenergic receptors following repeated injections of desmethylimipramine: permissive role of serotonergic axons. Neuropharmacology 21: 1145–1149

Ebstein RP, Hermoni M, Belmaker RH (1980) The effect of lithium on noradrenaline-induced cyclic AMP accumulation in rat brain: inhibition after chronic treatment and absence of supersensitivity. J Pharmacol Exp Ther 213: 161–167

Ebstein RP, Newman ME, Bennett ER, Lerer B (1989) Mechanisms of lithium and ECS action in affective disorders: modulation of postreceptor second messenger function. In: Tipton KF, Youdim MBH (eds) Biochemical and pharmacological aspects of depression. Taylor and Francis, London, pp 123–141

Engelmann W, Casper H (1984) Effect of RbCl on the circadian rhythm of locomotor activity in the cockroach. J Interdispl Cycle Res 15: 17–22

Fieve RR, Meltzer H, Donna DL, Levitt M, Mendlewicz J, Thomas A (1973) Rubidium: biochemical, behavioral and metabolic studies in humans. Am J Psychiatry 130: 55–66

Friedman E, Wang H-Y (1988) Effect of chronic lithium treatment on 5-hydroxytryptamine autoreceptors and release of 5-[^{3}H]hydroxytryptamine from rat brain cortical, hippocampal, and hypothalamic slices. J Neurochem 50: 195–201

Geisler A, Klysner K, Andersen PH (1984) Opposite effects of lithium and rubidium on neurohormone-stimulated cyclic AMP formation in rat brain. In: Corsini GU (Ed) Current trends in lithium and rubidium therapy. MTP Press, Lancaster, pp 37–57

Gilman AG (1989) G proteins and regulation of adenylyl cyclase. JAMA 262: 1819–1825

Gross G, Hanft G (1990) Does lithium in vitro and ex vivo alter the release of [^{3}H]noradrenaline from brain tissue and the sensitivity of presynaptic autoreceptors? Neuropharmacology 29: 831–835

Gross G, Dodt C, Hanft G (1988) Effect of chronic lithium administration on adrenoceptor binding and adrenoceptor regulation in rat cerebral cortex. Naunyn-Schmiedebergs Arch Pharmacol 337: 267–272

Hines G (1986) Effects of lithium and rubidium on shock-induced changes in open-field activity. Psychopharmacology 88: 209–212

Hotta I, Yamawaki S (1986) Lithium decreases 5-HT_1 receptors but increases 5-HT-sensitive adenylate cyclase activity in rat hippocampus. Biol Psychiatry 21: 1382–1390

Janowsky A, Okada KF, Manier D, Applegate CD, Sulser F (1982) Role of serotonergic input in the regulation of the β-adrenergic receptor-coupled adenylate cyclase system. Science 218: 900–901

Meltzer HL, Fieve RR (1975) Rubidium in psychiatry and medicine: An overview. In: Essman WB, Valzetti L (eds) Current developments in psychopharmacology, vol I. Spectrum, De Meern, pp 205–242

Messiha FS (1985) Cesium: an overview. In: Gabay S, Harrais J, Ho BT (eds) Metal ions in neurology and psychiatry. Neurology and neurobiology, vol 15. Liss, New York, pp 247–257

Mizuta T, Segawa T (1989) Chronic effects of imipramine and lithium on 5-HT receptor subtypes in rat frontal cortex, hippocampus, and choroid plexus: quantitative receptor autoradiographic analysis. Jpn J Pharmacol 50: 315–326

Mørk A (1990) Actions of lithium on second messenger activity in the brain: the adenylate cyclase and phosphoinositide systems. Lithium 1: 131–147

Mørk A, Geisler A (1987) Mode of action of lithium on the catalytic unit of adenylate cyclase from rat brain. Pharmacol Toxicol 60: 241–248

Mørk A, Geisler A (1989a) Effects of GTP on hormone-stimulated adenylate cyclase activity in cerebral cortex, striatum and hippocampus from rats treated chronically with lithium. Biol Psychiatry 26: 279–288

Mørk A, Geisler A (1989b) The effects of lithium in vitro and ex vivo on adenylate cyclase in brain are exerted by distinct mechanisms. Neuropharmacology 28: 307–311

Mørk A, Geisler A (1989c) Effects of lithium on GTP-mediated inhibition of calcium-stimulated adenylate cyclase activity in rat brain. Eur J Pharmacol 168: 347–354

Mørk A, Geisler A, Klysner R (1988) Isoprenaline- and guanosine triphosphate-stimulated cAMP accumulation in cerebral cortex from rats treated chronically with alprazolam and lithium. New Trends Exp Clin Psychiatry 4: 119–128

Newman ME, Belmaker RH (1987) Effects of lithium in vitro and ex vivo on components of the adenylate cyclase system in membranes from the cerebral cortex of the rat. Neuropharmacology 26: 211–217

Paschialis CC, Jenner FA, Lee CR (1978) Effects of rubidium chloride on the course of manic-depressive illness. J R Soc Med 71: 343–352

Placidi G, Lenzi A, Lazzerini F, Dell'Osso L, Cassano GB, Akiskal HS (1988) Exploration of the clinical profile of rubidium chloride in depression: a systematic open trial. J Clin Psychopharmacol 8: 184–188

Rosenthal NE, Goodwin FK (1982) The role of lithium ion in medicine. Annu Rev Med 33: 555–568

Spengler RN, Hollingsworth PJ, Smith CB (1986) Effects of long-term lithium and desipramine treatment upon clonidine-induced inhibition of ^{3}H-norepinephrine release from rat hippocampal slices. Fed Proc 45: 681

Stolk JM, Nowack WJ, Barchas JD (1970) Brain norepinephrine: enhanced turnover after rubidium treatment. Science 168: 501–503

Electrolytes, Renal Function, and Rubidium Chloride Therapy Side Effects

M. Tuoni, M. Taddei, C. Pasquini, A. Stefanelli, M. Meschi, A Bionda, B. Dal Pino and G.F. Placidi

Introduction

Rb was discovered by Kirchof and Bunsen in 1861. Widely distributed throughout nature (Perelman 1965) and animal tissues (Bertrand and Bertrand 1946) it belongs to the group 1A alkali metals just like potassium, sodium, cesium, and lithium. The first human clinical use of Rb and its effect on ten cardiac patients was described by Botkin in 1988; a subjective sense of well-being associated with increased blood pressure and decreased pulse rate was reported.

The therapeutic use of Rb salts in different pathological conditions (lue-epilepsy-etc..) lasted until 1918; after this date its use was discontinued.

More recently, Stolk's observation on Rb as an anti-lithium drug (Stolk et al. 1970) and the clinical activity of Rb reported by Meltzer and Fieve, Feive and coworkers (Fieve et al. 1971; Meltzer and Fieve 1975) suggested that Rb could be therapeutic for depression as lithium is for mania. The biochemical behaviour of these two salts is very different; Rb increases the release of norepinephrine from cellular storage (Eichelman et al. 1972, 1973; Kirpekar et al. 1972; Stolk et al. 1970; Tehrani et al. 1974) to enhance the O-methylation pathway without interfering with the other cerebral amines; lithium increases the uptake of norepinephrine into synaptosomes (Colburn et al. 1967) and it does not decrease adenyl cyclase activity (Kirpekar et al. 1972).

Physiologically, Rb is very similar to the potassium ion acting at the cellular level on membrane transport, affecting intracellular potassium metabolism (Hudson and Relman 1962; Kilpatrick et al. 1966; Relman et al. 1957; Sheehan and Renkin 1972). It is concentrated intracellularly in most living tissues and may cause histological changes in the suprarenal cortex, comparable to potassium-induced lesions. Lithium, on the other hand, may act either on sodium metabolism or on calcium channels (Hudson and Relman 1962; Kilpatrick et al. 1966; Relman et al. 1957; Sheehan and Renkin 1972).

About 4.2 mEq Rb is present in a normal man weighing 70 kg, while only 1% of this amount is present in the normal daily diet. The Rb completely absorbed after oral administration reaches its peak within 60–90 min and penetrates the liver, muscles, and the central nervous system (Bernstein and Israel 1970; Lieberman and Meltzer 1970); its biological half-life ranges from 30 to 60 days. Rb is mainly eliminated by the kidneys (Bernstein and Israel 1970; Fieve et al. 1971; Lieberman and Meltzer 1970; Rutigliano et al. 1980), but very little is known about the handling of Rb by the kidneys in humans, and the possible toxic or undesirable side effects after long-term Rb therapy remain to be investigated. Distal tubular degeneration (Tomizawa et al. 1974) has been histologically demonstrated in animal studies with toxic doses of Rb, moreover, the plasma Rb concentration in patients with chronic renal failure has been reported to be twice that of normal controls after the same loading dose; one area of potential concern, therefore, is the possibility that chronic Rb administration with a safe pharmacological dose might be potentially dangerous if, for a intercurrent nephrotoxicity, the plasma level concentration unexpectedly increases because of a reduced Rb urinary excretion.

The aim of the present study was to evaluate the nephrotoxic effects, if any, of medium- to long-term Rb therapy by the control of possible variations in renal function, and, moreover, the possible interaction between plasma Rb concentrations and plasma and urinary concentrations of the most common electrolytes.

Materials and Methods

A double-blind study was performed on 21 female patients (average age 56.2 years) of whom ten were affected by major depressive illness. The patients were subjected to a pharmacological washout for 1 week and thereafter they received 60–90 days of therapy with rubidium chloride (RC; 180 mg four times a day). All patients were maintained on normal caloric uptake and known amounts of dietary sodium and potassium (60 mEq/day). Before and during pharmacological therapy (15th, 30th, and 60th day) and 30 days after the treatment had been discontinued, the following chemical plasma and urine analyses were performed: BUN, creatinine, uric acid, sodium, potassium, calcium, and phosphate. Urea and creatinine clearance were also calculated. Because of potassium and uric acid renal interchangeability and since RC could affect potassium metabolism, we were also interested in calculating the uric acid clearance. Creatinine, BUN, uric acid (mg%), and electrolytes (Na, K, Ca, PO, mEq/l) were analyzed by an automated analyzer system. After the data were processed as mean value $\pm$ standard deviation ($\bar{M} \pm SD$) at all times of control, the double blind was removed, so that only in the ten patients known to be affected by major depressive illness the RC plasma concentration and its possible interaction with renal function were critically evaluated.

Results

Renal function, as evaluated by urea and creatinine clearance, appears to have reduced slightly during the treatment (even if the variation has to be considered not significant, while the uric acid clearance seems to have a neglecting increase, probably because of potassium-Rb tubular secretion interference. Anyway,

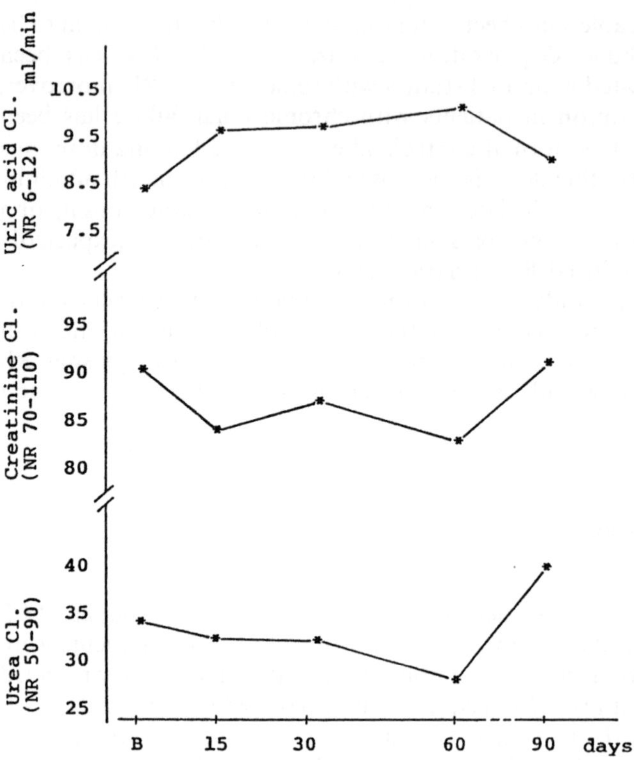

Fig. 1. Urea, creatinine, and uric acid clearance (*Cl.*) values (mean ± SD) before (*B*), during, and after RC therapy. *NR*, normal range

Table 1. Concentrations of Na^+, K^+, Ca^{2+}, and PO_4^{2-} in the blood (mEq/l, mean ± SD) before, during, and after RC therapy

Time (days of therapy)	Na^+	K^+	Ca^{2+}	PO_4^{2-}
Before	138.0 ± 3.8	4.0 ± 0.3	4.4 ± 0.4	2.1 ± 0.6
15	137.4 ± 3.6	4.3 ± 0.3	4.5 ± 0.2	1.9 ± 0.5
30	142.2 ± 2.8	4.5 ± 0.6	4.9 ± 0.5	2.1 ± 0.2
60	141.3 ± 6.8	4.1 ± 0.4	4.4 ± 0.3	2.1 ± 0.3
After (90)	132.0 ± 3.0	4.6 ± 0.2	4.5 ± 0.1	1.7 ± 0.1

when the RC therapy was discontinued, renal function, as well as urea, creatinine, and uric acid clearances, returned to the initial normal values (Fig. 1).

The data reported in Tables 1 and 2 and Figs. 2 and 3 show a common change, with a slight increase in the plasma and urinary concentration of electrolytes (particularly for potassium) with the RC plasma concentration (Table 3, Fig. 4); however it seems remarkable all the variations are within the normal range.

Table 2. Concentrations of Na^+, K^+, Ca^{2+}, and PO_4^{2-} in the urine (mEq/l, mean ± SD) before, during, and after RC therapy

Time (days of therapy)	Na^+	K^+	Ca^{2+}	PO_4^{2-}
Before	121.0 ± 36.6	53.2 ± 10.0	7.1 ± 2.0	27.2 ± 3.2
15	147.0 ± 31.0	56.6 ± 11.8	10.1 ± 1.8	37.4 ± 8.1
30	143.0 ± 14.0	60.6 ± 8.9	12.9 ± 2.9	33.0 ± 4.3
60	145.0 ± 3.7	51.0 ± 4.0	5.9 ± 1.5	27.6 ± 5.0
After (90)	124.0 ± 11.0	42.0 ± 1.0	5.1 ± 2.0	28.0 ± 4.5

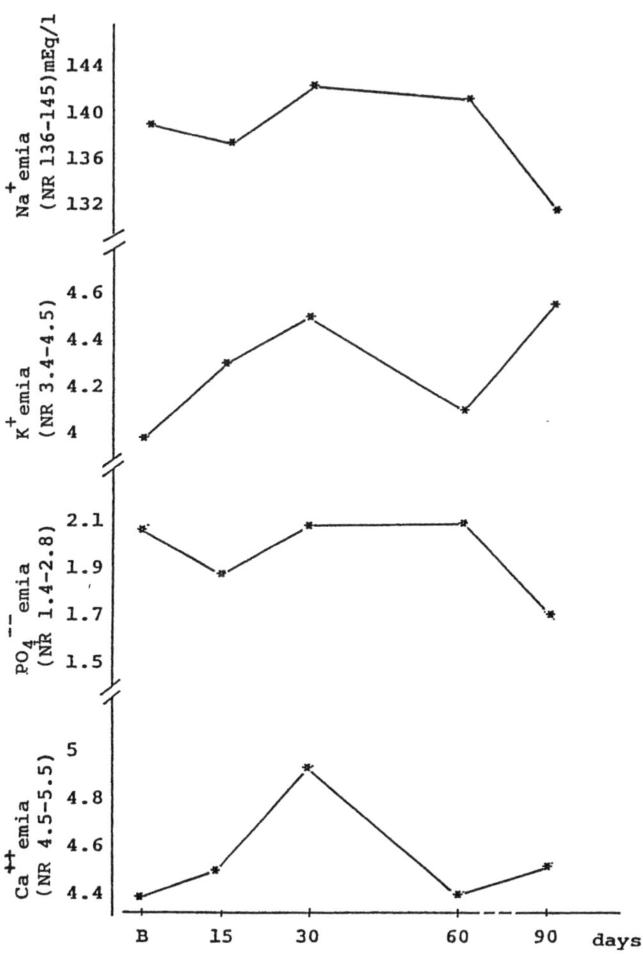

Fig. 2. Blood concentrations of Na^+, K^+, Ca^{2+}, and PO_4^{2-} (mean ± SD) before (*B*), during, and after RC therapy. *NR*, normal range

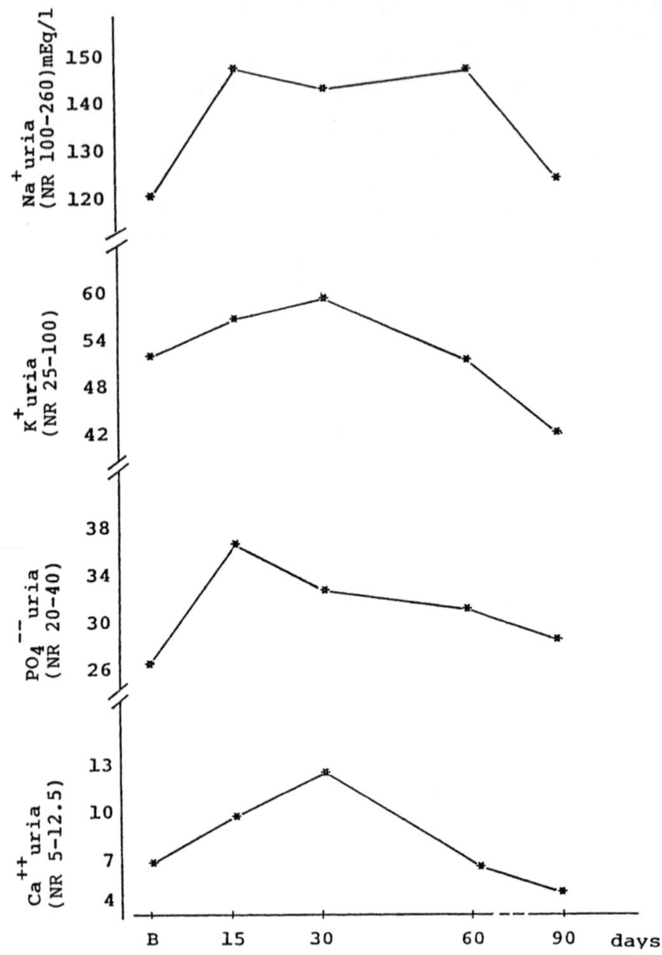

Fig. 3. Urinary concentrations of Na^+, K^+, Ca^{2+}, and PO_4^{2-} (mean $\pm$ SD) before (*B*), during, and after RC therapy. *NR*, normal range

Table 3. Plasma concentration of rubidium (mean $\pm$ SD) before and during RC therapy

Time (days of therapy)	Plasma concentration
Before	0.0047 ± 0.0026
15	0.087 ± 0.042
30	0.120 ± 0.054
60	0.139 ± 0.014

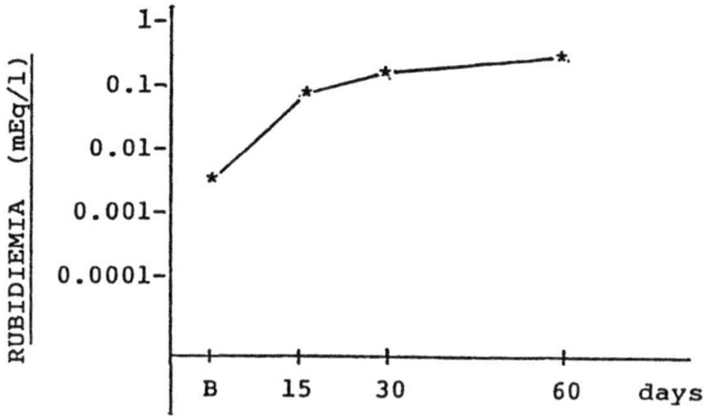

Fig. 4. Plasma concentrations of rubidium (mean ± SD) before (*B*), during, and after RC therapy

Conclusions

Our data show that there was no significant variation in renal function and plasma and urinary sodium, potassium, calcium, and phosphate concentrations.

The most important consideration, even if a small decrease in renal function has been noted and urinary and plasma uric acid and potassium mean values have increased during treatment, is that for all parameters considered the values always remained in the normal range.

It has been noted, moreover, that the RC plasma concentration seems to have some common correlation to human electrolytes (except for potassium, the Rb interchangeability of which is known) probably linked to a competitive mechanism of renal tubular secretion. This fact assumes particular significance if we consider that the therapeutic range of our ten patients (180 mg RC four times a day) has been normal–low, since the mean Rb plasma concentration was 0.12 and 0.14 mEq/1 at the 30th and 60th day of treatment, respectively (safe range 0.1–0.3 mEq/1).

In our previous study (Tuoni et al. 1987) we demonstrated that renal tolerance of RC, for a short period (15 days), was good and was without nephrotoxic effects. We may conclude now that in medium- to long-term Rb therapy no toxic or great adverse renal effects have been produced, but the slight variations in kidney function, as revealed by plasma and urinary levels (even though they are within normal range), seem to indicate the advisability of a more cautious approach in long-term Rb therapy and to suggest the periodic control of renal function and electrolytes monitoring.

References

Bernstein JC, Israel Y (1970) Active transport of 86-Rubidium in human red cells and rat brain slices. J Pharmacol Exp Ther 2: 323–329

Bertrand G, Bertrand D (1946) Sur la présence général du Rubidium chez les animaux. Ann Inst Pasteur 72: 805–809

Colburn R, Goodwin F, Bunney WE Jr (1967) Effect of lithium on the uptake of noradrenaline by synaptosomes. Nature 215: 1395–1397
Eichelman B, Thoa NB, Perez Cruet J (1972) Rubidium and Cesium: effects on aggression, adrenal enzymes and amine turnover. Fed Proc 2: 289
Eichelman B, Thoa NB, Perez-Cruet J (1973) Alkali metal cations: effects on aggression and adrenal enzymes. Pharmacol Biochem Behav 1: 121–123
Fieve RR, Meltzer HL, Taylor RM (1971) Rubidium chloride ingestion by volunteer subjects: initial experience. Psychopharmacology 20: 307–314
Hudson JB, Relman AS (1962) Effects of potassium and rubidium on muscle cell bicarbonate. Am J Physiol 203: 209–214
Kilpatrick R, Miller H, Munro DS et al. (1966) A comparison of the distribution of 42-potassium and 86-rubidium in rabbit and man. J Physiol 133: 194–201
Kirpekar SM, Prat CJ, Puig M, Wakade AR (1972) Modification of the evoked release of noradrenaline from the perfused rat spleen by various ions and agents. J Physiol (London) 3: 601–615
Lieberman KW, Meltzer HL (1970) Recognition of rubidium by the central nervous system. Brain Res 23: 124–127
Meltzer HL, Fieve RR (1975) Rubidium in psychiatry and medicine: an over view. In: Essman WB, Valzetti L (eds) Current developments in psychopharmacology, vol I. Spectrum, pp 205–242
Perelman FM (1965) Rubidium and cesium. MacMillan, New York
Relman AS, Lambie AT, Burrows BA (1957) Cation accumulation by muscle tissue. The displacement of K by Rb and Cs in the living animal. J Clin Invest 36: 1249–1256
Rutigliano G, Cerfeda S, Margari F (1980) Studio sulla cinetica e sulla biodisponibilità del cloruro di rubidio. Clin Ter 94: 679–686
Sheehan RM, Renkin EM (1972) Capillary, interstitial and cell membrane to blood-tissue transport of potassium and rubidium in mammalian skeletal muscle. Circulation Res 5: 588–607
Stolk JM, Nowack WJ, Barchas JD, Platman SR (1970) Brain norepinephrine: enhanced turnover after rubidium treatment. Science 168: 501–503
Tehrani JB, Rossi GV, Goldstein RJ (1974) Effect of lithium and rubidium on the ganglionic inhibitory action of norepinephrine. Life Sci 15: 525–537
Tomizawa S, Satoh P, Satoh H et al. (1974) Toxicity of rubidium chloride given orally to rats for a period of one month. Psychopharmacol Bull 10: 33–34
Tuoni M, Marchitiello M, Placidi GF, Meltzer HL et al. (1987) Renal tolerance of rubidium chloride: short term clinical evaluation. J Clin Pharmacol 27: 503–507

Antidepressive Action of Rubidium

D. De Maio, G. Buffa, D. Dorigo, and M. Laviani

The discovery of rubidium goes back to 1861 when Bunsen and Kirkhoff isolated it from rocks containing lepidolite. Therefore, its use in therapy only began in 1880, with its employment against epilepsy, syphilis, and cardiac insufficiency. Most patients treated with rubidium showed a reduction in heart rate, an increase in blood pressure and, above all, a psychic sense of well-being.

Thanks to its euphoria-inducing properties, rubidium was reevaluated in the early 1960s. Its pharmacotherapeutic identity was defined, on the one hand, as a consequence of the acknowledgement of the effectiveness of lithium in the therapy and prophylaxis of manic-depressive psychosis and on the other hand, by the highlighting of a biochemical and electroencephalographic (EEG) profile opposite to that of lithium.

Rubidium, an alkaline metal belonging to the same chemical group as lithium (Fig. 1), acts like potassium, sharing some metabolic properties with it. Rubidium can take its place and by taking advantage of its privileged transport system, it can accumulate inside the cell. Compared with lithium, which is similar to sodium in its physiological features, rubidium is more concentrated inside the cell and particularly sensitive to corporeal potassium variations.

Like other antidepressive drugs, rubidium strengthens the noradrenergic and dopaminergic transmission, probably through a mechanism of facilitating the release and turn-over of some specific neurotransmitters (Stolk et al. 1970). Moreover, unlike lithium, rubidium seems to increase the norepinephrine-sensitive cyclic adenosine monophosphate (cAMP) synthesis, amplifying the response of the target cell (Geisler et al. 1984; Belmaker et al. 1984). EEG alterations show an effect of activation and an increase in the basal rate in monkeys (Meltzer et al. 1969). As to its pharmacokinetic characteristics, rubidium reaches its steady state (average value 0.4 mEq/1) after a treatment of 3–4 days. The intraerythrocytic concentration of rubidium is far higher than its plasma concentration: the rubidium ratio (the relation between the intra-erythrocytic and plasma ion concentrations) reaches average values of 28–32 (Fieve and Meltzer 1974).

From a behavioral point of view, rubidium seems to produce a euphoric and disinhibiting effect, maybe through an amphetamine-like effect, at least in motor activity and hypnotic antagonism tests (Simon 1978). Hence the "specific" action of rubidium is mainly in situations of both psychic and motor slackening in parkinsonian akinesia and in the affective and emotional withdrawal in schizophrenic patients (Sarteschi et al. 1984). This same activating effect is responsible both for the aggressiveness and persecutory delusions which have arisen during

I	II	III	IV	V	VI	VII
Li +1	Be +2	B +3	C +4, +3, +2 +1,0, −1 −2, −3, −4	N +5 +3 −3	O −2 (−1)	F −1
Na +1	Mg +2	Al +3	Si +4	P +5, +3 +1, −3	S +6, +4 −2	Cl −1, +1 +3, +4 +5, +7
K +1	Ca +2		Ge +4	As +5, +3 −3	Se +6, +4 −2	Br −1, +1 +5
Rb +1	Sr +2		Sn +4, +2	Sb +5, +3 (−3)	Te +6, +4 −2	I −1, +1 +3, +5 +7
Cs +1	Ba +2		Pb +2,(+4)	Bi +5, +3 (−3)		

Fig. 1. Part of the periodic table

rubidium therapy in psychiatric patients (Sarteschi et al. 1984) and for an extension of the manic phase in bipolar patients (Sarteschi et al. 1984; Fieve et al. 1985). Because of its disinhibiting properties, rubidium should be specifically indicated in patients with recurrent major depression and in schizoaffective disorders. The investigation carried out at our center was undertaken (1) to verify the general antidepressive property of rubidium and (2) to ascertain whether rubidium has any selective activity.

Patients and Methods

34 patients, 22 men and 12 women, were investigated: their average age was 40.3 (20–62) years.

The patients can be divided into two groups: the first consisting of 16 patients whose therapy was started during their stay in hospital and then clinically continued and the second consisting of 18 patients whose therapy was undertaken on an outpatient basis, without any previous hospitalization, and checked regularly throughout their treatment period.

The patients belonging to the first group had the following diagnoses according to DSM III-R: recurrent major depression ($n = 11$), dysthymia ($n = 4$), and cyclothymia ($n = 1$). Patients were treated with variable dosages, from 180 to 540 mg/day, for a period not less than 30 days. This was repeated, when necessary, for another 30 days after a drug-free period of 2 weeks. Five of 16 patients were on antidepressive treatment with tricyclic antidepressants (TCA), often in association with benzodiazepines (BDZ); one was undergoing treatment with BDZ only, which used to be taken in excess. After 2–3 weeks in hospital, patients were followed up in the outpatient clinic during the whole treatment period and were subjected to laboratory analysis both at the beginning and at the end of any pharmacological treatment. Their cardiac, hepatic, and renal functions were investigated, as were blood glucose, electrolytes, and uricemia. Patients were tested at the beginning of their treatment, on the 15th and 30th day after commencement, and at the end of therapy.

Every patient, when the treatment was over, was subjected to a final evaluation, including both drug tolerability (compliance and side effects) and clinical efficacy (according to the patient and in the experimenter's opinion).

As regards the second group, patients were enrolled and followed up in our lithium center and submitted to the same control procedures as above. Eighteen patients, 10 men and 8 women, have been observed. Ten of them were affected by recurrent major depression, six by dysthymia, and two by cyclothymic disorder (DSM III-R diagnostic criteria). For these patients too, variable dosages (180–540 mg/day were adopted, for a 30-day period, which could be extended to 60 days (with a drug-free interval of 2 weeks) if their clinical conditions required. The same biochemical parameters were investigated and the same clinical checks were carried out as in the first group.

The evolution of the depressive condition causing pharmacological treatment was evaluated using the Hamilton Rating Scale for Depression (HRSD), according to the modalities already described for the first group.

Results

Four patients dropped out and six showed no signs of improvement. In the remaining 24 we noticed an appreciable improvement: in 16 cases of recurrent major depression, in five cases of dysthymia, and in three cases of cyclothymic disorder.

In those patients who responded favorably to therapy it was possible to observe selective activity on some items of HRSD. Particularly, its direct action on the depressive nucleus, characterized by sadness and the inability to react and plan, demonstrates the specific activating properties of rubidium.

The 24 patients who completed their treatment reported a total remission of their depressive condition; in 13 cases, a new interest for work arose and their guilt and feelings of inadequacy disappeared. Nine of the 10 patients who had expressed suicidal ideas displayed better adaptability to their conditions of existence. The specific disinhibiting effect of the drug induced an improvement in psychomotor slackening and emotional withdrawal in 17 patients.

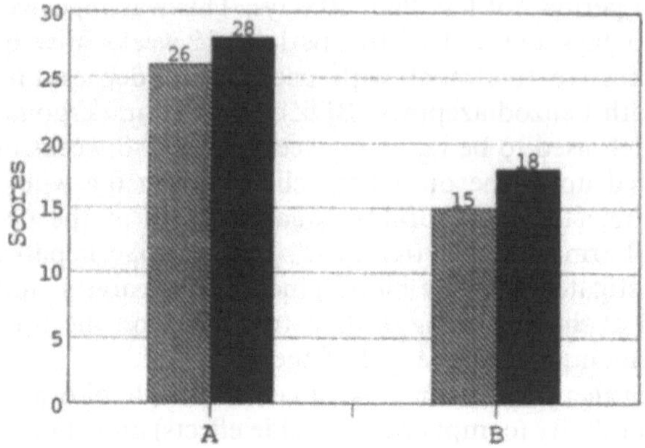

Fig. 2. Average HRSD scores at the beginning (*A*) and the end (*B*) of therapy. ▧ males; ■ females

In contrast, rubidium showed a poor therapeutic effect on anxiety and insomnia. That is why symptoms linked with anxiety somatization were relatively refractory to therapy.

Moreover, we must take into account the fact that the evaluation of these items is generally invalidated by the concurrent administration of anxiolytic and hypnoinductive drugs. This also happens with lithium: the greater its action, the lower the anxiety level associated to the depressive nucleus.

Taking into consideration, on the one hand, the role and meaning of anxiety and on the other hand, the biological-asituational profile of major depression, rubidium can be supposed to be a drug with a more activating than thymoleptic role. In this sense, rubidium is much more similar to monoamine oxidase inhibitors than to TCA, as demonstrated also by its latency period. The time necessary to obtain an improvement in symptoms was about 7 days.

Drug tolerability proved good; the only side effects reported by patients were headaches in six cases and dizziness in two cases. Laboratory analyses have always been normal from the beginning to the end of treatment.

Figure 2 shows the HRSD scores in the two sexes at the beginning and at the end of treatment.

Conclusions

This investigation of the therapeutic activity of rubidium in affective disorders is one of the aspects of the research and clinical activity at our lithium center for the therapy of periodical psychic afflictions.

The main activity of our center is the diagnosis and therapy of affective disorders (bipolar disorders and recurrent major depression), behavioral anomalies characterized by impulsiveness and aggressiveness, and eating disorders such as anorexia nervosa.

In the last 5 years at our center, 134 patients have been observed and treated: in the last year more research work has been carried out regarding the use of rubidium in 18 patients affected by depressive symptoms. Rubidium has proved to have a good antidepressive effect mainly as an activating and disinhibiting drug, confirming literature data (Casacchia et al. 1984: Corsini et al. 1984).

The clinical-therapeutic value of this drug lies in its power to positively influence depressed mood, guilt feelings, loss of interests, working aptitude, and psychomotor slackening. We have paid particular attention to the ideational-behavioral aspects, as we have noticed before talking about anxiety.

The world of a depressed person is full of renunciations and regrets, ruminations, lost chances, and desires that die even before they are expressed. This is the fear to do anything attitude, marked by fear and lack of "fight", which is so typical of depressed patients. Rubidium, owing to the qualitative and quantitative modifications of mood, acts as a drug that helps to do things since it improves one's "fighting" attitude. It has proved its usefulness in the therapy of endogenous recurrent depressive episodes (16 cases out of 34). It acts quickly (within about 1 week), so it can be used in emergency cases, unlike TCA, which need a longer time. No significant side effects or alterations in the main metabolic functions have been noted.

An important indication emerging from our study is the poor predictive value of the blood rubidium level. This observation confirms the emerging opinion that the blood lithium level is not useful in predicting therapeutic efficacy but is useful in predicting drug tolerability. Recently Abou-Saleh and Coppen (1989), comparing two groups of patients with blood lithium levels of 0.45 mEq/l and 0.60 mEq/l or more, reported substantial similarity of the therapeutic efficacy in the two groups in spite of the sizeable difference in the concentration of the ion in the blood. Our experience, too, seems to confirm the poor therapeutic predictiveness of this parameter yet, on the contrary, the good reliability of the lithium ratio as a predictor of toxicity (De Maio et al. 1989).

So the evaluation of the blood concentration of rubidium does not yield any useful clinical information. We even noted that the half-life of rubidium is not to be overemphasized. This is a pharmacokinetic finding, which is useful for differentiation between drugs of the same group (i.e., BDZ), but it does not add any information concerning the therapeutic efficacy or side effects.

As to plasma concentrations of alkali metals in manic-depressive psychosis, an extremely interesting field, we are setting up a device (an atomic absorption spectrophotometer) for monitoring blood concentrations of vanadium, which is

Table 1. Some metals and their therapeutic activity

	Prophylactic	Antidepressive	Antimanic
Lithium	Yes	Yes	Yes
Rubidium	No	Yes	No
Vanadium	–	–	–
Selenium	–	–	–
Cesium	–	?	–

supposed to increase the depressive phase. Lithium seems to have the power to oppose this increase, acting in a therapeutic role. As to the overall therapeutic aspect in bipolar disorders, we have started a new study in which rubidium is used in the depressive phase while lithium is used after its resolution, taking advantage of the prophylactic properties of this ion (Table 1). The preliminary results seem to indicate that rubidium does not cause any switch from the depressive to the manic phase. If this finding is confirmed in the future, we shall have new methods in contrast to traditional antidepressive drugs. Finally, rubidium, in spite of its psychostimulating action, does not induce a "rebound" effect or drug dependency causing the beginning of the complex "drug's orphan" syndrome.

References

Abou-Saleh MT, Coppen A (1989) The efficacy of low-dose lithium: clinical, physiological and biological correlates. J Psychiatr Res 23/2: 157–162

Belmaker RA, Hamburger-Barr R et al. (1984) The effect of rubidium and lithium on adenylate cyclase and neurotransmitter receptors. In: Corsini GU (ed) Current trends in lithium and rubidium therapy. MTP Press, Lancaster, pp 59–75

Casacchia M, Rossi A, Marola V et al. (1984) The use of rubidium chloride in depressive disorder: clinical aspects. In: Corsini GU (ed) Current trends in lithium and rubidium therapy. MTP Press, Lancaster, pp 255–259

Corsini GU, Reda M, Burrai C et al. (1984) Preliminary results with rubidium in depressed patients. In: Corsini GU (ed) Current trends in lithium and rubidium therapy. MTP Press, Lancaster, pp 247–253

De Maio D et al. (1989) Metabolismo del litio e liposomi di fosfolipidi ipotalamici. In: Atti del 37 congresso nazionale della Societa Italiana di Psichiatria, 6–11 Feb 1989, Rome. CIC Internazionali, Rome, Suppl II, pp 243–251

Fieve RR, Meltzer HL (1974) Rubidium salts: toxic effects in human and clinical effects as an antidepressant drug. Psychopharmacol Bull 1: 38–50.

Fieve RR, Jamison KR, Goodnick PJ (1985) The use of lithium and experimental rubidium in psychiatry. In: Gabay S et al. (eds) Metal ions in neurology and psychiatry. Liss, New York, pp 107–120

Geisler A, Klysner R, Andersen PH (1984) Opposite effects of lithium and rubidium on neurohormone-stimulating cyclic-AMP accumulation in rat brain homogenates. In: Corsini GU (ed) Current trends in lithium and rubidium therapy. MTP Press, Lancaster, pp 37–55

Meltzer HL, Taylor RM, Platman SR, Fieve RR (1969) Rubidium; a potential modifier of affect and behavior. Nature 233: 321–322

Sarteschi P, Placidi GF, Lanzi A et al. (1984) Rubidium salts in depressed patients. An open pilot study standardized techniques. In: Corsini GU (ed) Current trends in lithium and rubidium therapy. MTP Press, Lancaster, pp 225–246

Simon P (1978) Que peut apporter la pharmacologie experimentale à l'étude des antidepresseurs ? In: Pichot P (ed) Les voies normelles de la depression. Masson, Paris, pp 162–168

Stolk JM, Nowack WJ, Baargas JD (1970) Brain norepinephrine: enhanced turnover after rubidium treatment. Science 168: 501–503

Treatment of Depressive Disorders with Rubidium Chloride

M. Nardini, G. Bonelli, N. Magnani, and M. Mancuso

Introduction

Rubidium is an alkali metal present in small quantities inside the organism in physiological conditions. Its clinical use was reserved for organic pathologies – cardiac insufficiency, epilepsy, syphilis (Belmaker et al. 1984) from the middle of the nineteenth century to the beginning of the twentieth century. In 1969 Meltzer and colleagues (1969) localized the effectiveness of the drug on mood disorders (Fieve and Meltzer 1974; Fieve et al. 1973, 1980; Paschalis et al. 1978; Stolk et al. 1971). The pharmacokinetics (by oral administration) show a plasma peak within 45–90 min, and Rb is largely retained in the intracellular compartment after repeated administration (Relman et al. 1957). The half-life is variable between 50 and 70 days and is related to the quantity of potassium passed in the urine (Fieve 1976; Mendel and Closson 1906). Elimination is basically urinary and is improved by the administration of lithium salt. The toxicity of the drug is related to the Rb/K ratio (toxic effects if >0.1) (Calandra and Nicolosi 1980) and is outside the therapeutic range (0.1–0.3 mEq/l).

The effect on neurotransmitters is to improve noradrenergic and dopaminergic action (Stolk et al. 1970) with biochemical effects (improvement of cyclic adenosine monophosphate, cAMP, by norepinephrine) (Belmaker et al. 1984; Geisler et al. 1984), modifications of the EEG and of the behavior opposite to that of lithium salt (Calandra et al. 1989; Corsini et al. 1984; Dell'Osso et al. 1989; Moja et al. 1984; Nicolosi et al. 1984). The latency of the observed effect is variable among the different studies, between 7–10 days (Carolei et al. 1975; Casacchia et al. 1984) and 15 days (Corsini et al. 1984; Sarteschi et al. 1984). Side effects are few and insignificant. The effectiveness of the drug has been evaluated in many clinical studies on subjects afflicted with recurrent major depression, bipolar disorder, and depressive major episode (Fieve and Meltzer 1974). Authors have noted a selective action on symptoms such as "retardation", "depressive mood", and "loss of interest" (Carolei et al. 1975; Sarteschi et al. 1984) similar to other antidepressive drugs such as chlorimipramine (Calandra et al. 1989). Use of the drug in bipolar patients (Paschalis et al. 1978) has shown a marked reduction (in duration and gravity) of depressive episodes, with elongation of the manic periods.

The majority of studies have shown neither important side effects nor significant changes in renal functions at therapeutic dosages.

The aim of our study is to investigate the effectiveness of rubidium chloride on 30 depressed patients, in relation to their clinical and psychopathological characteristics, and to compare its antidepressant action to that of chlorimipramine, fluoxetine, and amineptine.

Material and Methods

Our study is based on an investigation of 30 patients aged 18–65 years suffering from mood disorder diagnosed by DSM III-R criteria, and having (at baseline) a score ≥ 15 for the first 17 items of the Hamilton Rating Scale for Depression (HAM-D) (Hamilton 1960). Excluded from this study were patients during pregnancy or while breast feeding, patients who had interrupted monoamine oxidase inhibitors (I-MAO) for 15 days or less; patients with depression secondary to other organic or psychiatric illnesses, patients with serious organic pathologies or taking drugs which could interfere with Rb, subjects refusing treatment, drug addicts, and alcoholics. After a wash-out of at least 3 days, treatment with rubidium chloride was started at a fixed dose of 540 mg/day divided into three administrations. It was possible to reduce anxiety symptoms or insomnia using clordemetildiazepam (free dosage). Checks have been made at baseline (T0) and at the 7th, 14th, 21st, and 28th days of treatment. Clinical history data have been investigated by Adult Personal Data Inventory (APDI). The gravity of symptomatology as well as therapeutic effect have been evaluated by HAM-D and Clinical Global Improvement (CGI). Dosage Record Treatment Emergent Symptoms Scale (DOTES) and Tess Write In Scale (TWIS) were used to check for side effects. At T0, and on the 28th day of therapy, ECG and plasma analysis [azotemia creatinine, GOT, GPT, gammaGT, K, Na] were made. Upon termination of treatment, the Psychiatric Termination Record (PTR) was used.

All patients who refused treatment were considered as drop-outs; however, we included those who discontinued treatment because it proved ineffective after a minimum of 2 weeks' therapy, or due to serious side effects. In these cases the PTR was used as well. We have randomly compared ten of the above-mentioned patients to three groups of depressed patients who were treated with amineptine, chlorimipramine, and fluoxetine (free dosage), respectively, investigating the scores of HAM-D and CGI at baseline and 45 days after beginning the treatment.

Finally, a statistical analysis by chi-square and Student's *t* test was made.

Results and Discussion

The 30 patients we studied had a mean age ($\pm$ standard deviation, SD) of 55.7 ± 12.3 years and were predominantly female (20 patients). A high percentage (25 patients, 83.4%) had no positive familial clinical history of psychiatric disorders, but many themselves had a record of previous depressive and/or manic episodes (23 subjects, 76.6%), previous hyperthymic and/or depressive temperament (15 patients, 50%).

In relation to the actual test, 73.3% (22 subjects) of the patients were diagnosed as suffering from major depressive episode (recurrent in 50% of the patients – 15 subjects), 26.7% (8 patients) were diagnosed as bipolar disorder of depressive type. Melancholia was present in 26.6% (17 subjects) of the cases. Duration of the episode was between 1 and 6 months for 73.4% of the patients (22 subjects).

60% of the patients (18 subjects) have been treated with rubidium chloride without benzodiazepines. Association with benzodiazepines has been necessary in 40% of the patients (12 subjects) due to the presence of marked anxiety symptoms and insomnia since the beginning of the study. The appearance of agitation/excitement could not be controlled by anxiolytic drugs. All patients were treated on an outpatient basis. In one case only we observed, by PTR, an irregularity in the intake of the drug. We did not notice the side effects described

Table 1. Side effects of treatment

Side effects	Rubidium (30 pat.)		Rubidium (10 pat.)		Amineptine (10 pat.)		Chlorimipramine (10 pat.)		Fluoxetine (10 pat.)	
	n	%	*n*	%	*n*	%	*n*	%	*n*	%
Excitement/ agitation	2	6.6	1	10	–	–	–	–	–	–
Mania	1	3.3	–	–	–	–	–	–	–	–
Diarrhea	1	3.3	–	–	–	–	–	–	–	–
Confusion	–	–	–	–	3	30	–	–	–	–
Neurovegetative symptoms	–	–	–	–	4	40	8	80	3	30
Cardiovascular symptoms	–	–	–	–	–	–	–	–	2	20
Anorexia	–	–	–	–	–	–	–	–	1	10
Hypotension	–	–	–	–	–	–	–	–	1	10

pat., patients

Table 2. Average scores ± standard deviation for Clinical Global Improvement at baseline and on days 7, 14, 21, and 28 of treatment

CGI	T0	T7	T14	T21	T28	Significance
Gravity of the illness	4.96 ± 0.6	4.80 ± 0.5	4.04 ± 0.6	3.44 ± 1.0	2.60 ± 1.1	T0/T14**
Global improvement	–	3.72 ± 0.6	2.84 ± 0.7	2.16 ± 0.9	1.72 ± 1.1	T7/T14**

T0, baseline; T, day of treatment
** $p < 0.001$.

in the literature (such as epigastric pain, insomnia, dryness of the fauces, nausea, and constipation), except in one case of diarrhea, and excitement/agitation of a serious to moderate gravity in four subjects on the 7th day of therapy. Two of these patients interrupted therapy due to the appearance of manic symptoms on days 14 and 21, respectively (Table 1).

Table 3. Total average scores ± standard deviation of HAM-D scores, at various times of observation

Day of observations	Mean ± SD	Significance
Baseline	28.04 ± 6.3	**
7	24.12 ± 6.2	**
14	18.52 ± 5.9	**
21	12.73 ± 5.1	**
28	9.21 ± 4.7	**

** $p < 0.001$ for baseline vs following days of observation.

Table 4. Average scores ± standard deviation, of items of HAM-D at baseline and day 28 of therapy

Items	Baseline	Day 28	Significance
DM	3.48 ± 0.5	1.30 ± 0.7	**
G	2.2 ± 1.1	0.69 ± 0.8	**
S	1.6 ± 0.7	0.17 ± 0.3	**
IN1	1.04 ± 0.5	0.26 ± 0.5	**
IN2	1.08 ± 0.9	0.0 ± 0.0	**
IN3	1.16 ± 0.6	0.34 ± 0.5	**
WI	2.28 ± 0.7	1.13 ± 0.4	**
R	0.92 ± 0.9	0.04 ± 0.2	**
A	0.72 ± 1.0	0.43 ± 0.6	
PA	2.68 ± 0.7	1.04 ± 0.4	**
SA	1.8 ± 0.8	0.87 ± 0.6	**
GIS	1.36 ± 0.6	0.52 ± 0.5	**
GSS	1.48 ± 0.5	0.56 ± 0.5	*
GS	0.84 ± 0.6	0.43 ± 0.5	*
HY	1.16 ± 0.8	0.21 ± 0.7	**
W	0.6 ± 0.7	0.21 ± 0.7	*
I	0.32 ± 0.4	0.0 ± 0.0	**
DV	0.56 ± 0.5	0.08 ± 0.2	**
D	0.64 ± 0.6	0.21 ± 0.4	*
PS	0.12 ± 0.4	0.04 ± 0.2	
OCS	0.64 ± 0.4	0.65 ± 0.4	

DM, depressed mood; G, guilt; S, suicide; IN1, initial insomnia; IN2, central insomnia; IN3, delayed insomnia; WI, work and interest; R, retardation; A, agitation; PA, psychic anxiety; SA, somatic anxiety; GIS, gastrointestinal somatic symptoms; GSS, general somatic symptoms; GS, genital symptoms; HY, hypochondria; W, loss of weight; I, insight; DV, diurnal variation; D, depersonalization; PS, paranoiac symptoms; OCS, obsessive-compulsive symptoms.
* $p < 0.05$; ** $p < 0.001$.

Therefore, in relation to the above mentioned criteria, no patients have been considered drop-outs. No alterations were observed in the ECG or the plasma values.

Considering the therapeutic response investigated by CGI, we observed a significant difference between the gravity of the investigated clinical condition and a remarkable improvement thereof at day 14 of the treatment ($p < 0.001$) (Table 2).

Table 5. Average scores ± standard deviation of the items of HAM - D at baseline and day 28 of therapy for two groups of patients treated with (A) rubidium and (B) rubidium + benzodiazepines

Items	Group A		Group B	
	Baseline	Day 28	Baseline	Day 28
DM	3.53 + 0.5	1.22 + 0.8**	3.40 + 0.9	1.20 + 0.8‡
G	2.33 + 1.1	0.77 + 0.8**	2.00 + 1.0	0.77 + 0.8†
S	1.73 + 0.7	0.11 + 0.3**	1.40 + 0.6	0.11 + 0.3‡
IN1	1.13 + 0.5	0.11 + 0.3*	0.90 + 0.5	0.11 + 0.3†
IN2	1.06 + 0.9	0.00 + 0.0*	1.10 + 0.8	0.00 + 0.0†
IN3	1.26 + 0.7	0.55 + 0.5*	1.00 + 0.6	0.55 + 0.5†
WI	2.33 + 0.7	1.11 + 0.3**	2.20 + 0.7	1.10 + 0.3†
R	1.13 + 1.0	0.00 + 0.0*	0.60 + 0.5	0.00 + 0.0†
A	0.73 + 1.0	0.66 + 0.7	0.70 + 1.0	0.66 + 0.7
PA	2.66 + 0.8	1.11 + 0.6*	2.70 + 0.6	1.11 + 0.6‡
SA	1.53 + 0.8	1.11 + 0.7	2.20 + 0.7	1.10 + 0.7†
GIS	1.46 + 0.6	0.66 + 0.5*	1.20 + 0.6	0.66 + 0.5†
GSS	1.40 + 0.5	0.66 + 0.5*	1.60 + 0.5	0.66 + 0.5†
GS	0.73 + 0.5	0.66 + 0.5	1.00 + 0.8	0.66 + 0.5
HY	1.20 + 0.7	0.33 + 1.0	1.10 + 0.8	0.33 + 1.0†
W	0.66 + 0.8	0.00 + 0.0*	0.50 + 0.5	0.00 + 0.0†
I	0.33 + 0.4	0.00 + 0.0	0.30 + 0.4	0.00 + 0.0
DV	0.53 + 0.5	0.00 + 0.0*	0.60 + 0.5	0.00 + 0.0†
D	0.60 + 0.6	0.20 + 0.4*	0.61 + 0.6	0.22 + 0.4†
PS	0.12 + 0.4	0.04 + 0.2	0.10 + 0.4	0.03 + 0.2
OCS	0.64 + 0.4	0.65 + 0.4	0.65 + 0.4	0.64 + 0.4

See Table 4 for abbreviations.
* $p < 0.05$; ** $p < 0.001$; † $p < 0.05$; ‡ $p < 0.001$.

Table 6. Average scores ± standard deviation for Clinical Global Improvement – Gravity of Illness at baseline and day 45 of therapy for patients treated with rubidium, amineptine, chlorimipramine, and fluoxetine

CGI	Baseline	Day 45	Significance
Rubidium	5.0 ± 0.66	3.3 ± 0.94	**
Amineptine	4.6 ± 1.64	1.9 ± 1.28	**
Chlorimipramine	4.8 ± 0.63	4.1 ± 0.87	*
Fluoxetine	5.2 ± 0.42	2.9 ± 1.19	**

* $p < 0.05$; ** $p < 0.001$.

Table 7. Average scores ± standard deviation for Clinical Global Improvement for patients treated with rubidium, amineptine, chlorimipramine, and fluoxetine

CGI	Average score	Significance of rubidium vs other groups
Rubidium	2.4 ± 1.17	–
Amineptine	2.8 ± 1.13	**
Chlorimipramine	1.2 ± 0.63	–
Fluoxetine	1.9 ± 0.73	–

** $p < 0.001$.

Table 8. Average scores ± standard deviation of the items of HAM-D at baseline and day 45 for patients treated with rubidium

Items	Baseline	Day 45	Significance
DM	3.2 ± 0.63	1.3 ± 1.50	**
G	1.7 ± 1.41	0.6 ± 1.07	*
S	1.2 ± 0.78	0.2 ± 0.42	*
IN1	0.8 ± 0.63	0.4 ± 0.69	
IN2	0.9 ± 0.99	0.4 ± 0.69	
IN3	1.1 ± 0.73	0.0 ± 0.00	**
WI	2.4 ± 0.69	1.2 ± 0.63	**
R	1.1 ± 1.10	0.1 ± 0.31	
A	1.0 ± 0.94	0.5 ± 0.70	
PA	2.4 ± 0.96	1.0 ± 0.66	**
SA	1.6 ± 1.35	0.9 ± 0.73	*
GIS	1.1 ± 0.73	0.6 ± 0.51	
GSS	1.6 ± 0.51	0.6 ± 0.51	**
GS	1.1 ± 0.87	0.7 ± 0.67	
HY	1.7 ± 0.82	0.5 ± 1.08	*
W	0.5 ± 0.97	0.5 ± 1.08	
I	0.2 ± 0.42	0.0 ± 0.00	
DV	0.6 ± 0.51	0.2 ± 0.42	
D	0.7 ± 0.82	0.1 ± 0.31	*
PS	0.2 ± 0.63	0.0 ± 0.00	
OCS	0.3 ± 0.48	0.4 ± 0.51	

See Table 4 for abbreviations.
* $p < 0.05$; ** $p < 0.001$.

Finally, the HAM-D analysis showed a significant reduction ($p < 0.001$) in the total score as early as day 7 of therapy, with a further improvement at later observations (Table 3).

A significant reduction was observed in all symptoms, except for agitation, paranoiac and obsessive–compulsive symptoms (Table 4). The patients were divided into two groups. One group was treated exclusively with rubidium chloride (18 patients) and the other group was treated with rubidium + benzodiazepines (12 patients). We thus obtained a distribution, indicating good response to the drug without benzodiazepines, but with less reduction in anxiety symptoms (agitation, psychic and somatic anxiety). Somatic anxiety in particular was significantly reduced only in association with benzodiazepines (Table 5).

In order to allow a comparison between the various methods of treatment, ten patients were treated with Rb, ten with amineptine, ten with chlorimipramine, and ten with fluoxetine. These patients had a respective mean age of 55.9 ± 9.8, 62.8 ± 6.3, 55 ± 7.95, and 62.4 ± 14.58 years, respectively. Seven of the patients treated with Rb and amineptine were female, six of those treated with chlorimipramine and fluoxetine were male.

The average dosages of amineptine, chlorimipramine, and fluoxetine (±SD) were 200 mg ± 44.72, 85 mg ± 27.83 and 22 mg ± 6, respectively. The fixed dosage for Rb was 540 mg/day. The predominant diagnosis was major depressive episodes for the ten patients treated with chlorimipramine and for the nine patients treated with fluoxetine. One of the subjects treated with fluoxetine presented dysthymia.

Of the ten patients treated with amineptine, five exhibited major depressive episodes and the other five dysthymia. Of the ten patients treated with Rb, five had a major depressive episode and five a major depressive episode in bipolar disorder.

Considering CGI, on the 45th day from the beginning of therapy, we observed a significant reduction in the gravity of the illness in patients treated

Table 9. Average scores ± standard deviation of the items of HAM-D at baseline and day 45 of therapy for patients treated with amineptine

Items	Baseline	Day 45	Significance
DM	3.3 ± 0.94	2.0 ± 1.15	*
G	0.7 ± 0.82	0.5 ± 0.70	
S	0.7 ± 0.94	0.2 ± 0.63	
IN1	0.5 ± 0.70	0.7 ± 0.94	
IN2	0.6 ± 0.84	0.5 ± 0.70	
IN3	0.7 ± 0.82	0.8 ± 0.91	
WI	1.5 ± 1.08	0.9 ± 0.99	
R	0.3 ± 0.48	0.1 ± 0.31	
A	0.8 ± 0.78	0.5 ± 0.70	
PA	2.9 ± 0.31	1.8 ± 0.91	*
SA	2.1 ± 1.28	1.5 ± 0.97	
GIS	0.4 ± 0.51	0.2 ± 0.63	
GSS	1.3 ± 0.82	1.3 ± 0.48	
GS	1.4 ± 0.69	1.2 ± 0.63	
HY	1.8 ± 0.78	1.3 ± 1.05	
W	0.6 ± 0.96	0.0 ± 0.00	
I	0.2 ± 0.40	0.2 ± 0.40	
DV	1.5 ± 0.52	0.6 ± 0.69	**
D	0.0 ± 0.00	0.0 ± 0.00	
PS	1.0 ± 1.33	0.8 ± 0.91	
OCS	0.7 ± 0.82	0.3 ± 0.48	

See Table 4 for abbreviations.
* $p < 0.05$; ** $p < 0.001$.

with Rb, chlorimipramine, fluoxetine ($p < 0.001$), and amineptine ($p < 0.05$) (Table 6).

Finally only those patients treated with chlorimipramine showed a more significant improvement versus those treated with Rb ($p < 0.001$), merely a trend towards a more positive improvement for patients receiving fluoxetine versus Rb therapy, and a lesser improvement for those patients treated with amineptine (Table 7). The total score ($\pm$SD) obtained at HAM-D decreased significantly for those patients treated with Rb (from 26.3 ± 6.05 to 10.6 ± 5.79), chlorimipramine (from 24.7 ± 3.12 to 8.3 ± 5.41), fluoxetine (from 23.1 ± 3.63 to 9.3 ± 4.94, $p < 0.001$) and amineptine (from 25.7 ± 5.14 to 17.3 ± 6.65, $p < 0.05$).

The scores obtained for each item of HAM-D at baseline and on the 45th day of therapy showed the following results:

– For patients treated with Rb: a reduction in nuclear symptoms (depressed mood, guilt, suicidal tendency, work and interest, retardation, somatic and psychic anxiety, and hypochondria)

– For patients treated with chlorimipramine: in addition to the reduction in the above-mentioned symptoms, we also found a reduction in the somatic symptoms (gastrointestinal and general, genital)

– For patients treated with fluoxetine a distribution similar to that of the patients treated with Rb

Table 10. Average scores ± standard deviation of the items of HAM-D at baseline and at day 45 of therapy for patients treated with chlorimipramine

Items	Baseline	Day 45	Significance
DM	3.5 ± 0.52	0.6 ± 0.84	**
G	0.7 ± 0.82	0.2 ± 0.42	*
S	1.6 ± 1.07	0.4 ± 0.69	*
IN1	1.4 ± 0.84	0.1 ± 0.38	**
IN2	0.6 ± 0.84	0.4 ± 0.69	
IN3	1.1 ± 0.73	0.2 ± 0.42	*
WI	2.5 ± 0.52	0.6 ± 0.69	**
R	0.9 ± 0.73	0.2 ± 0.42	*
A	1.7 ± 0.82	0.5 ± 0.52	*
PA	2.4 ± 0.96	1.0 ± 0.66	**
SA	1.4 ± 0.69	1.1 ± 0.56	
GIS	0.8 ± 0.42	0.2 ± 0.42	*
GSS	1.1 ± 0.56	0.5 ± 0.52	*
GS	1.2 ± 0.78	0.5 ± 0.52	*
HY	1.1 ± 0.99	0.6 ± 0.69	
W	0.1 ± 0.31	0.0 ± 0.00	
I	0.0 ± 0.00	0.0 ± 0.00	
DV	1.6 ± 1.26	0.6 ± 0.96	*
D	0.3 ± 0.67	0.0 ± 0.00	
PS	0.2 ± 0.42	0.0 ± 0.00	
OCS	0.7 ± 0.67	0.3 ± 0.48	

See Table 4 for abbreviations.
* $p < 0.05$; ** $p < 0.001$.

Table 11. Average scores ± standard deviation of the items of HAM-D at baseline and day 45 of therapy for patients treated with fluoxetine

Items	Baseline	Day 45	Significance
DM	3.1 ± 0.73	1.1 ± 0.73	**
G	1.4 ± 1.26	0.4 ± 0.69	
S	1.6 ± 1.43	0.0 ± 0.00	*
IN1	1.2 ± 0.78	0.2 ± 0.42	
IN2	0.4 ± 0.69	0.2 ± 0.42	
IN3	0.4 ± 0.51	0.1 ± 0.31	
WI	2.7 ± 1.33	1.1 ± 0.73	*
R	1.1 ± 1.10	0.6 ± 0.84	*
A	0.7 ± 0.94	0.3 ± 0.48	
PA	2.0 ± 0.94	0.8 ± 0.78	*
SA	1.7 ± 0.67	1.1 ± 0.73	*
GIS	0.8 ± 0.42	0.4 ± 0.51	*
GSS	1.0 ± 0.66	0.7 ± 0.67	
GS	0.6 ± 0.69	0.4 ± 0.69	
HY	1.5 ± 0.97	0.5 ± 0.85	*
W	0.5 ± 0.70	0.0 ± 0.00	*
I	0.3 ± 0.67	0.0 ± 0.00	
DV	1.1 ± 0.87	0.8 ± 0.91	
D	0.1 ± 0.31	0.1 ± 0.31	
PS	0.4 ± 0.84	0.2 ± 0.42	
OCS	0.4 ± 0.51	0.3 ± 0.67	

See Table 4 for abbreviations.
* $p < 0.05$; ** $p < 0.001$.

– For patients treated with amineptine a significant reduction only in the items "depressed mood" and "psychic anxiety" (Tables 8–11).

The presence of side effects was significantly less for those patients treated with Rb (one subject presented excitement/agitation) than for the other investigated groups (Table 1).

Conclusions

The treatment with rubidium chloride for patients with mood disorders showed a marked response by the 14th day of therapy, a lack of change in ECG, of plasma analysis and of serious side effects (only excitement/agitation, in four patients, of whom two interrupted the therapy due to manic symptoms). According to our study, the activity of Rb was significantly less only to that of chlorimipramine, but with a smaller number of side effects.

The effectiveness of Rb was similar to that of chlorimipramine and fluoxetine relative to nuclear symptoms (depressed mood, guilt, suicidal tendency, insomnia, retardation, work and interest, psychic and somatic anxiety, hypochondria) although chlorimipramine produced a major reduction in the somatic symptoms (gastrointestinal and general somatic symptoms, genital symptoms). The activity observed for amineptine was minor.

Moreover, with the patients treated with rubidium chloride and having recurrent mood disorder (monopolar or bipolar) and/or previous hyperthymic or depressive temperament, the fact that some responded well to the drug could justify the effectiveness of Rb on the affective disorders of the "Bipolar Spectrum" (Cassano et al. 1986; Placidi et al. 1988).

This hypothesis should be confirmed by experiments on the pharmacokinetics of the salt and on its prolonged administration

References

Belmaker RH, Hamburger-Bar R, Newman M, Bannet J (1984) The effect of rubidium and lithium on adenylate cyclase and neurotransmitter receptors. In: Corsini GU (ed) Current trends in lithium and rubidium therapy. MTP Press, Lancaster, p 59

Calandra C, Nicolosi M (1980) Confronto tra due farmaci ad azione antidepressiva: rubidio Cloruro e clorimipramina. In: XXXIV congresso nazionale della Società Italiana di Psichiatria. 24–29 April, Catania, pp 1–45

Calandra C et al (1989) Valutazione clinica dell'efficacia terapeutica del rubidio cloruro nel trattamento di pazienti depressi. In: Atti del XXXVII congresso nazionale della Societa Italiana di Psichiatria, standard diagnostici ed epidemiologia. CIC Internazionali, Rome

Carolei A, Sonsini U, Casacchia M, Agnoli A, Fazio C (1975) Azione farmacologica del cloruro di rubidio. Effetto antidepressivo: confronto con l'imipramina. Clin Ter 75: 469–478

Casacchia M, Rossi A, Marola V, Meco G (1984) The use of rubidium chloride in depressive disorders Clinical aspects. In: Corsini GU (ed) Current trends in lithium and rubidium therapy MTP Press, Lancaster

Cassano CB, Dell'Osso L, Musetti L (1986) Lo spettro bipolare: implicazioni diagnostiche e terapeutiche. Q Ital Psichiatr

Corsini GU, Reda M, Burrai C, Poddighe A, Rudas N (1984) Preliminary results with rubidium in depressed patients. In: Corsini GU (ed) Current trends in lithium and rubidium therapy. MTP Press, Lancaster

Dell'Osso L et al (1989) Sali di rubidio nel trattamento della depressione: contributo clinico. In: Atti del XXXVII congresso nazionale della Sacietà Italiana di Psichiatria, standard diagnostici ed epidemiologia. CIC Internazionali, Rome

Fieve RR (1976) Drug treatment of mental disorders. In: Simpson LL (ed) Raven, New York, p 193

Fieve RR, Meltzer HL (1974) Is there any clinical evidence that rubidium exerts an antidepressant action? J Pharmacol (Paris) 5 [Suppl 1]: 80–81

Fieve RR, Meltzer RL, Donner DL, Levitt M, Mendlewicz J, Thomas A (1973) Rubidium: biochemical, behavioural and metabolic studies in humans. Am J Psychiatry 130/1: 55–61

Fieve RR, Meltzer HL, Dunner DL (1980) Clinical trials with rubidium chloride in depressed patients. An update and review of evidence for antidepressant action from four psychiatric centers. Rev Dep Psichiatr Facult Med Barcelona VIII: 3

Geisler A, Klysner R, Andersen PH (1984) Opposite effects of lithium and rubidium on neurohormone-stimulated cyclic AMP accumulation in rat brain homogenates. In: Corsini GU (ed) Current trends in lithium and rubidium therapy. MTP Press, Lancaster, p 37

Hamilton M (1960) A rating scale for depression. J Neurol Neurosurg Psychiatry 23: 56–62

Meltzer HL, Taylor RM, Platman SR, Fieve RR (1969) Rubidium: a potential modifier of affect and behaviour. Nature 223: 321–322

Mendel LB, Closson DE (1906) The paths of excretion for inorganic compounds: III The excretion of rubidium. J Physiol 16: 152–159

Moja E et al. (1984) In: Corsini GU (ed) Current trends in lithium and rubidium therapy. MTP Press, Lancaster
Nicolosi M et al. (1984) In: Corsini GU (ed) Current trends in lithium and rubidium therapy. MTP Press, Lancaster
Paschalis C, Jenner FA, Lee CR (1978) Effects of rubidium chloride on the course of maniac-depressive illness. J R Soc Med 71: 343–352
Relman AS, Lambie AT, Burrows SA (1957) Cation accumulation by muscle tissue: the displacement of K by Rb and Cs in the living animal. J Clin Invest 36: 1249
Sarteschi P, Placidi GF, Lenzi A, Rampello E, Cassano GB (1984) Rubidium salts in depressed patients. An open pilot study using standardized techniques. In: Corsini GU (ed) Current trends in lithium and rubidium therapy. MTP Press, Lancaster
Stolk JM, Nowack WJ, Barchas JD (1970) Brain norepinephrine: enhanced turnover after rubidium treatment. Science 168: 501–503
Stolk JM, Conner RL, Barchas JD (1971) Rubidium-induced increase in shock-elicited aggression in rats. Psychopharmacologia 22: 250–260

Clinical Investigations on the Efficacy and Tolerability of Rubidium Chloride

V. Rapisarda, G.A. Sorge, and A. Virzì

Rubidium (atomic number 37, atomic weight 85.47), discovered in 1861 by Kirchof and Bunsen, is an alkali metal belonging to the same periodic series as sodium, potassium, cesium, and lithium (Meltzer et al. 1969). It is widespread in nature, being present in the earth's crust and in vegetable and animal organisms. There are also physiological traces of rubidium in man (Rutigliano et al. 1980).

Biologically rubidium acts like potassium and it has a high degree of metabolic interchange. It tends to occur much more in intracellular fluids than in extracellular ones (Olsson et al. 1959), intervening in the transport of membrane mechanism. It can also replace potassium in the sodium pump mechanism. It would seem to act on some of the adenosine triphosphatase (ATP) activity but remains inactive on the potassium-dependent phosphatase (Farska and Krulik 1975). Instead it inhibits the action of lithium similar to that of sodium (Del Vecchio et al. 1979).

Not long after its discovery, at the end of the nineteenth century, rubidium was being used in the treatment of sicknesses such as syphilis and epilepsy, but not in mental illness (Botkin 1888). Eighty years later, Meltzer and coworkers' studies (1969) gave precise data on its antidepressant activity. In monkeys treated with this cation, they noticed a more intensive activity in the electroencephalographic tracing and an increased reactivity. These effects are contrary to those of lithium, whose known antimanic action suggested the possibility of utilizing rubidium (in the form of rubidium chloride) as an antidepressant. From then rubidium's antidepressant effect has been confirmed by many experimental results on animals and man (Fieve et al. 1971; Fieve and Meltzer, 1974).

Clinical experiments have shown the efficacy of RbCl as an antidepressant drug in about 65%–70% of the patients treated, and no notable toxic effects have been found at the stated doses. As its action is strictly related to mood, it is also capable of prolonging manic episodes in bipolar subjects, and therefore is useless in this group of patients (Paschalis et al. 1978).

In Canada, only in two studies by Chouinard and Annable (1977) did RbCl, administered at doses of 1g/day to schizophrenic patients together with common neuroleptics, show an improvement in the psychomotor retardation, albeit with increased hostility and intensification of delusions of persecution.

More recently RbCl's antidepressant activity was confirmed during the International Symposium on Lithium and Rubidium Therapies (29 Sep-1 Oct 1983, Venice) and the Thirty-Seventh National Congress of the Italian Society of Psychiatry (6–12 Feb 1989, Rome) (Calandra et al. 1989; Casacchia et al. 1984; Corsini et al. 1984; Dell'Osso et al. 1989; Sarteschi et al. 1984; Sorge et al. 1989).

However, it must be remembered that RbCl's precise mechanism is not yet entirely clear.

At a neurotransmitter level, this cation seems to determine an increase in norephinephrine turnover and an increment in tyrosine-hydroxylase activity in the central nervous system, but it does not alter the number of beta-adrenergic, serotoninergic, GABAergic, and cholinergic receptors (Stalk et al. 1970; Gessa 1983). Of particular interest would seem to be its stimulating and potentiating action on central dopaminergic activity (Judd et al. 1975), confirmed by increased synthesis and release of dopamine and a large increase in its principal metabolite concentrations (DOPAC). RbCl does not exert any action on monoamine oxidase (MAO) and cathecol-o-methyl-transferase (COMT) activity and unlike lithium, does not influence adenylate cyclase activity (Placidi et al. 1988).

RbCl is completely absorbed after oral administration, reaching the plasma level peak in 60–90 min. It penetrates slowly into the intracellular level and it moves into the liver, muscular tissue, and central nervous system. It has a half-life of about 42 days and its elimination is principally renal.

Clinical Experiments Performed in the Psychiatric Clinical Institute, University of Catania, Italy

Rubidium chloride has been used in our Psychiatric Institute for 10 years. In one of the first studies (Calandra and Nicolosi 1980), performed double-blind on 28 patients, the therapeutic activity of RbCl was compared with that of clomipramine in the treatment of depression.

All patients, six males and 22 females (average age 47.95 years), received RbCl (540 mg/day) or clomipramine (100 mg/day) for 30 days after a wash-out period of 7 days. Before the treatment and at 7, 15, and 30 days of therapy,

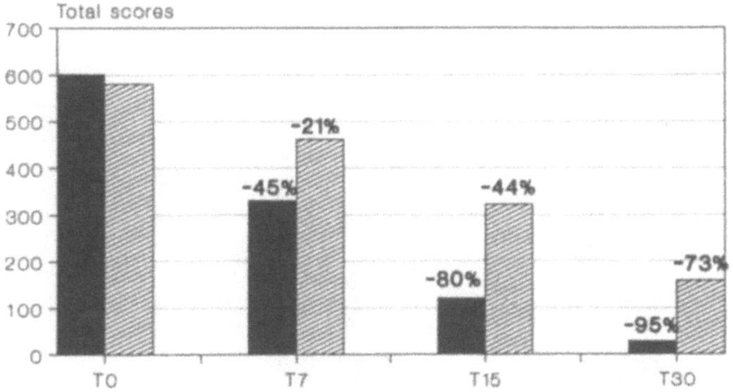

Fig. 1. Comparison of HAM-D scores in patients treated with RbCl or clomipramine. ■, rubidium; ▨, clomipramine; *T*, days after treatment began

Hamilton's scales for depression (HAM-D) and anxiety (HAM-A) were applied. Wittenborn's scale was applied before treatment and at 15 and 30 days of treatment. Any side effects were registered weekly for each patient. After the basic evaluation at the beginning of treatment, weekly during the treatment of RbCl the principal laboratory tests were carried out and electrolytes and RbCl plasma levels were determined.

Data analysis of Hamilton's scales using Fisher's method and of Wittenborn's scale using the Mann-Whitney method was performed. Patients treated with RbCl showed a significantly greater reduction in HAM-D and HAM-A than did patients treated with clomipramine (72.6% HAM-D and 74.1% HAM-A, vs 95.2% HAM-D and 95.7% HAM-A, $p < 0.01$; Figs. 1 and 2). A particularly significant score reduction in scale items of HAM-D was observed in patients who had exhibited depressed mood, suicidal ideas, work problems, psychomotor retardation, and hypochondria, confirming the antidepressant action of RbCl. On Wittenborn's scale in patients treated with RbCl a

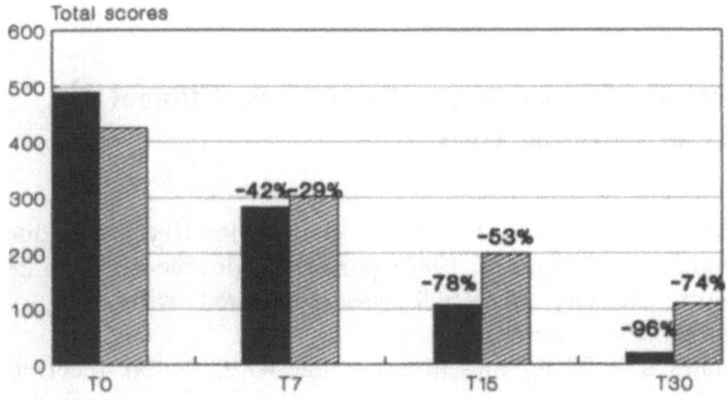

Fig. 2. Comparison of HAM-A scores in patients treated with RbCl or clomipramine. ■, rubidium; ▨, clomipramine; *T*, days after treatment began

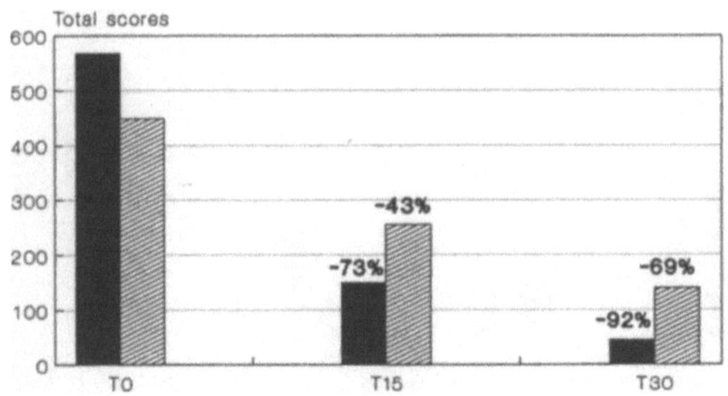

Fig. 3. Scores on Wittenborn's scale in patients treated with RbCl or clomipramine. ■, rubidium; ▨, clomipramine; *T*, days after treatment began

significant reduction in percentage of the score ($p < 0.01$) was observed on 30th day of treatment, compared to that seen in patients treated with clomipramine (68.8% vs 92.1%; Fig. 3).

Plasma levels of RbCl which coincided with the therapeutic effect were between 0.102 and 0.320 mEq/l. The principal laboratory tests and electrolytes were normal during treatment.

The absence of toxic manifestations and significant side effects, the short latency time of the therapeutic efficacy of RbCl, from 5 to 10 days, and the clinical effect suggest a therapeutic superiority of RbCl over clomipramine.

Recently we carried out an open study on 30 patients whose general data were collected using the Adult Personal Data Inventory (APDI) scale. Our group was composed of 12 men and 18 women (Fig. 4), mean age 44.66 years, of whom 15 were married, 12 had never been married, two were separated or

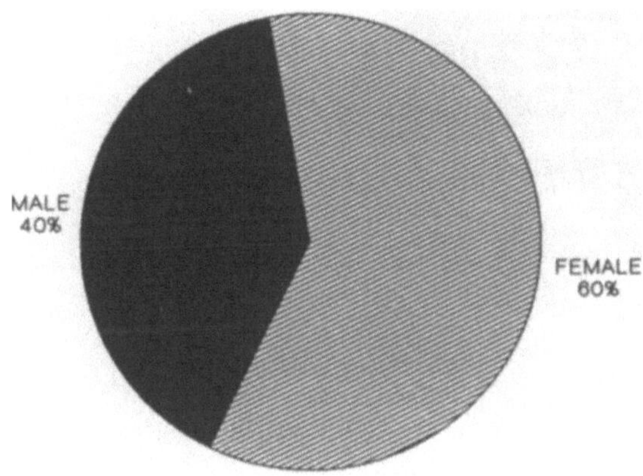

Fig. 4. Sex of patients treated with RbCl

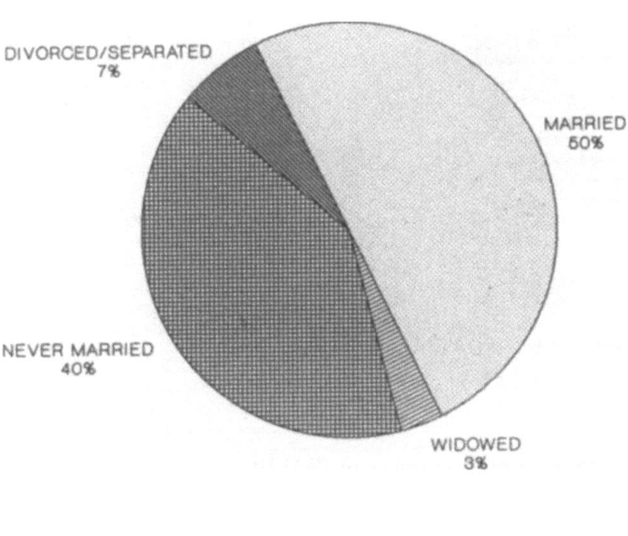

Fig. 5. Marital status of patients treated with RbCl

divorced, and one was a widower (Fig. 5). The educational levels are shown in Fig. 6.

Forty percent were affected by major depression and 60% by dysthymic disorders according to DSM III criteria (Fig. 7). On the HAM-D each patient presented a score ≥ 15 in the first 17 test items. All the patients were given 540 mg/day RbCl; for a maximum of 28 days after a 3-day wash-out period the dosage could be increased up to 900 mg/day in the absence of clinical response. The only other therapy allowed from the third day of treatment onwards was freely dosed chlordemethyldiazepam.

The clinical response was measured using Clinical Global Improvement (CGI) and HAM-D. The side effects and the doses were recorded with Dosage

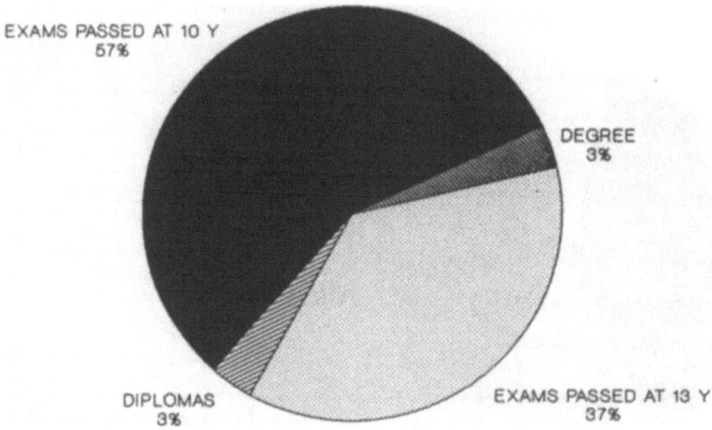

Fig. 6. Educational levels of patients treated with RbCl

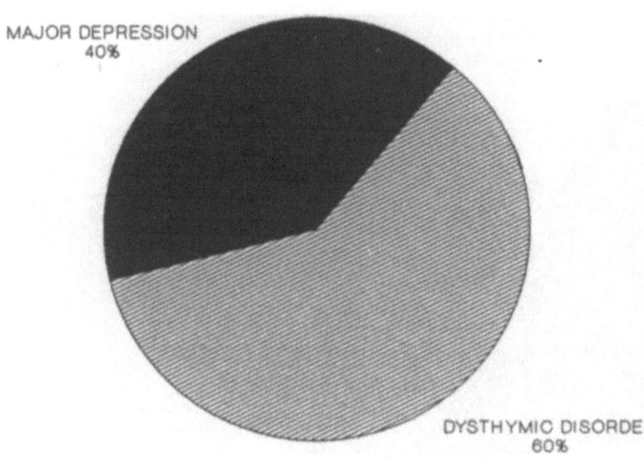

Fig. 7. Diagnosis of patients treated with RbCl according to DSM III criteria

Record Treatment Emergent Symptoms Scale (DOTES) and the Tess Writein Scale (TWIS). All the above-mentioned evaluations were carried out and monitored before the start of the therapy and weekly thereafter until completion.

At the beginning and at the end of treatment, RbCl plasma level and electrocardiographic and blood parameters were determined and renal and liver functions were tested. In 20 patients, the study was completed by evaluating plasma prolactin (PRL) concentrations in basic conditions on the 7th and 15th day of treatment, to verify eventual alterations induced by RbCl on PRL release, which as we know is controlled by the dopaminergic system.

The statistical analysis of data with Student's t Test showed a significant improvement in depressive symptoms after 7 days of therapy ($p < 0.01$), with a reduction of 33.01% in HAM-D scores. Such an improvement was stable for the entire period of treatment (Fig. 8). The analysis of Hamilton's scale factors – anxiety-somatization, cognitive disturbances, psychomotor retardation, sleep disturbance, loss of weight from the seventh day of treatment onwards – showed a significant reduction in the average scores ($p < 0.01$, Figs. 9–13).

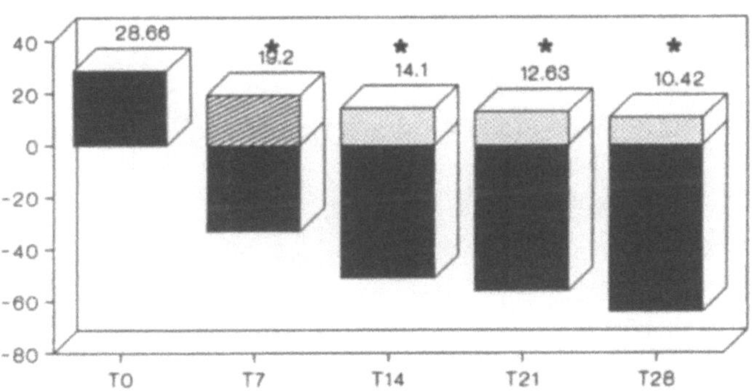

Fig. 8. HAM-D scores before and during treatment with RbCl. ■, mean; ▨, mean; ▦, mean; ■ % decrease; *, $p < 0.01$; T, days after treatment began

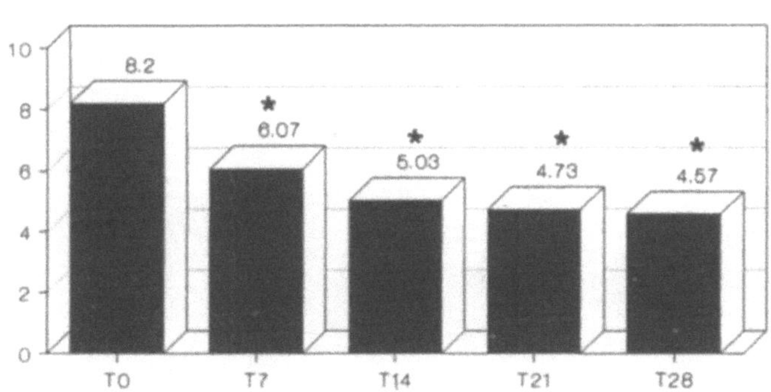

Fig. 9. Analysis of HAM-D relating to anxiety-somatization factor. ■, mean; *, $p < 0.001$ vs T0; T, days after treatment began

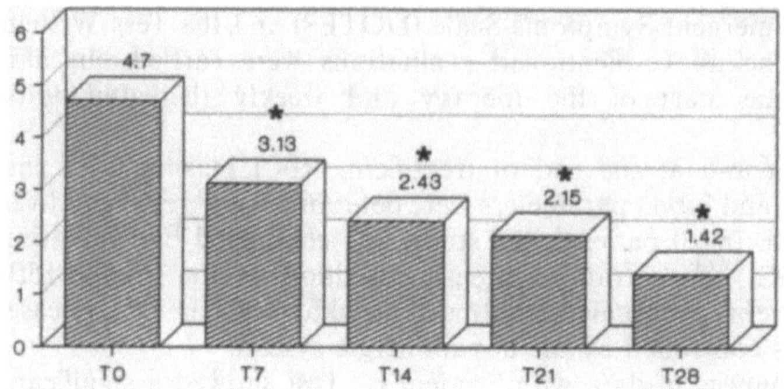

Fig. 10. Analysis of HAM-D relating to cognitive disturbances factor. ▨, mean; *, $p < 0.001$ vs T0; *T*, days after treatment began

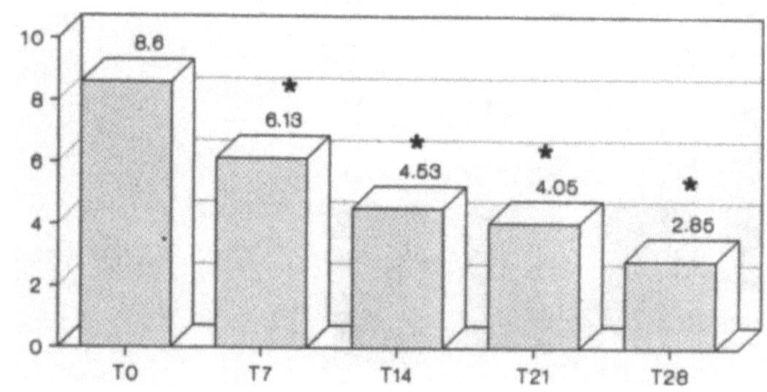

Fig. 11. Analysis of HAM-D relating to retardation factor. ▩, mean; *, $p < 0.001$ vs T0; *T*, days after treatment began

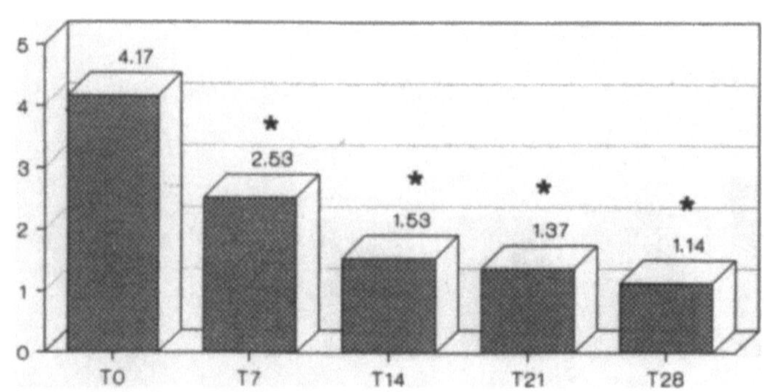

Fig. 12. Analysis of HAM-D relating to sleep disturbances factor. ▩, mean; *, $p < 0.001$ vs T0; *T*, days after treatment began

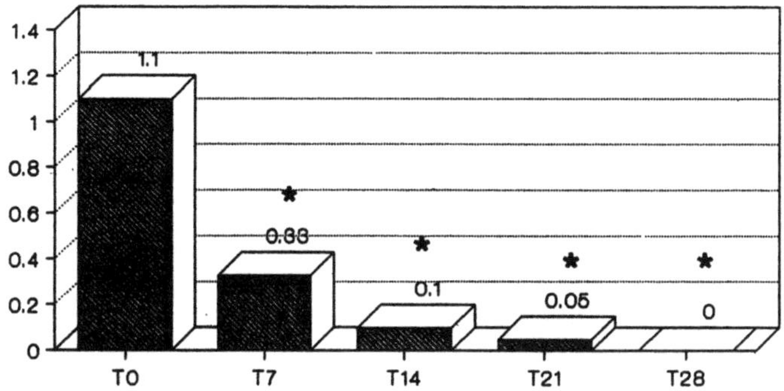

Fig. 13. Analysis of HAM-D relating to loss of weight factor. ▨, mean; *, $p < 0.001$ vs T0; *T*, days after treatment began

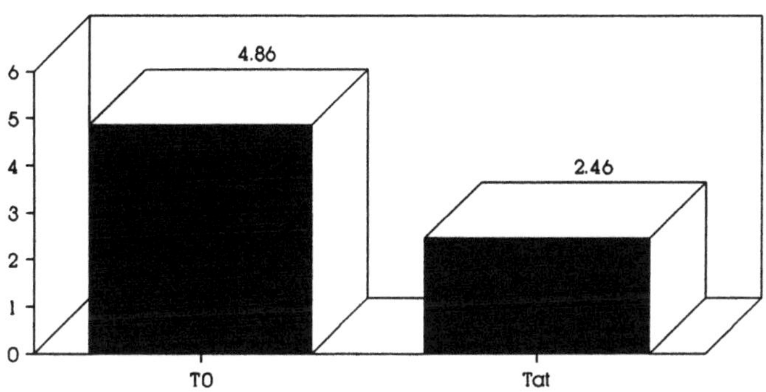

Fig. 14. Clinical global improvement: severity of illness. ■, mean; *Tat*, ▮▮; *T*, days after treatment began. $p < 0.01$

The parameter Severity of Illness, one item of CGI, decreased significantly ($p < 0.01$) from an initial mean value of 4.86 to a final 2.46, proof of clinical improvement (Fig. 14). Basal plasma levels of RbCl (0.0236 mEq/l) increased significantly at the end of the therapy (0.205 mEq/l, $p < 0.01$; Fig. 15). The statistical analysis of Spearman's test did not show any significant correlation ($p = 0.78$) between plasma concentrations of RbCl reached at the end of treatment and HAM-D scores.

The basal concentrations of PRL varied greatly (probably due to sex and to patients' ages) but were within the normal range (9.96 ± 6.3 ng/ml), except in three patients whose values were slightly increased. No statistically significant variations in PRL levels were seen in two blood tests carried out on days 7 and 15 of the therapy compared to basal values, in contrast to the findings of researchers investigating other antidepressants (Ben Hadj 1987) (Fig. 16).

These data appeared contradictory, as we had in fact expected a PRL decrease due to RbCl-induced dopaminergic hypertone exerted at lactotrophic cell level. The absence of a PRL decrease in our patients might result from a

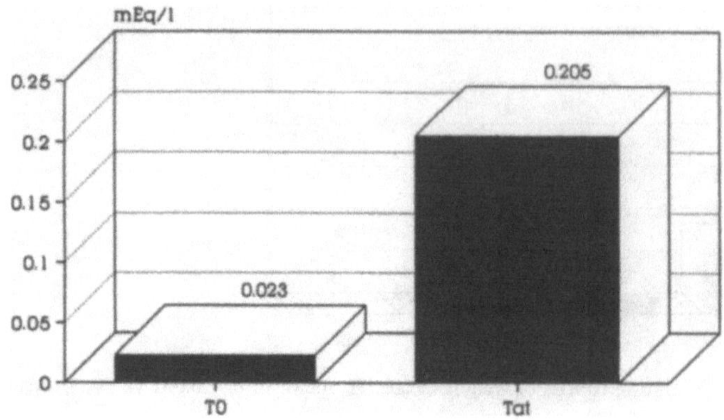

Fig. 15. Plasma levels of rubidium. ■, mean; *Tat*, ▮▮; *T*, days after treatment began. $p < 0.01$

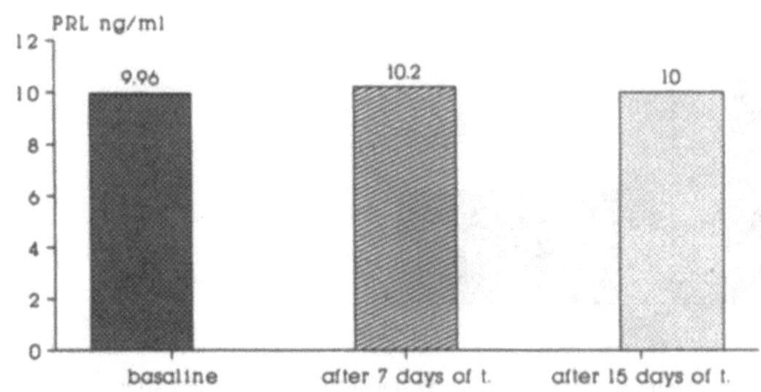

Fig. 16. Treatment with RbCl: hormonal evaluation. *t*, treatment

reduced effect of RbCl on the dopaminergic transmission, suggesting that the clinical efficacy of RbCl is attributed to a selective effect at the level of other neurotransmission systems.

With regard to side effects, in 18 patients generally at the highest daily doses (720–900 mg/day) we found that symptoms due to the neurovegetative system constituted 31.48%, cardiovascular 25.93%, psychic disorders and behavior disorders 12.96%, and other symptoms, including those using the TWIS scale, 29.63%. No neurological symptoms were found (Fig. 17).

Neurovegetative disorders (dry mouth, blurred vision, nausea/vomiting, and diarrhea) were generally slight. Some cases of diarrhea required drugs but this did not affect the treatment. Cardiovascular symptoms such as hypotension, hypertension, and dizziness/lipothymia were very slight. Electrocardiographic variations included a negative T wave in D II, D III, and A VF. There were also signs of cardiac anterior ischemia but it is unlikely there was any link with drug administration. Among psychic and behavioral disorders (insomnia, drowsiness,

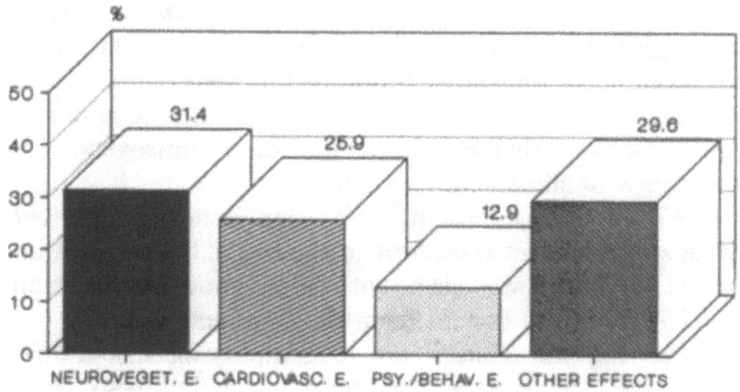

Fig. 17. Side effects during treatment with RbCl

Table 1. Side effects during treatment with RbCl

Symptoms	Mild	Moderate	Severe	Total
Autonomic nervous system				
Diarrhea	4	3	0	7
Nausea/vomiting	5	1	0	6
Dry mouth	2	0	0	2
Blurred vision	2	0	0	2
Cardiovascular system				
Dizziness/lipothymia	5	0	0	5
Hypotension	4	0	0	4
Hypertension	1	0	0	1
Changes in ECG	2	0	2	4
Neurotic/behavioral symptoms				
Insomnia	3	1	0	4
Drowsiness	2	0	0	2
Excitement/agitation	0	1	0	1
Other symptoms				
Headache	3	4	0	7
Gastric distress	2	1	0	3
Weight gain	2	0	0	2
Weight loss	2	0	0	2
Perimalleolar edema	1	0	0	1
Increase of thyroid nodule	1	0	0	1

excitement-agitation) only one case of psychomotor agitation was seen that required the use of corrective drugs.

Other symptoms, all of minor importance, included headache, cleared with analgesic drugs, gastric distress, disappeared with the administration of RbCl on a full stomach, weight variations (gain and loss), perimalleolar edema, and an increase in size of a small preexisting thyroid nodule (Table 1). In two cases we saw hypomanic symptomatology: in one it disappeared on the suspension of the treatment, while in the other it increased, involving a manic episode.

In 14 of the 30 patients in our study it was necessary to raise the daily doses to 720 or 900 mg/day, beginning on the 7th or 14th day of treatment. Seven (23.33%) of the patients completed the study, 12 (40%) followed therapy for 21 days, and 11 (36.67%) for 14 days. (Fig. 18). The end of the therapeutic trial, which was brought forward, was defined by a significant improvement in symptoms or by obvious lack of efficacy of treatment.

In conclusion, 20 (66.67%) of the 30 patients had a complete remission with no signs of mental disease on psychic examination at the end of the therapy, and three (10%) had a partial remission was seen, with fairly good improvement. Only seven patients (23.33%) had no benefit from the treatment (Fig. 19).

At present we are studying the efficacy and tolerability of this drug in outpatients at dosages of 360–540 mg/day. The preliminary findings overlap with those of our previous studies. Our data confirm that, among the thymoleptics, RbCl is to be considered one of the first-choice drugs because of its short latency time, its remarkable antidepressant activity, and its only moderate side effects.

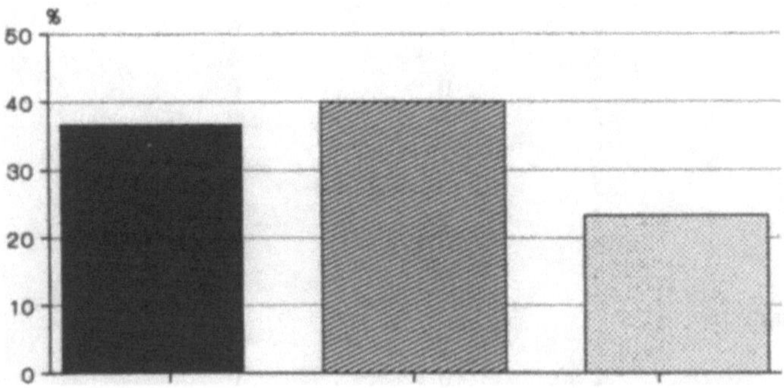

Fig. 18. Duration of treatment. ■, day 14 of therapy; ▨, day 21 of therapy; ▦, day 28 of therapy

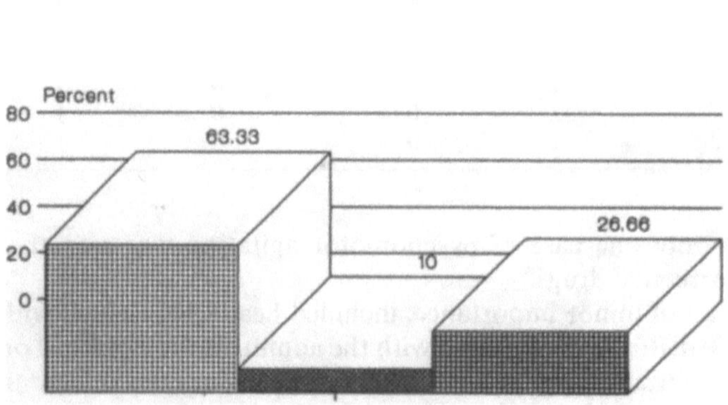

Fig. 19. Clinical evaluation at the end of the trial. ▦, complete remission; ■, partial remission; ▦, ineffective

References

Ben Hadj Ali D (1987) Prolactine, dépressions et antidépresseurs. Encéphale XIII: 101–112

Botkin SS (1888) The influence of the salts of rubidium and cesium upon the heart and circulation in connection with the laws of physiological action of alkali metals. Doctoral dissertation, St. Petersburg Military Academy

Calandra C, Nicolosi M (1980) Confronto tra due farmaci ad azione antidepressiva: rubidio cloruro e clorimipramina. In: Atti del XXXIV congresso nazionale della Società Italiana di Psichiatria, 24–29 April 1980, Catania

Calandra C, Costanza G, Pavone R, Sorge GA, Virzì A (1989) Valutazione dell'efficacia terapeutica del Rubidio Cloruro nel trattamento di pazienti depressi. In: Atti del XXXVII congresso nazionale della Società Italiana di Psichiatria. CIC Internazionali, Rome

Casacchia M, Rossi A, Marola V, Meco G (1984) The use of rubidium chloride in depressive disorders: clinical aspects. In: Corsini GU (ed) Current trends in lithium and rubidium therapy. MTP Press, Boston, pp 255–259

Chouinard G, Annable L (1977) The effect of rubidium in schizophrenia. Commun Psychopharmacol. 1: 373–383

Corsini GU, Reda M, Burrai C, Poddighe A, Rudas N (1984) Preliminary results with rubidium in depressed patients. In: Corsini GU (ed) Current trends in lithium and rubidium therapy. MTP Press, Boston, pp 247–254

Dell'Osso L, Meschi M, Pellegrini L, Massimetti G, Placidi GF (1989) I sali di Rubidio nel trattamento della depressione: contributo clinico. In: Atti del XXXVII congresso nazionale della Società Italiana di Psichiatria. CIC Internazionali, Rome

Del Vecchio M, Famiglietti LA, May M, Zizolfi S, Borriello R, Sciaudone G (1979) Kinetics of Lithium and Rubidium after a single administration. Acta Neurol XXXIV 3: 204–213

Farska I, Krulik R (1975) The effect of rubidium on Mg and Na K ATPase and on K-dependent phosphatase. Act Nerv Super 4: 251

Fieve RR, Meltzer HL (1974) Is there clinical evidence that rubidium exerts an antidepressant action? J Pharmacol [Suppl] 1: 80

Fieve RR, Meltzer HL, Taylor RM (1971) Rubidium chloride ingestion by volunteer subjects: initial experience. Psychopharmacologia 20: 307–314

Gessa GL (1983) Relazione farmaco-tossicologica sul prodotto "Rubidium". 30 June 1983, Cagliari

Judd A, Parker J, Jenner FA (1975) The role of noradrenaline, dopamine and 5-hydroxytryptamine in the hyperactivity response resulting from the administration of tranylcypromine to rats pretreated with lithium or rubidium. Psychopharmacologia 42: 73–77

Meltzer HL, Taylor RM, Platman SR, Fieve RR (1969) Rubidium: a potential modifier of effect and behaviour. Nature 223: 321–322

Olsson KA, Soremark R, Wing KR (1959) Uptake and distribution of rubidium and potassium-43 in mice and rats. An autoradiographic study. Acta Physiol Scand 77: 322–332

Paschalis C, Jenner FA, Lee CR (1978) Effects of rubidium chloride on the course of manic-depressive illness. J R Soc Med 71: 343–352

Placidi GF, Lenzi A, Lazzerini F, Dell'Osso L, Cassano GB, Akiskal HS (1988) Exploration of the clinical profile of rubidium chloride in depression: a systematic open trial. J Clin Psychopharmacol 8: 184–188

Rutigliano G, Cerfeda S, Margari F (1980) Studio sulla cinetica e sulla biodisponibilità del cloruro rubidio. Clin Ter: 1–8

Sarteschi P, Placidi GF, Lenzi A, Rampello E, Cassano GB (1984) Rubidium salts in depressed patients. An open pilot study using standardized techniques. In: Corsini GU (ed) Current trends in lithium and rubidium therapy. MPT Press, Boston, pp 225–246

Sorge GA, Calandra C, Pavone R, Virzi A, Mongioi A (1989) Valutazione della prolattinemia in pazienti depressi trattati con Rubidio Cloruro. In: Atti del XXXVII congresso nazionale della Società Italiana di Psichiatria. CIC Internazionali, Rome

Stalk JM, Nowack WJ, Barchas JD et al. (1970) Brain norepinephrine: enhanced turnover after rubidium treatment. Science 168: 501–503

Rubidium Chloride in Recurrent Depression: Clinical and Biological Correlates

E. Aguglia, I. Allegranti, G. Conti, and M. De Vanna

Introduction

Rubidium, an alkali metal, has been used for over a century in human therapy in the form of rubidium salts, but it has only recently been introduced in psychiatric pharmacology (DeAngelis et al. 1988). Physiologically, rubidium is very similar to potassium, with which it can easily be substituted at a metabolic level.

Interest in rubidium as an antidepressant revived after its neurochemical, neurophysiological, and behavioral effects proved to be opposite to that of lithium (Meltzer et al. 1969; Fieve et al. 1971; Plant 1986; Shukla 1987), whose therapeutic and prophylactic effectiveness in manic-depressive patients had already been established. Stolk et al.'s observation (1970) that rubidium could be viewed as "antilithium" suggested that rubidium might have an antidepressant effect just as lithium has an antimanic one.

From a biochemical point of view rubidium affects cerebral neurotransmitters, causing an increase in norepinephrine turnover without changing the number of beta-adrenergic, serotoninergic, GABAergic and cholinergic receptors (Gessa 1983); moreover, it stimulates and enhances dopaminergic activity in the CNS (Judd et al. 1975).

During the last 20 years various double-blind (Table 1) and open (Table 2) clinical studies have been carried out to assess the effectiveness of RbCl as an antidepressant.

Unfortunately, the data available in literature cannot be easily compared as there is no methodological homogeneity, either in diagnostic criteria of case selection or in study performance, especially in less recent studies. Rubidium's potential as an antidepressant, suggested by Fieve in the 1970's (Fieve et al. 1971; Fieve et al. 1973; Fieve and Meltzer 1974; Fieve 1980), was confirmed in over 300 cases reported in literature, in which 60%–75% of depressed patients showed an improvement (see Tables 1 and 2). The drug's therapeutic effectiveness proved to be equivalent, and sometimes superior to that of tricyclic antidepressants (imipramime, chlorimipramine, and amitriptyline), with a mean latency of 7–15 days. The reported side effects of dry mouth, nausea, diarrhea, headache, and insomnia seem scarcely significant; in any case they are less relevant than the ones produced by tricyclics.

It is not yet absolutely clear which depression types respond more favorably to rubidium salts, although major recurrent depressive disorders, or single episodes, seem to do so. In bipolar forms reductions in the severity and duration

Table 1. Double-blind studies on RbCl antidepressant effect

Authors	Type of study	Duration (days)	Cases	Latency (days)	Plasma rubidium (mEq/1)	Significant side effects	Results
Fieve et al. (1974)	Vs. placebo	15–86	Nonspecifically depressed patients	/	/	/	Significant improvement
Fieve and Meltzer (1974)	Vs. placebo	41	15 patients with "dysthymic disorders"	/	/	/	Improvement
Meltzer and Fieve (1975)	Cross-over	28	25 bipolar and unipolar dysthymics, depressed patients	/	0.440 (max.)	/	70% positive response (55% after 21 days) (15% after 14 days)
Carolei et al. (1975)	RbCl (540 mg/day) vs. impriamine (200 mg/day)	28	30 endogenous, reactive, neurotic, involutional depressed patients	10	/	0	65% positive response
Calandra and Nicolosi (1980)	RbCl (540 mg/day) vs. chlorimipramine (100 mg/day)	30	28 endogenous, neurotic, reactive secondary depressed patients	5–10	0.102–0.320	0	Positive effect significantly greater than with chlorimiplamine[a]
Dell'Osso et al. (1989)	RbCl (540 mg/day) vs. imipramine (75 mg/day)	28	20 patients: 10 major depression 10 dysthymic depression	7–14	/	0	Improvement with both drugs
Dell'Osso et al. (1989)	RbCl (540–720 mg/day) vs. amitriptyline (75–100 mg/day)	28	34 patients: 16 major depression 18 dysthymic depression	7–14	/	0	Improvement with both drugs

[a] RbCl dosage ranging between 360 and 720 mg/day.

Table 2. Open trial studies on RbCl antidepressant effect

Authors	Type of study	Duration (days)	Cases	Latency (days)	Plasma rubidium (mEq/1)	Significant side effects	Results
Casacchia et al. (1984)	RbCl (540 mg/day) vs. impiramine (150 mg/day)	28	40 major depressive episodes or dysthymic disorder (DSM III)	7	0.150–0.430	0	Improvement > 50% for both drugs
Corsini et al. (1984)	RbCl (180–540 mg/day)	28	10 depressed patients (DSM III)	10–14	/	0	Improvement > 50%
Sarteschi et al. (1984)	RbCl (180–540 mg/day)	21	21 depressed patients (DSM III)	7–15	1.5–3.7 (whole blood)	0	61.9% positive response
Placidi et al. (1988)	RbCl (180–720 mg/day)	21	30 patients: 18 major depression 5 dysthymic depression 3 cyclothymic depression 4 bipolar depression	7	0.150–0.370	0	70% definite improvement
Dell 'Osso et al. (1989)	RbCl (540–900 mg/day)	28	162 patients: 108 major depression 29 bipolar depression 25 dysthymic depression	7	/	Yes	73% improvement 20% no change 7% worse
Bonelli et al. (1989)	RbCl (540 mg/day)	28	30 major depression or bipolar depression	14	/	0	43.3% definite improvement
Calandra et al. (1989)	RbCl (540–900 mg/day)	15–28	30 depressed patients (DSM III)	7	0.205 (maximum)	0	63.33%[a] complete remission

[a] 10% fair improvement, 26.66% no improvement.

of depressive episodes have been reported with a longer duration, however, of manic episodes (Paschalis et al. 1978).

In the light of these data, we carried out a study on RbCl antidepressant effects in patients affected by recurrent depression; on the possible relationships among dosage, plasma rubidium levels, and side effects; and on possible correlations between antidepressant effects and plasma rubidemia.

Subjects and Methods

Our study was carried out on ten patients affected by recurrent depression and hospitalized at the Psychiatric Clinical Institute of the University of Trieste, Italy; their diagnosis was produced according to DSM III-R criteria. We excluded subjects with arterial hypertension treated with diuretics, subjects with hypopotassemia, subjects with cardiovascular disorders requiring digital therapy, subjects with substance abuse disorders or organic cerebral damage, and pregnant women.

The expected duration of the study was 8 weeks (56 days); after a 3- to 4- day wash-out period, patients were administered RbCl in doses ranging from 720 to 1080 mg/day (180-mg capsules), fractioned over the day but always at least 1 h before or after a meal. In some cases association with benzodiazepines was allowed.

At day 0, day 28, and day 56 (and when treatment was discontinued in drop-out cases) complete blood count, liver and kidney function test, electrolytes, urine analysis, and ECG were performed. Plasma rubidium and potassium levels were monitored weekly. Plasma rubidium was also tested in willing patients 7, 21, and 35 days after the trial had ended. The plasma level of rubidium was determined by atomic absorption and spectrophotometry according to Sutter et al. (1970).

At days 0, 14, 28, 42, and 56 (and when treatment was discontinued in drop-out cases) all subjects were evaluated using the Clinical Global Improvement (CGI) to give a global clinical assessment, the Hamilton Psychiatric Rating Scale for Depression (HAM-D) to quantify depression conditions (our study included only subjects with an initial rough score of 15 or higher) the Dosage and Treatment Emergent Symptoms Scale (DOTES) to assess side effects, and the Tess Write In Scale (TWIS), to assess symptoms which appeared during treatment.

At day 56 and when the drug was discontinued in drop-out cases, a Patient Termination Record (PTR) was filled out.

Results

Out of ten patients, three men and seven women, age ranging from 43 to 67 years (Table 3 reports social and biographical data), eight had recurrent major depression and two had dysthymic disorder with a past history of recurrent

Table 3. Study sample social and biographical data

	Men ($n = 3$)	Women ($n = 7$)
Mean age (years)	55	57.3
Marital status		
– single	0	0
– married	2	5
– widowed	1	0
– separated/divorced	0	2
Lives alone	1	2
Lives with family	2	5

$n = 10$, mean age = 56.6 years, age range = 43–67 years.

Table 4. Diagnoses according to DSM III-R

	n
Axis I (clinical syndromes):	
– recurrent major depression	8
– dysthymic disorder	2
Axis II (personality disorders):	
– none	7
– compulsive	1
– dependent	1
– avoidant	1
Axis III (organic disorders):	
– absent	10
Axis IV (psychosocial stressors):	
– absent	7
– present	3
Axis V (adaptation level in previous year):	
– good	3
– fair	4
– poor	3

hospitalization at our institute. Personality disorders had never been diagnosed in seven cases, whereas in three cases obsessive–compulsive, dependent, and avoidant personality disorders were reported respectively (Table 4).

Two drop-outs were recorded at day 14, one because of depressive impairment and the other because of side effects, and five at day 28 – two patients did not show up for their check-ups and in three patients treatment was discontinued because of vomiting and diarrhea which had no other cause than RbCl administration. Only three patients (30%) completed the 8-week treatment period (56 days) envisaged by the case study, whose mean duration time was 33.6 days (Table 5 shows total PaTR data). Two of the drop-outs were affected by dysthymic disorder; both discontinued treatment at day 14.

Table 5. PTR golbal assessment

Items assessed	Data
Total number of patients	10
Expected study duration (days)	56
Mean study duration (days)	33.6
Therapy discontinued:	
– patients not present at check-up	2
– side effects	4
– ineffective or impaired	1
Patients who discontinued treatment	7 (70%)
Patients who completed treatment	3 (30%)
Drug intake:	
– irregularity	0
– no irregularity	10
Nonpharmacological treatment:	
– none	4
– environmental therapy	4[a]
– individual psychotherapy	3[a]

[a] Including one patient who received both support therapies.

As regards CGI the severity of illness began to decrease at the 14th day, reaching the lowest level after 42 days (one of the remaining three patients reported "normal", one reported a mild illness, and one a moderate illness). The improvement rate was 60% (six patients) after 2 weeks of treatment, 75% (six patients) after 4 weeks, 100% (three patients) after 6 weeks and 66% (two patients) after 8 weeks (Tables 6 and 7). The severity mean score dropped from 4.7 (day 0) to 2.6 (day 42), then increased to 3.3 (day 56). The final mean CGI score was 3.0.

There was a parallel decrease in HAM-D scores, at day 14, 50% of patients already had a score lower than 15; at day 42, 66% of patients were below 15 and 33% varied between 15 and 20 at day 42 (Table 8). At day 0, the mean score was 24.7; at day 28, 11.8; at day 42, 6.4; and at day 56, 16.6. All factors except for insomnia and gastrointestinal symptoms contributed to the decrease in score.

Table 9 shows the reported side effects; according to DOTES they were all mild except for insomnia, nausea, vomiting, and diarrhea – the latter three accounting for four drop-outs. Weight loss and loss of appetite were probably associated with gastrointestinal disorders rather than RbCl intake. The mean DOTES score did not change greatly during the study: at day 14 it was 12.4 and at day 56 it was 12.6.

All blood test results were within the normal range, including potassium level, which was monitored weekly and which did not vary from reference values (4.0–6.0 mEq/l). No ECG tracing alterations were reported.

Mean plasma rubidium levels varied between 0.124 mEq/l (standard deviation, SD, 0.04) after 1 week of treatment and 0.585 (SD 0.013) after 8 weeks. At

Table 6. Clinical Global Improvement: severity of illness

Day of treatment	No. of patients	Severity of illness				
		Very severe	Severe	Moderate	Mild	Normal
0	10	3	1	6	0	0
14	10	0	2	6	2	0
28	8	0	0	4	2	2
42	3	0	0	1	1	1
56	3	0	1	1	0	1

Table 7. Clinical Global Improvement: global improvement

Day of treatment	No. of patients	Global improvement					
		Greatly improved	Moderately improved	Slightly improved	No change	Slightly impaired	Moderately impaired
14	10	0	4	2	2	1	1
28	8	2	2	2	2	0	0
42	3	1	1	1	0	0	0
56	3	1	1	0	0	0	1

the sixth week, when the highest improvement rate was reported, the mean plasma rubidium level was 0.503 mEq/l (SD 0.012). Two patients in whom plasma rubidium was tested after the 56-day period of drug intake, had a mean level of 0.562 mEq/l after 1 week, 0.485 mEq/l after 3 weeks, and 0.339 mEq/l after 5 weeks.

Discussion

The findings of our case study, though based on a small sample with a high drop-out rate, confirm the reports in the literature regarding the antidepressant efficacy of RbCl (improvement in 75% of patients after 4 weeks of treatment) and latency – 2 weeks on average.

The doses we administered (720–1080 mg/day) and the total study duration time (56 days) were higher and longer than in other studies and although the second month of therapy was completed by only 3 of the 10 patients, we can assume that a treatment prolonged to 6 weeks might be more effective. In fact our findings show clinical improvement in all three patients at day 42. This dropped to two out of three in the following period, probably because of

Table 8. HAM-D scores reported by patients at various study stages

Score	Day 0 (n = 10)	Day 14 (n = 10)	Day 28 (n = 8)	Day 42 (n = 3)	Day 56 (n = 3)
> 30	2	0	0	0	1
30–25	0	1	0	0	0
25–20	2	2	0	0	0
20–15	6	2	4	1	0
<15	0	5	4	2	2

Table 9. Side effects reported by patients at various study stages

Side effects	Day 14 (n = 10)	Day 28 (n = 8)	Day 42 (n = 3)	Day 56 (n = 3)
State of mental confusion	4	2	1	1
Excitement/restlessness	4	3	0	1
Insomnia	5	4	3	3
Dry mouth	1	0	0	0
Blurred vision	2	0	0	0
Sweating	3	1	0	1
Nausea/vomiting	5	2	1	1
Diarrhea	4	2	1	1
Lipothymia/dizziness	1	0	0	0
Tachycardia	1	0	0	0
Weight loss	2	2	2	1
Anorexia/loss of appetite	3	2	2	1
Headache	3	0	0	0

accumulation due to the drug's half-life (50 days) (Rutigliano et al. 1980). Accumulation, enhancing side effects, probably lowers the drug tolerability and thereby impairs the general clinical picture.

There seems to be a positive correlation between plasma rubidium levels and antidepressant efficacy; however, the correlation became negative after the first 6 weeks of treatment, when mean rubidemia levels were above 0.503 mEq/l.

The side effects reported in our study were more severe than those reported in the literature, probably due to the high RbCl doses administered. Although the dosage was 1080 mg/day for a prolonged period, it was comforting to note that no pathologic alterations in potassium levels, ECG tracings, or liver and kidney function levels were reported.

It is interesting to note that 5 weeks after the therapy ended plasma rubidium levels were still within the therapeutic range, a further confirmation that rubidium may be considered as a long-acting drug.

In conclusion we may say that our findings support the data reported in the literature regarding the efficacy and safety of RbCl, even administered in high doses for a period of 4–6 weeks. Longer periods enhance the severity of side effects, to the detriment of the therapeutic efficacy, in proportion to plasma level increase.

It is advisable that more double-blind case studies be carried out on larger samples of patients and for longer treatment periods, with follow-ups allowing the verification of the assumed mood-modulating effect of rubidium.

References

Bonelli G, Magnani N, Mancuso M, Nardini M (1989) Trattamento dei disturbi depressivi con rubidio cloruro. Recent Med XXVIII: 19–34

Calandra C, Nicolosi M (1980) Confronto fra due farmaci ad azione antidepressiva: rubidio cloruro e clorimipramina. In: Atti del XXXIV congresso nazionale della Società Italianà di Psichiatria. 24–29 April 1980. Catania, pp 1–45

Calandra C, Costanza G, Pavone R, Sorge GA, Virzì A (1989) Valutazione clinica dell'efficacia terapeutica del rubidio cloruro nel trattamento dei pazienti depressi. Recent Med XXVIII: 99–108

Carolei A, Soncini V, Casacchia M, Agnoli A, Fazio C (1975) Azione farmacologica del cloruro di rubidio. Effetto antidepressivo: confronto con l'imipramina. Clin Ter 75: 469–478

Casacchia M, Rossi A, Marola V, Meco G (1984) The use of chloride rubidium in depressive disorders: clinical aspects. In: Corsini GU (ed) Current trends in lithium and rubidium therapy. MTP Press, Lancaster, pp 225–259

Corsini GU, Reda M, Burrai C, Poddiche A, Rudas N (1984) Preliminary result with Rb in depressed patients. In: Corsini GU (ed) Current trends in lithium and rubidium therapy. MTP Press, Lancaster, pp 247–253

De Angelis L, Aguglia E, Allegranti I, Ventre L (1988) Rubidium chloride: current status of the present research. Drugs Today 24: 733–741

Dell'Osso L, Meschi M, Pellegrini L, Sebastiani P, Scarpellini G, Massimetti G, Placidi GF (1989) Sali di rubidio nel trattamento della depressione: contributo clinico. In: Atti del XXXVII congresso nazionale della Società Italiana di Psichiatria. CIC Internazionali, Rome

Ermentini A, Fazzari G, Robotti CA, Vampini C (eds) (1985) Litio e rubidio: farmacologia e terapia. Moretto, Brescia

Fieve RR (1980) Litio e rubidio: promesse dell'era moderna. Aggiornamenti 1: 43

Fieve RR, Meltzer HL (1974) Is the clinical evidence that rubidium exerts an antidepressive action ? J Pharmacol [Suppl] 1: 80

Fieve RR, Meltzer HL, Taylor RM (1971) Rubidium chloride ingestion by volunteer subjects: initial experience. Psychopharmacologia 4: 307–316

Fieve RR, Meltzer HL, Dunner DL, Levitt M, Mendlewicz L, Thomas A (1973) Rubidium: biochemical, behavioural, and metabolic studies in humans. Am J Psychiatry 1: 55–61

Gessa GL (1983) Relazione farmaco-tossicologica sul prodotto "Rubidium". 30 June 1983, Cagliari

Judd A, Parker J, Jenner FA (1975) The role of noradrenaline, dopamine, and 5-hydroxytryptamine in the hyperactivity response resulting from the administration of tranylcypromine to rats pretreated with lithium or rubidium. Psychopharmacologia 42: 73–77

Meltzer HL, Fieve RR (1975) Rubidium in psychiatry and medicine: an overview. In: Essman WB, Valzelli L (eds) Current developments in psychopharmacology, Vol. 1. Spectrum, Jamaica NY, pp 205–211

Meltzer HL, Taylor RM, Platman SR, Fieve RR (1969) Rubidium: a potential modifier of affect and behaviour. Nature 223: 321–322

Paschalis C, Jenner FA, Lee CR (1978) Effects of rubidium chloride on the course of manic depressive illness. J R Soc Med 71: 343–352

Placidi GF, Lenzi A, Lazzerini F, Dell'Osso L, Cassano GB, Akiskal HS (1988) Exploration of the clinical profile of rubidium chloride in depression: a systematic open trial. J Clin Psychopharmacol 8: 184–188

Plant TD (1986) The effect of Rb ions components of the potassium conduction in the frog node of Ranvier. J Physiol (Paris) 37: 81–105

Rutigliano G, Ceferda S, Margari F (1980) Studio sulla cinetica e sulla biodisponibilità del cloruro di Rubidio. Clin Ter 46: 679
Sarteschi P, Placidi GF, Lenzi A, Rampello E, Cassano GB (1984) Rubidium salts in depressed patients. An open pilot study using standardized techniques. In: Corsini GU (ed) Current trends in lithium and rubidium therapy. MTP press, Lancaster, pp 225–247
Shukla GS (1987) Mechanics of lithium action. Pharmacol Biochem Behav 26: 235–240
Stolk JM, Nowack WJ, Barchas JD (1970) Brain norepinephrine: enhanced turnover after rubidium treatment. Science 168: 501–503
Sutter E, Platman SR, Fieve RR (1970) Atomic absorption and spectrophotometry of rubidium in the biological fluids. Clin Chem 16: 602–605

Rubidium Chloride in Chronic Mood Disorders

M. Casacchia, S. de Cataldo, and P. Stratta

Diagnostic Issues

The introduction of the concepts of "Dysthymic Disorder" in DSM III and "Dysthymia" in DSM III-R excited relevant interest and some doubts. Dysthymic disorder is the new diagnostic category that substituted the concept of neurotic depression and depressive personality in the American Psychiatric Association official nomenclature.

The essential features of the dysthymic disorder according to DSM III can be schematized as follows: (1) chronicity, (2) persistent or intermittent depressive manifestations, (3) subsyndromic severity, (4) absence of psychotic manifestations, and (5) frequent association with a personality disturbance.

Because of the heterogeneity of the disorder, DSM III-R dysthymia has been categorized as "secondary", if it develops in the setting of another major psychiatric disorder, or "primary" as "early onset" or "late onset" dysthymia – onset of the disturbance before or after age 21 years.

The prototypic dysthymic category in DSM III-R refers to the primary early-onset subtype characterized by an insidious origin which is often in childhood or adolescence, hyperbolic descriptions such as "I was born depressed", or "I am the most miserable creature on earth", and low-grade symptomatology.

Akiskal (1983), utilizing the strategy of pharmacological dissection championed by Klein et al. (1980), undertook a systematic study of this early-onset low-grade depressive subtype. The findings led to the suggestion that these patients could be divided into predominantly affective ("subaffective dysthymic") and characterologic ("character-spectrum") groups on the basis of the response to rigorous pharmacological trials.

The "subaffective dysthymia" subgroup of patients showed a depressive temperament with a favorable response to tricyclic antidepressants (TCAs), lithium, or both.

They also displayed subtle bipolar tendencies such as family history similar to bipolar patients and brief hypomanic switches on TCA challenge. The "character-spectrum disorder" delineates patients presenting a mélange of dependent, hystrionic, and antisocial personality traits. Often this disorder is characterized as a dysphoric condition developing in the context of an early unstable familial environment. Although the patients of this subgroup failed to show an appreciable response to systematic clinical trials, a benefit from low-dose stimulants, imipramine or monoamine oxidase inhibitors (MAOIs) has been suggested. This benefited above all those patients particularly sensitive to romantic disappointment and other types of separation events in adult life.

Even in the presence of better defined operational diagnostic criteria, the proposed symptomatology for dysthymia is quite polymorphic, as demonstrated by the contemporaneous presence of symptomatic criteria that can be in opposition, (e.g., insomnia–hypersomnia, poor appetite–overeating). Some of these reversed symptoms characterize a form defined as "atypical depression." Commonly this term is used to indicate a subgroup of depressive patients with remarkable anxious and/or phobic symptomatology, or patients with vegetative symptoms like hypersomnia and hyperphagia, and diurnal variations which worsen in the evening.

Although all these symptoms are found within the diagnostic criteria for dysthymia, several authors have suggested describing this as a distinct non-melancholic atypical depressive syndrome that responds preferentially to MAOIs even though this categorization, according to Quitkin (1979) criteria, has proven to be somewhat elusive.

Atypical depression is also a heterogenous disorder which probably embraces several subtypes. Two forms of atypical depression are usually described: one characterized by marked anxiety (A-type) and the other by vegetative symptomatology (V-type), in which reversed vegetative change has occurred, (e.g., hyperphagia, hypersomnia, weight gain, and increased libido) (Davidson and Pelton 1985).

In order to define those patients who could positively respond to MAOIs, (Shader 1984; Shader and Greenblatt 1984) proposed the acronym "TROUBLEs" (transient, regressive, overanxious, unstable, bulimic, labile episodes) which describes the most characteristic clinical presentations of these patients. Liebowitz and colleagues (1988) proposed similar criteria for atypical depression and demonstrated the usefulness of phenelzine in treating this condition.

These observations seem to justify the nosographic autonomy of atypical depression not only from a clinical viewpoint but also on the basis of a better response to MAOIs (Nies and Robinson 1982). Psychobiological hypotheses also seem to support the clinical autonomy of atypical depression.

As shown in Fig. 1, Klein et al. (1980) proposed that endogenous depressives suffer from a dysregulation of a "consumatory pleasure center" that mediates the ability to enjoy consuming food, sex, etc., while atypical depressives suffer from a dysregulation of two other systems: the first, an "appetitive pleasure center", which is thought to mediate the anticipatory pleasure capacity, and the second a center that would mediate the reactivity to social approval. These centers have been proposed to be mediated by endogenous substances with amphetamine-like properties. Stimulation of the systems by social approval or the possibility of goal attainment would produce euphoria, excitement, high energy, decrease of appetite, etc. Rapid fall-off of activity in this system, caused by social disapproval or the impossibility of goal attainment, produces, on the other hand, lethargy, hopelessness, and overeating. The endogenous amine phenylethylamine has been proposed as a possible mediator of anticipatory pleasure and

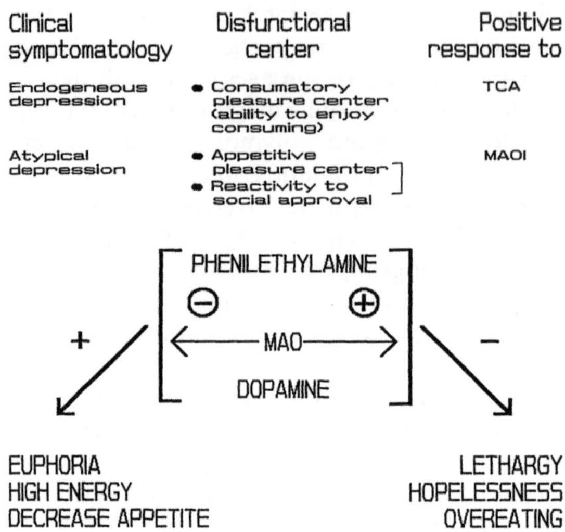

Fig. 1. Psychobiological hypotheses. *TCA*, tricyclic antidepressant; *MAOI*, monoamine oxidase inhibitor; *MAO*, monoamine oxidase. (From Klein et al. 1980)

interpersonal reactivity. Phenylethylamine is a prime substrate of MAO-B, and levels are greatly elevated by MAOIs (Fig. 1).

The reconceptualization of these syndromic manifestations is not simply a terminological revision: in fact these syndromes are not conceived any more as an expression of a stable character disorder or conflictual dynamics, but as real mood disorders modifiable with adequate pharmacological treatment, even if this approach is not completely standardized.

Clinical Observations

On the basis of previous clinical experiences about the effects of rubidium on affective disorders available in the literature (Casacchia et al. 1983; De Angelis et al. 1988; Placidi et al. 1988), and taking into account the mechanism of action of this salt and effects on the central nervous system:

- Increase in the turnover of norepinephrine in rats
- Increase in the dopamine-stimulated adenylate cyclase activity
- Amphetamine-like effects: reducing food intake; weight loss in mice

we undertook an open trial using standardized clinical evaluations in depressive patients.

The study was carried out on ten outpatients (eight women and two men), diagnosed according to Shader (1984) as affected by atypical depression, who were referred to the Department of Clinical Psychiatry at the University of L'Aquila. The mean ($\pm$standard deviation, SD) index age of patients was 34.80 $\pm$ 10.24 years. The characteristics of the studied sample are reported in Table 1.

All patients were treated with rubidium chloride (540 mg daily in three doses) over 6 weeks. Inclusion criteria were based on the Atypical Depression

Table 1. Sample characteristics

Total no. of samples:	10
– males	2
– females	8
Age (years)	34.80 ± 10.24
Length of illness (years)	9.23 ± 8.41
Length of current episode (weeks)	15.20 ± 6.89
Height (cm)	165.16 ± 9.17
Pre-study weight (kg)	78.18 ± 17.42
Post-study weight (kg)	77.41 ± 15.18[a]

Variables expressed as mean ± SD.
[a] Paved t-test (pre- vs post-study weight) not significant.

Table 2. HDRS and SCL-61 weekly total scores during the trial (mean ± SD)

Weeks	HDRS	SCL-61
Baseline	16.46 ± 3.51	123.41 ± 23.22
1st	16.03 ± 2.97	122.97 ± 21.43
2nd	15.78 ± 3.03	120.45 ± 20.33
3rd	15.48 ± 2.74	118.17 ± 22.37
4th	14.60 ± 3.95	116.88 ± 23.34
5th	14.87 ± 4.05	114.80 ± 24.67
6th	13.20 ± 4.42	112.70 ± 24.18

Scale (ADS; Quitkin, personal communication); at baseline and at weekly intervals during the trial, psychopathology was evaluated with the Hamilton Depression Rating Scale (HDRS; Hamilton 1960), the Symptoms Check List (SCL-61; Derogatis et al. 1976), and ADS.

As shown in Table 2, the total score of the psychopathological rating instruments decreased significantly. Interestingly a relevant positive effect of the drug on atypical symptomatology (sleep, appetite, social relationships) was observed (Table 3). Examination of treatment-emergent symptomatology did not disclose the presence of any severe reactions.

The results of the present study are encouraging and provide good but preliminary evidence of rubidium efficacy in the treatment of depressed patients with atypical symptomatology. From the above data it was shown that rubidium chloride at 540 mg daily can be administered safely and no undesirable clinical side effects are shown.

The usefulness of new drugs such as rubidium salts in patients with atypical symptomatology could be of heuristic value in confirming atypical depression as a distinct diagnostic subtype and delineating its boundaries fully.

However, further phenomenological, clinical, psychobiologic, familial, and psychopharmacologic studies are needed. This is likely to improve diagnostic precision at a time when to do so has become of great importance in psychiatry.

Table 3. ADS weekly scores during the trial (mean ± SD)

Week	ADS		
	Sleep	Appetite	Social relationships
Baseline	19.7 ± 7.4	8.9 ± 2.7	16.2 ± 5.7
1st	19.7 ± 6.4	7.8 ± 2.9	16.4 ± 6.7
2nd	17.6 ± 6.8	6.6 ± 3.0	14.8 ± 5.7
3rd	16.9 ± 7.8	6.7 ± 2.5	12.6 ± 6.3
4th	14.6 ± 6.3	5.8 ± 2.3	12.4 ± 7.0
5th	13.4 ± 4.7	4.2 ± 2.4	10.4 ± 6.3
6th	13.2 ± 4.2	3.4 ± 3.0	9.6 ± 6.5

References

Akiskal HS (1983) Dysthymic disorder: psychopathology of proposed chronic depressive subtypes. Am J Psychiatry 140: 11–20

Casacchia M, Rossi A, Marola V, Meco G (1983) The use of rubidium chloride in depressive disorders: clinical aspects. In: Corsini GU (ed) Current trends in lithium and rubidium therapy. MTP Press, Lancaster, pp 255–259

Davidson J, Pelton S (1985) Forms of atypical depression and their response to antidepressant drugs. Psychiatry Res 17: 87–95

De Angelis L, Aguglia E, Allegranti I, Ventre L (1988) Rubidium chloride: current status of the present research. Drugs Today 24: 733–741

Derogatis LR, Rickels K, Rock AF (1976) The SCL-90 and the MMPI: A step in the validation of a new self-report scale. Br J Psychiatry 128: 280–289

Hamilton M (1960) A rating scale for depression. J Neurol Neurosurg Psychiatry 23: 56–62

Liebowitz MR, Quitkin FM, Stewart JW, McGrath PJ, Harrison WM, Markowitz JS, Rabkin JG, Tricamo E, Goetz DM, Klein DF (1988) Antidepressant specificity in atypical depression. Arch Gen Psychiatry 15: 129–137

Klein DF, Gittelman R, Quitkin FM, Rifkin A (1980) Diagnosis and drug treatment of psychiatric disorders: adults and children, 2nd edn. Williams and Wilkins, Baltimore

Nies A, Robinson DS (1982) Monoamine oxidase inhibitors. In: Paykel ES (ed) Handbook of affective disorders. Churchill Livingstone, Edinburgh, pp 246–261

Placidi G, Lenzi A, Lazzerini F, Dell'Osso L, Cassano GB, Akiskal HS (1988) Exploration of the clinical profile of rubidium chloride in depression: a systemic open trial. J Clin Psychopharmacol 8: 184–188

Quitkin FM, Rifkin A, Klein DF (1979) Monoamine oxidase inhibitors: a review of antidepressant effectiveness. Arch Gen Psychiatry 36: 749–760

Shader RI (1984) Monoamine oxidase inhibitors. Presented at Tufts University School of Medicine's Psychopharmacology Update Conference, Boston

Shader RI, Greenblatt DJ (1984) A new axis II diagnosis: troubles. J Clin Psychopharmacol 4: 241

Rubidium Chloride Versus Imipramine: A Double-Blind Study

G.F. Placidi, M. Meschi, L. Pellegrini, P. Freer, and L. Dell'Osso

In the late 1960s interest in the clinical activity of rubidium was stimulated by the reports of Meltzer and coworkers (Meltzer et al. 1973; Meltzer and Fieve 1975; Fieve 1976; Fieve and Meltzer 1974a, b; Fieve et al. 1973). Since then various open and a few controlled studies have been published on the antidepressant efficacy of this compound (Calandra and Nicolosi 1980; Casacchia et al. 1984; Corsini et al. 1984; Belmaker et al. 1984; Geisler et al. 1984; Sarteschi et al. 1984; Vampini and Robotti 1985).

However, despite the encouraging findings for its use in depressive disorders, research on rubidium has remained limited. Recently, in a multicenter open trial on over 350 depressed in- and outpatients (Dell'Osso et al. 1989), a 65%–70% response rate was found.

In order to explore the clinical correlates of response to rubidium chloride, we previously examined the effects of this salt in depressive disorders in an open study (Placidi et al. 1988). The study was carried out on 31 female inpatients. After an average wash-out period of one week, patients received rubidium chloride in a flexible dosage schedule ranging from 180 to 720 mg/day; a benzodiazepine, lorazepam, was allowed. By DSM III-R criteria (American Psychiatric Association 1987) diagnosis on Axis I was major depression and chronic mood disorders. The mean duration of the treatment was 14.3 (standard deviation, SD, 5.4) days. Only 16 (52%) of the 31 patients completed the 21-day trial. Premature interruptions were due to adverse reaction, inefficacy, and switch from depression to mania. During the treatment with rubidium, the score for severity of illness decreased significantly from "marked to severe" to "moderate". Of the 16 patients who completed 3 weeks of the trial, 11 (69%) showed a significant improvement, which appeared greater during the second week (86%) than during the first week (67%) and the third week (80%).

Regression analysis suggested that anhedonia, social withdrawal, lost of interest in sex, gastrointestinal symptoms, anorexia, and suicidal ideation were predictive of a good response to rubidium chloride, whereas depressed mood, constipation, and depersonalization–derealization were predictive of a poor response. Rubidium blood level was between 0.15 and 0.37 mEq/l, and no significant correlation was found between blood concentration and clinical improvement. The most common side effects that needed a downward adjustment in dosage or treatment interruption included diarrhea, polyuria, confusional state, and/or excitement.

On the basis of such findings, we planned a double-blind study to compare rubidium chloride to an active tricylic antidepressant, imipramine. Preliminary results of this ongoing study on 24 patients (11 on rubidium and 13 on imipramine) in the first 3 weeks of treatment are reported.

Methods

A 4-week double-blind randomized controlled study was carried out on female inpatients aged 18–70 years suffering from a major depressive episode, with a score of at least 18 in the first 17 items of the Hamilton Rating Scale for Depression (HRSD).

Assessment of Psychopathology. Diagnosis was made according to DSM III-R criteria. Demographic data were collected with the Adult Personal Data Inventory (APDI). At baseline and at weekly intervals during the trial, psychopathology was evaluated by the following rating scales: Clinical Global Impression (CGI) and HRSD. Dosage and side effects were recorded weekly using Dosage and Treatment Emergent Symptoms Scale (DOTES). The Patient Termination Record (PTR) was administered at the end of the trial or when a patient dropped out.

The data were analyzed by means of the standard procedures of the biometric laboratory information processing system (BLIPS) and biomedical computer programs (BMDP).

Experimental Design. Patients with organic brain damage, cardiovascular disease, alcoholism, drug abuse, pregnancy, or treatment with monoamine oxidase (MAO) inhibitors or electroconvulsive therapy (ECT) in the last 2 months were excluded.

After 7-days placebo wash-out, the patients were randomly assigned to rubidium or to imipramine. In case of insomnia 2–4 mg of a benzodiazepine, chlordemethyldiazepam, was allowed. The doses were 360–720 mg/day rubidium and 50–100 mg/day imipramine.

Laboratory Examinations. At baseline and at the end of treatment, the following examinations were carried out: ECG, complete blood count, serum glutamic oxaloacetic transaminase, blood urea nitrogen, serum glucose, gamma-glutamyltranspeptidase, alkaline phosphatase, creatinine, bilirubin, and electrolytes. The renal function was studied by urea, creatinine, and uric acid clearances; urinary Na, K, Ca, and P concentrations; urinary enzymes (NAG, gamma-GT); and urinary beta$_2$-microglobulin.

The plasma level of rubidium was determined by atomic absorption and spectrophotometry according to Sutter et al. (1970).

Results

Demographic Data. No significant differences were found in mean age (rubidium group 56.2 years, imipramine group 53.5 years), marital or socio-economic status, present and prior treatment, or duration of the present episode of both groups.

Duration of present episode was 7.4 (±14.4) months in the rubidium group and 5.6 (±4.5) months in the imipramine group. Mean number of previous hospitalizations for psychiatric illnessess was 3.5 in both groups. Mean total duration of previous psychiatric hospitalization was 7.7 months in patients on rubidium and 5.6 months in patients on imipramine (Table 1).

Diagnoses according to DSM III-R criteria were major depression, single episode (one patient on rubidium); major depression, recurrent (six rubidium and 11 imipramine); and bipolar disorder, depressive episode (four rubidium and two imipramine) (Table 2).

Termination Data. According to PTR the mean duration of treatment was 19.1 days in the rubidium group and 19.9 days in the imipramine group. Ineffectiveness was the reason for premature termination for three patients on rubidium and two patients in the imipramine group (Table 3).

Table 1. Characteristics of the sample[a]

	Rubidium	Imipramine
No. of subjects	11	13
Mean age: years (SD)	56.2 (8.1)	53.5 (11.1)
Duration of present episode: months (SD)	7.4 (14.4)	5.6 (4.5)
No. of hospitalizations: mean (SD)	3.5 (3.7)	3.5 (2.6)
Total duration of hospitalization: months (SD)	7.7 (17.5)	5.6 (7.3)

[a] According to the Adult Personal Data Inventory.

Table 2. Diagnosis (DSM III-R)

	Rubidium		Imipramine	
	n	%	*n*	%
Major depressive single episode	1	9.1	–	
Major depressive recurrent:				
– severe or melancholic	5	45.5	10	76.9
– mood-congruent psychotic features	1	9.1	1	7.7
Bipolar disorder depressed:				
– severe or melancholic	2	18.2	2	15.4
– mood-congruent psychotic features	2	18.2	–	

Table 3. Patient termination record at the third week

	Rubidium	Imipramine
Total number of patients	11	13
Mean total days in study	19.1	19.9
Premature termination:		
– adverse reaction	0	0
– ineffectiveness	3	2

Dosage Data. The minimum and the maximum doses given were 50 and 100 mg for imipramine and 360 and 720 mg for rubidium. When needed, chlordemethyldiazepam was given at night, from 2 to 4 mg/day. Rubidium plasma level was between 0.06 and 0.16 mEq/l, and no significant correlation was found between blood concentration and clinical improvement.

Clinical Global Impression. During treatment the score for the severity of illness decreased in both groups (Table 4). The initial score for severity of illness was similar in the two groups of treatment: 5.5 for rubidium and 5.6 for imipramine, between "severely ill" and "markedly ill". At the third week of treatment the score decreased to 4.8 (between "markedly ill" and "moderately ill") in the rubidium group and to 4.3 (between "markedly ill" and "moderately ill", in the imipramine group.

End point covariance analysis (using pretreatment scores as covariates) showed that in both groups the final severity of illness score was not significantly different.

The "global improvement" item from the CGI was evaluated weekly for each patient. At the end of treatment the mean global improvement score was 3.2 ("minimally improved") for rubidium- and 2.7 (close to "minimally improved") for imipramine-treated patients.

Hamilton Rating Scale for Depression. The analysis of the weekly scores of HRSD demonstrated a significant decrease in both groups during treatment. No significant differences were observed between the two drugs (Table 5).

Table 4. Clinical Global Improvement: severity scores (last observable data carried forward)

Week	Rubidium (n)	Imipramine (n)	p
Baseline	5.5 (11)	5.6 (13)	ns
1	5.1 (11)	4.8 (13)	ns
2	4.5 (11)	4.6 (13)	ns
3	4.8 (8)	4.3 (11)	ns

Baseline vs weeks 1, 2, 3: $p < 0.05$ in both treatment groups.

Table 5. HRSD weekly total scores (last observable data carried forward)

Week	Rubidium (n)	Imipramine (n)	p
Baseline	26.7 (11)	26.6 (13)	ns
1	21.7 (11)	20.6 (13)	ns
2	20.1 (11)	18.5 (13)	ns
3	22.5 (8)	18.4 (11)	ns

Baseline vs weeks 1, 2, 3: $p < 0.05$ in both treatment groups.

Table 6. Side effects (DOTES)

Symptom	Rubidium	Imipramine
Excitement/agitation	3	0
Insomnia	1	0
tremor	0	1
Dry mouth	8	10
Constipation	0	5
Nausea/vomiting	1	0
Diarrhea	1	0
Hypotension	1	1
Hypertension	0	1
Headache	3	1

Side Effects. The pattern of unwanted emergent symptoms considered at least "moderate" during imipramine treatment showed the well-known anticholinergic effects such as dry mouth and constipation, while effects such as agitation, insomnia, nausea, and headache were prominent with rubidium, with its activating and disinhibiting properties (Table 6).

Discussion

In this trial two drugs were compared: the standard one was selected so that its profile of action would be similar to that of the investigational drug. By comparing the newer drug, rubidium, which is characterized by activating-disinhibiting properties and a lack of anxiolytic, sedating, and sleep-inducing effects, with the older tricyclic antidepressant imipramine, we assumed there would not be a risk of "breaking the blind". Indeed during the double-blind study the raters were unable to find any difference between the two compounds.

The preliminary results of the double-blind study seem to confirm our previous findings. A rate of about 70% positive responses to rubidium chloride, similar to that found in our previous open study (Placidi et al. 1989), can be compared to that reported with standard tricyclic antidepressants. Due to the characteristics of the sample, which consisted of inpatients, and particularly of the responders group characterized by mainly endogenous symptomatology, the placebo effects would be unremarkable. The prevalent activity of rubidium on retardation, which is typical of bipolar depression, allows us to hypothesize for this compound an effect similar and yet opposite to that of lithium salts.

The preliminary results of this double-blind study, both as regards premature termination due to ineffectiveness and psychopathology ratings, showed, at the third week, no significant differences between rubidium and imipramine; mean scores of HRSD and CGI decreased significantly and equally on both drugs.

Although there was no significant difference in terms of safety and side effects, more patients on imipramine showed anticholinergic effects, while under rubidium the number of patients who experienced agitation, nausea, or headaches was higher. However, such effects were not so severe as to need downward adjustment of dosage or interruption of treatment in either group.

Our findings tend to support the literature indicating the safety and efficacy of rubidium chloride in mood disorders. However, more extensive controlled clinical trials over longer periods are necessary. Such studies could aim to achieve a more accurate definition of its clinical profile, which, considering its pharmacological characteristics, could be quite different from those of other antidepressant drugs.

References

American Psychiatric Association (1987) Diagnostic and statistical manual of mental disorders, 3rd ed, revised. American Psychiatric Association, Washington

Belmaker RH, Hamburger-Barr R, Newman M, Bannet J (1984) The effect of rubidium and lithium on adenylate cyclase and neurotransmitter receptors. In: Corsini GU (ed) Current trends in lithium and rubidium therapy. MTP Press, Lancaster, pp 59–75

Calandra C, Nicolosi M (1980) Confronto tra due farmaci ad azione antidepressiva: rubidio cloruro e clorimipramina. In: Atti del 34° congresso nazionale della Società Italiana di Psichiatria, 24–29 April 1980, Catania

Casacchia M, Rossi A, Marola V, Meco G (1984) The use of rubidium chloride in depressive disorders: clinical aspects. In: Corsini GU (ed) Current trends in lithium and rubidium therapy. MTP Press, Lancaster, pp 255–259

Corsini GU, Reda M, Burrai C, Poddighe A, Rudas N (1984) Preliminary results with rubidium in depressed patients. In: Corsini GU (ed) Current trends in lithium and rubidium therapy. MTP Press, Lancaster, pp 247–253

Dell'Osso L, Meschi M, Pellegrini L, Sebastiani P, Scarpellini G, Massimetti G, Placidi GF (1989) Sali di rubidio nel trattamento della depressione: contributo clinico. In: Atti del XXXVII congresso nazionale della Società Italiana di Psichiatria. CIC Internazionali, Rome

Fieve RR (1976) In: Simpson LL (ed) Drug treatment of mental disorders. Raven, New York, pp 193–215

Fieve RR, Meltzer HL (1974a) Is there clinical evidence that rubidium exerts an antidepressant action? J Pharmacol [Suppl] 1: 80–87

Fieve RR, Meltzer HL (1974b) Rubidium salts: toxic effects in human and clinical effects as an antidepressant drug. Psychopharmacol Bull 1: 38–42

Fieve RR, Meltzer HL, Dunner DL, Levitt M, Mendlewicz J, Thomas A (1973) Rubidium: biochemical, behavioural, and metabolic studies in humans. Am J Psychiatry 1: 55–61

Geisler A, Klysner R, Andersen PH (1984) Opposite effects of lithium and rubidium on neurohormone-stimulated cyclic AMP accumulation in rat brain homogenates. In: Corsini GU (ed) Current trends in lithium and rubidium therapy. MTP Press, Lancaster, pp 37–55

Meltzer HL, Fieve RR (1975) Rubidium in psychiatry and medicine: an overview. In: Essman WB, Valzelli L (eds) Current developments in psychopharmacology, vol 1. Spectrum, Jamaica, NY, pp 205–211

Meltzer HL, Lieberman KW, Shelley EM, Stallone F, Fieve RR (1973) Metabolism of naturally occurring rubidium in the human: the constancy of urinary Rb-K. Biochem Med 7: 218–223

Placidi GF, Lenzi A, Lazzerini F, Dell'Osso L, Cassano GB, Akiskal HS (1988) Exploration of the clinical profile of rubidium chloride in depression: a systematic open trial. J Clin Psychopharmacol 8: 184–188

Sarteschi P, Placidi GF, Lenzi A, Rampello E, Cassano GB (1984) Rubidium salts in depressed patients. An open pilot study using standardized techniques. In: Corsini GU (ed) Current trends in lithium and rubidium therapy. MTP Press, Lancaster, pp 225–246
Sutter E, Platman SR, Fieve RR (1970) Atomic absorption and spectrophotometry of rubidium in the biological fluids. Clin Chem 16: 602–605
Vampini C, Robotti CA (1985) Il rubidio. In: Ermentini A, Fazzari G, Robotti CA, Vampini C (eds) Litio e rubidio: farmacologia e terapia. Psychopatologia. Tipografia Artigiana, Brescia, pp 33–52

Psychotherapeutic Problems in Chronic and Resistant Depressions

V. Volterra and G. Martini

The planning of a psychotherapy intervention strategy in the treatment of subjects suffering from chronic and resistant depressions always involves the consideration that the depressive disorder should not be taken for the depressive affect.

It is in fact a global psychosomatic response of the organism that petrifies mental activity and prevents the patients struggling against the painful experience of loss. Now, it is the role of drugs to prevent or to counter this fixation, to suppress the sterile rumination and the inhibition which strike mental activity and to restore the means necessary to revive an active struggle. Only after this stage, i.e., after the recovery from the depressive fixation, can the economic balance of conflicts and defenses be managed and the analysis of and detachment from the depressive position become possible and accessible to psychotherapy.

This means that an indispensable and valid integrated treatment, obviously varying from case to case and intended to avoid both reductionism and eclecticism, must be based on the assumption that theories, even if they are reference points for a correct, targeted, and articulated therapeutic work, risk becoming reasons for separation, for detachment from the patient's mental world and creation of a safe distance between the psychiatrist and the depressed patient's suffering, in which the former does not want to be involved.

It can happen, in fact, that the therapist profits from the chronicization, feeling sufficiently satisfied with the pharmacological results and thus partially avoiding – may be against his usual work practice – clarifying and identifying the basic conflicts.

It is thus important to first ascertain the exact moment during the clinical course when the depressed patient is accessible to psychotherapy, and then to define the goals and patterns of such an intervention.

The purpose of psychotherapy is actually based on different criteria than that of pharmacotherapy and its aim is not the recovery defined as mere disappearance of symptoms. The successive steps that the therapist should take are the following:

1. A "holding" action to contain the devastating pervasiveness of the depressive feeling.

2. To detach the patient from the system of thoughts in which he is imprisoned.

3. To make the patient understand that this system is only a part of his person and assure him that he will recover his usual way of living and thinking very soon.

4. To develop some systems of thought different from the depressive ones. To do that, he can resort either to analytical psychotherapy with focal goals or to behavioral–cognitivistic psychotherapy, giving the patient progressively involving daily tasks.

5. To attenuate the patient's depressive vulnerability, bearing in mind that depressive vulnerability and depressive personality can be either superimposed or distinct.

6. To modify the traits that permanently feed his psychopathological condition and are at its basis:

a) the affective dependence, linked to the feeling of abandonment, the nucleus of depression
b) the excessive narcissistic self-esteem that in situations of defeat and frustration becomes belittlement and renouncement
c) the sadomasochistic game, linked to the aggressive component and to multiple identification

7. To paradoxically teach the patient to be depressed and to make him able to become depressed; the chronically depressed patient is chronically depressed because he has not been able to "draw" from the depressive situation.

8. To share with the patient his depressive feeling, bearing in mind that this is not easy for a therapist.

9. To renounce or deny this disquieting similitude through mechanism of detachment – pharmacological means may be employed – and to petrify the disease's negative fatality and freeze the similitude, depriving it of any dialectics.

10. To adopt some technical contrivances, such as a variable setting and a "pedagogic" attitude, to foster a stable and positive transference, a warm and flexible atmosphere, constantly encouraging the patient to verbalize (provided this is not perceived as an aggressive action), and finally to help the patient live with his depression.

11. To accept one's own impotence, instead of becoming part of a game centered on "narcissistic complementarity", pushed by the patient who, bent on his negative omnipotence, triggers a "positive" one.

12. To avoid the opposite risk of falling into "therapeutic despair", through the acceptance of one's own depression as a work instrument, given that only the feelings of nostalgia and of depressive elaboration can shield the therapist from collusion with the patient's despair.

13. To realize how, in a dynamic sense, the real chronic and resistant depression is the one from which, implicitly or manifestly, the refusal to relate leaks out; this can arise from the patient, when he is no longer able to make any contribution, not even on the therapist, but can also be triggered by the therapist's attitude of pessimism and defeat.

14. To bear in mind that the intervention must be timely and prior to the completion of the chronicization process and that it is necessary to tackle the

problem of suicide, when it has not yet taken hold of the mind of the depressed person in an obsessive and obscuring way. If this happens, the patient will know that there is someone who knows his ideas and who will be able, if not to exorcise them, at least to share and understand them.

15. To check the countertransference or counterattitudes with respect to the feelings of rage and boredom that the chronically depressed person transmits, with the several risks this involves, such as the improper response by the therapist – for instance a peremptory, ironical, or simply impatient tone – with a subject who is absolutely unable to accept such a response.

16. To limit himself, especially at the beginning, to accepting the deep suffering of the patient, and to utilize the interpretative instrument only successively when it can be perceived as being bereft of those aggressive values which it can involve – contrary to the therapist's intentions – during the first stage.

17. To transmit to the patient that depression is not equal to regression, to total loss. This can be done only when the therapist has come through his personal elaboration, to the "depressive position". The roots of this feeling are in fact the roots of creativity and change. Every process of thought passes through the pain of depression; both the serious mental illness and the existential elaboration with good results bring with them the roots of life and death, which cannot be sorted out, which contrast and face each other in a dialectic game (not always, yet!) and represent the essence of human existence.

The therapy of a chronically depressed patient can thus only be the beginning of a process which is, by definition, interminable and can lead to different solutions, not excluding tragedy. The avoidance of pain cannot be in itself an index of therapeutic success: it can represent the interruption and closing of a static condition (i.e., the chronicity dimension), but also the unavoidable opening of new incertitudes.

Bibliography

Volterra V (1982) Il recupero psicosociale del depresso. In: La condizione depressiva. Masson, Milan, p 251

Volterra V, Martini G (1984) Interventi psicoterapici nelle depressioni. In: Cazzullo CL (ed) La depressione: condizione esistenziale o insidia biologica. Pensiero Scientifico, Rome, p 119

Volterra V, Martini G (1989a) La depressione: tappa fondamentale del viaggio nella psicosi. Psich Gen Evol 27: 517

Volterra V, Martini G (1989b) Contributo clinico allo studio delle depressioni croniche e resistenti. Riv Neurol Psichiatr Sci Umane [Suppl] IX: 21

Volterra V, Martini G (1989c) La depressione nei disturbi dell'adattamento. In: Atti del XXXVII congresso della Società SIP, Italiana di Psichiatria. CIC Internazionali, Rome, suppl. II, p 515

Volterra V, Martini G (1990) Problemi nella definizione e nell'affrontamento delle depressioni resistenti. In: Psicofarmacoresistenza: problemi e prospettive. Idelson, Napoli, p 99

Bright Light Treatment of Seasonal Affective Disorder and Nonseasonal Bipolar and Unipolar Affective Syndromes

J.A. Deltito

Seasonal affective disorder, which has been described in our earliest published observations of pathological mood states (Jones and Withington 1923–1931; Ross 1953), has gained particular attention and definition over the past decade (Rosenthal et al. 1984; Wirz-Justice et al. 1986; Lewy et al. 1982; Kripke et al. 1983). The prototypic syndrome has been described as consisting of a depressive episode beginning in the fall or winter and remitting the following spring or summer. This occurs on a regular yearly cycle. During the winter depressive episode these patients complain of concentration difficulties, hypersomnia, daytime fatigue and drowsiness, and overeating, usually with intense carbohydrate craving. Although the picture of an atypical depression is most common, we also see patients with either typical or mixed syndromes of neurovegatative symptoms. These patients oftentimes show mild hypomanias in the summertime period. Most qualify for a DSM-III-R diagnosis of bipolar disorder, NOS, although they may also be classified as having bipolar disorder (when there is associated lifetime history of mania), recurrent major depression (when there is no summertime hypomania), or depressive disorder, NOS.

The DSM-III-R does not contain an individual diagnosis of seasonal affective disorder, but allows the subclassification of the above-mentioned four diagnoses as having a "seasonal pattern."

The criteria for seasonal pattern in the DSM-III-R require the onset of the depressive disorder to occur during a particular 60-day period of the year (not obviously related to regular seasonal stresses, such as being unemployed every winter); a full remission from the depressive episode within a particular 60-day period of the year; a lifetime history of at least 3 separate years that demonstrated this pattern with at least 2 of those years being consecutive; and the seasonal episodes of mood disorder as defined outnumber the lifetime nonseasonal episodes (if they have occurred) by at least three to one (American Psychiatric Association 1987).

Although the winter pattern of seasonal affective disorder is the most common, there are also individuals who show a summertime pattern. It has been estimated that approximately 5% of individuals with seasonal affective disorder have a summertime variant. These patients usually show summertime depressions with associated typical and not atypical neurovegatative symptoms.

One interesting patient seen at the Anxiety and Depression Clinic at Cornell University Medical Center has shown a regularly occurring summertime and wintertime depression. Her wintertime depression was quite distinctive from her summertime depression. Beginning in November, she shows a picture of a retarded depression with prominent fatigue, hypersomnia, overeating, and weight gain. This syndrome goes into remission in late April. In late June, she then goes into a state of agitated depression with prominent restlessness, insomnia, anorexia, and weight loss; this usually resolves by mid September. Whether or not these summertime depressions may really represent dysphoric hypomanias remains an open question. Interestingly, the family history of this patient reveals a mother with severe bipolar disorder and a sister with cyclothymia, both of whom do quite well on lithium treatment. This patient with "double seasonal affective disorder" did not clinically resolve with either high-intensity light treatment, tricyclic antidepressants, or lithium carbonate. She has done quite well on therapeutic doses of monoamine oxidase inhibitors.

Bright light therapy (>2500 lx) has been shown to be consistently successful in patients suffering from the full and classic wintertime syndrome of SAD (Rosenthal et al. 1988). In fact, we have seen essentially a 100% success rate in our SAD patients treated at the Cornell University Medical Center, Westchester Division within 1 week of daily treatment (2 h). Characteristically, these patients will relapse within 4–10 days of stopping treatment. SAD patients have universally responded to reinstitution of bright light treatment within 4–7 days. Such patients are now routinely maintained on daily doses of bright light which they receive at home with special portable light boxes made for home use. We have instructed these patients to discontinue these treatments at the time of the year they normally go into remission, usually mid to late May. In such patients we now recommend starting similar light treatments the following autumn, about 1 week before their SAD symptoms usually occur. At the latitude of New York City, this is about late October for most patients.

It appears that while certain individuals may suffer from a full syndrome of SAD, a sizeable percentage of the population at certain latitudes may show an attenuated or subsyndromal form of SAD. These patients may show some combination of low energy, depression, overeating, weight gain, and increased need for sleep (Kaspar et al. 1989). These changes occur with a cyclicity and time course identical to that seen in SAD. Such patients seem to also be sensitive to treatment with high-intensity light. Some estimates have suggested that up to 20% of the population at the latitude of New York City might suffer from such conditions. The implications for public health, industry, and educational systems are tremendous, considering the large number of individuals potentially adversely affected by wintertime oscillation in mood, energy, concentration, sleep, and appetite and the potentially available treatment with high-intensity lights.

The rates of both SAD and subsyndromal SAD appears to be distributed according to latitude in North America. It has been estimated that at latitude 45°–50° (e.g., Minnesota, Maine, Ontario) SAD may affect 10% of the population and subsyndromal forms 20%, while at latitude 20°–30° (e.g., Texas, Florida, Mexico) SAD may affect only 1.5% of the population and the subsyndromal form may be in evidence in only 7.5% of the population (Rosenthal 1989). Intermediate latitudes have proven to show intermediate percentages of SAD and subsyndromal SAD. Should these figures estimated in North America be translatable to Europe, they would have even more significance as the latitudes of 50°–55° are heavily populated in Europe (e.g., British Isles, Czechoslovakia) as compared with sparsely populated areas in the United States and Canada.

The efficacy of bright light treatment of nonseasonal depressive disorders has yet to be established. Yerevanian et al. 1986 showed a distinct difference in efficacy of bright light in seasonal vs nonseasonal depressives. Kripke and colleagues in treating primarily male nonseasonal affective disorders have shown definite but small improvements in these patients comparing high-intensity with low-intensity light treatment (Kripke et al. 1987). The interpretations of these studies are problematic due to the high number of patients having comorbidity for alcoholism and patients not being drug-free during this study.

We are currently conducting research on the use of high-intensity light treatment (>2500 lx) on patients who do not conform to the syndrome of SAD, but who have a wintertime depression. Our patients are drug-free and have been divided into a bipolar spectrum vs a unipolar spectrum of disorders. The bipolar spectrum includes patients with bipolar disorder (lifetime history of mania) or bipolar NOS (major depressive disorder with either history of hypomania or hyperthymic personality). The unipolar patients have either major depressive episode or dysthymia. Patients receive 1 week of bright light treatment under controlled situations. Preliminary analysis of our first 19 patients shows marked improvement in the bipolar patients as compared with unipolars. Further analyses and study are needed to substantiate this finding.

It may be that bipolarity and not seasonality is the main predictor of treatment outcome in recurrent mood disorders under treatment with bright light therapy. Currently there is a great deal of ongoing clinical and basic research on the definition and treatment of seasonal affective disorder and its variants.

References

American Psychiatric Association (1987) Diagnostic and statistical manual of mental disorders, 3rd edn, revised. American Psychiatric Association, Washington DC

Jones WHS, Withington ET (eds) (1923–1931) Works of Hippocrates. Harvard University Press, Cambridge

Kaspar S, Robers SL, Yancey A, Schuly PM, Skwerer RG, Rosenthal NE (1989) Phototherapy in individuals with and without sybsyndromal seasonal affective disorder. Arch Gen Psychiatry 46: 837–844

Kripke DF, Risch SC, Janowsky D (1983) Bright white light alleviates depression. Psychiatry Res 10: 105–112

Kripke DF, Gillin JC, Mullaney DJ, Risch SC, Janowsky DS (1987) Treatment of major depressive disorders by bright white light for five days. In: Halaris A (ed) Chronobiology and neuropsychiatric disorders. Elsevier, New York, pp 207–218

Lewy AJ, Kern HA, Rosenthal NE, Wehr TA (1982) Bright artificial light treatment of a manic-depressive patient with a seasonal mood cycle. Am J Psychiatry 139: 1496–1498

Rosenthal NE (1989) Seasons of the mind. Bantam, New York

Rosenthal NE, Sack DA, Gillin JC, Lewy AJ, Goodwin FK, Davenport Y, Mueller PS, Newsome DA, Wehr TA (1984) Seasonal affective disorder: a description of the syndrome and preliminary findings with light treatment. Arch Gen Psychiatry 41: 72–80

Rosenthal NE, Sack DA, Skwerer RG, Jacobsen FM, Wehr TA (1988) Phototherapy of seasonal affective disorder. J Biol Rhythms 3: 101–120

Ross WD (ed) (1953) Aristotle: problemata, book XXX, problem 1, translated into English by E.S. Forster, Oxford University Press, Oxford (The works of Aristotle, vol 7)

Wirz-Justice A, Buchelli C, Graw P, Kielholz P, Fish HU, Woggon B (1986) Light treatment of seasonal affective disorder in Switzerland. Acta Psychiatry Scand 74: 193–204

Yerevanian BI, Anderson JL, Grota LJ, Bray M (1986) Effects of bright incandescent light on seasonal and nonseasonal major depressive disorder. Psychiatry Res 18: 355–364

Springer-Verlag and the Environment

We at Springer-Verlag firmly believe that an international science publisher has a special obligation to the environment, and our corporate policies consistently reflect this conviction.

We also expect our business partners – paper mills, printers, packaging manufacturers, etc. – to commit themselves to using environmentally friendly materials and production processes.

The paper in this book is made from low- or no-chlorine pulp and is acid free, in conformance with international standards for paper permanency.

MIX
Papier aus verantwortungsvollen Quellen
Paper from responsible sources
FSC® C105338

If you have any concerns about our products,
you can contact us on
ProductSafety@springernature.com

In case Publisher is established outside the EU,
the EU authorized representative is:
Springer Nature Customer Service Center GmbH
Europaplatz 3, 69115 Heidelberg, Germany

Printed by Libri Plureos GmbH
in Hamburg, Germany